INBORN ERRORS OF METABOLISM

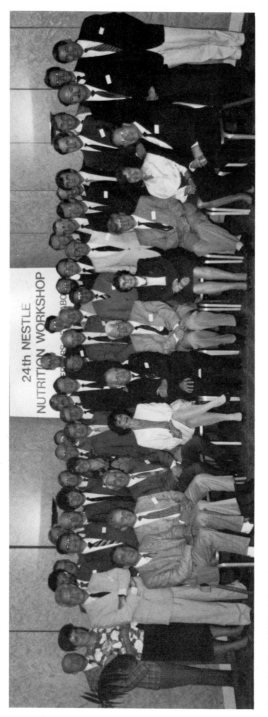

The 24th Nestlé Nutrition Workshop, Inborn Errors of Metabolism, was held in Brussels, Belgium, from September 24–28, 1989.

Workshop participants (*left to right*): Seated—J. L. Dhondt, J. P. Farriaux, J. Schaub, L. Dufour, F. Van Hoof, H. L. Vis, M. Hamosh, E. Eggermont, E. Vamos, J. Brodehl. Standing—K. De Block, M. J. Mozin, A. Kahn, M. Nordin-Mohan, C. Roe, T. R. Wang, W. Endres, J. P. van Biervliet, D. Brasseur, E. Harms, L. De Meirleir, K. Baerlocher, A. Otten, P. Tantibhedhyangkul, G. Mannaerts, U. Wendel, K. Barlett, R. J. A. Wanders, D. Carton, A. P. Mowat, L. van Maldergem, M. Odièvre, B. Bhandari, T. Friedmann, J. H. Broehles, L. Corbeel, J. Hobbs, J. Jaeken, M. Duran, G. van den Berghe, S. Krywawych, A. Verloes, J. Holton, K. Widhalm, C. de Prèlle, J. M. Saudubray.

Inborn Errors of Metabolism

Editors

Jürgen Schaub, M.D.
Professor of Pediatrics
University of Kiel
Kiel, Federal Republic of Germany

François Van Hoof, M.D.
Professor of Biochemistry
Université Catholique de Louvain
Faculté de Médecine
Brussels, Belgium

Henri L. Vis, M.D.
Professor of Pediatrics
Hôpital Universitaire des Enfants
Brussels, Belgium

Nestlé Nutrition
Workshop Series
Volume 24

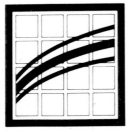

NESTLÉ NUTRITION

RAVEN PRESS ■ NEW YORK

Nestec Ltd., 55 Avenue Nestlé, CH-1800 Vevey, Switzerland
Raven Press, Ltd., 1185 Avenue of the Americas, New York,
New York 10036

Made in the United States of America

Library of Congress Cataloging-in-Publication Data

Inborn errors of metabolism / editors, Jürgen Schaub, François Van
   Hoof, Henri L. Vis.
        p.   cm. — (Nestlé Nutrition workshop series ; v. 24)
     Based on papers presented at the 24th Nestlé Nutrition workshop
   held in Brussels, Belgium Sept. 24–28, 1989.
     Includes bibliographical references.
     Includes index.
     ISBN 0-88167-752-3
     1. Metabolism, Inborn errors of—Congresses. I. Schaub, Jürgen.
   II. Van Hoof, François, [date].   III. Vis, H. L. (Henri L.)
   IV. Nestlé Nutrition S.A.   V. Series.
     [DNLM: 1. Metabolism. Inborn Errors—congresses.   W1 NE228 v. 24
   / WD 205 I3563 1989]
   RJ286.I53   1991
   618.92'39—dc20
   DNLM/DLC
   for Library of Congress   90-9098

Preface

For those of us who were actively involved in medicine forty years ago, and later on in pediatrics in the 1950s, it was evident that a solid knowledge of biochemistry was necessary for a full understanding of various pathological conditions.

The middle of the twentieth century was a period of profound changes for pediatric medicine, during which the understanding of the pathophysiology of illnesses in general, and of genetic diseases in particular, has been totally modified.

At the end of the 1940s and during the 1950s, the advances in our knowledge were due in part to the biological applications of extraordinary technical developments such as electrophoresis and chromatography. The availability of these new techniques provided strong support for Garrod's theory on inborn errors of metabolism.

Gibson described in 1948 the first well-documented enzyme deficiency in "familial methemoglobinemia": the NADH-dependent reductase. In 1949, Pauling and coworkers showed that normal and sickle cell hemoglobin migrated in different ways on paper electrophoresis, and Ingram demonstrated in 1956 that this different behavior was due to the substitution of a valine residue for a glutamic acid residue in position 6 of the β chain of the globin.

Garrod's theory in 1908 was based on his observations on alcaptonuria; only fifty years later, the underlying mechanisms of the disease were discovered by LaDu and coworkers: a deficiency of homogentisic acid oxidase. Cori and Cori pointed out in 1952 that glucose-6-phosphatase deficiency was responsible for the glycogenosis type I described by von Gierke in 1929. As early as 1934, Følling suspected that phenylketonuria was an inborn error or metabolism, but it took about 20 years to elucidate the mechanisms of the classic form of the disease: the deficiency of phenylalanine hydroxylase (Jervis, 1953).

However, hyperphenylalaninemia, which was thought to be a very simple metabolic disease, became with time a very complicated one with different variants. Phenylketonuria is a classic example of an inborn error of metabolism, not only because dietetic treatment can prevent mental retardation (as long as it is administered soon enough after birth), but also because a generalized screening program could be set up. This enables early diagnosis, which is one of the most important prerequisites for the efficacy of the dietetic treatment.

At that time, the only therapeutic possibilities were dietetic manipulations or a few palliative interventions (e.g., blood transfusion in sickle cell anemia or thalassemia). In a small number of diseases, some success could also be achieved by giving large amounts of some substances such as pyridoxine or, more recently, carnitine.

Simultaneously with the exponential increase of our knowledge concerning metabolic phenomena, very important developments occurred during the last decade in many fields of pediatrics. Widespread utilization of organ and bone marrow transplantation has been facilitated by the discovery of cyclosporin in 1973 and its use in clinical practice since 1978.

The prognosis of many pathologic conditions in the 1970s has been modified by organ and tissue transplantation. In transplanting tissues or organs, our target is to replace an organ that has been destroyed by a pathological process (kidney transplantation), or to correct metabolic deficits (e.g., by auxilliary transplantation). Not only can one organ or tissue (kidney, liver, bone marrow) be grafted, but transplantations of several organs at the same time are also performed (e.g., heart–lung transplantation in cystic fibrosis or kidney–liver transplantation in hyperoxaluria type I).

In the last decade it is in the field of molecular genetics that the most spectacular and important advances have taken place. The time lapse between the clinical description of an inherited anomaly and the discovery of the underlying metabolic error has been strikingly shortened.

The efflorescence of research in this particular field is leading to an enormous increase in our knowledge. The way we look at inborn errors of metabolism has been profoundly modified as a result of the combined development of genetics and molecular biology. At the present time, for instance, we refer to genetic diseases rather than to inborn errors of metabolism. One is fascinated when looking back at the progress made since Lejeune and his coworkers, in 1957, discovered the exact number of chromosomes in the human cell. Now the analysis of specific sequences among restriction DNA fragments, separated by gel electrophoresis, gives us the possibility of analyzing human genes responsible for diseases. In 1978, Kan and Dozy were the first to identify a restriction fragment length polymorphism (RFLP) at the globin locus.

I am personally very much impressed, when looking at the chapters dealing with molecular genetics in the current editions of most textbooks of pediatrics, by the enormous gaps that exist between the information that can be found in these textbooks and the information available from more specialized publications in this area.

We know that inborn errors of metabolism are not infrequent. For instance, the incidence of Følling disease more than doubled in certain countries once a clear clinical description of the illness could be given, and simple diagnostic procedures were made available. The same certainly applies to more recently described illnesses, such as peroxisomal or mitochondrial defects of fatty acid oxidation, or to the fragile X syndrome.

Nevertheless, it is becoming more and more difficult for the practicing clinician to keep his knowledge up-to-date in this field. Clinical diagnosis is usually extremely difficult because the initial symptoms of these illnesses are often very nonspecific—vomiting, convulsions, changes in behavior, hypoglycemia, and so on—while the demonstration of the defect is usually very subtle and frequently requires highly sophisticated techniques.

This volume will contribute to the practicing pediatrician's insight into one of the major challenges of modern medicine: diagnosis, treatment and prevention of inherited metabolic diseases.

HENRI L. VIS, M.D.

As a biochemically-trained physician, I was struck from the beginning of my career by the paradox of inborn metabolic diseases. Those diseases, which represent a burden of pain and distress for the patients and their parents, constitute at the same time, an irreplaceable opportunity for the scientist to understand the mysteries of life, the functioning of human cells, and the biochemical by-passes and regulation processes without which there would be no life on earth.

If one calls for the best specialist to repair an old astronomical clock, he will start by removing the pieces of this complex mechanism one after the other, and then analyze systematically the effects of each component. Only after that, will he know the exact function of each piece and, eventually, be able to repair the entire clock. The mechanisms of life are orders of magnitude more complex than an astronomical clock, and the inherited disorders of metabolism constitute experiments of nature comparable to the removal of a single piece from the complex mechanism of a clock. Thus is generated the excitement of the biochemist when confronted with disease, and the sorrow of the physician, who though appreciating the progress in the diagnosis and understanding of the pathogenesis of these disorders, remains so frequently devoid of therapeutic tools.

Among the 334 inborn errors of metabolism listed in 1988 by Victor McKusick (*Mendelian Inheritance in Man*, The Johns Hopkins University Press, Baltimore and London, pp. 1626), disorders responding to dietary manipulations unfortunately constitute only a minority, and for a long time antenatal diagnosis and genetic counseling have been the most efficient weapons against the others. Hardy and Weinberg's law, however, tells us that if there is one phenylketonuric (PKU) baby out of every 10,000 newborns, the PKU gene is carried by one out of every 50 adults. The overwhelming majority of mutated genes thus belong to the clinically normal population, and all our efforts concerning the families with an affected child will not significantly diminish the frequency of appearance of new patients in other families.

Fortunately, the paradox has now been partially solved. For more than a decade, great hope has risen from the progress made, first in cell, and later in organ transplantation. Without underestimating the many drawbacks of this technique, orthotopic liver transplantation appears to be a major breakthrough in the cure of inborn disorders of metabolism, because the liver is the principal, if not the only site of so many essential metabolic steps. If a new car does not start even though the electrical system is working satisfactorily, you ask for the motor to be changed. That is just what the surgeon does by orthotopic liver transplantation in Crigler-Najjar disease and in many other inborn disorders of liver metabolism.

The future lies not only in replacing, but in repairing. When will we be able to repair a defective gene? This is the challenge of the last contribution to this exciting symposium and the present book.

FRANÇOIS VAN HOOF, M.D.

Acknowledgments

We thank the Nestlé Company (Nestlé Belgilux and Nestec), and especially Drs. Pierre R. Guesry and Laila Dufour who brilliantly organized the symposium and managed, in a timely manner, the difficult task of publishing its contributions and discussions as a book in the Nestlé Nutrition Workshop Series.

JÜRGEN SCHAUB
FRANÇOIS VAN HOOF
HENRI L. VIS

Foreword

Inborn errors of metabolism are among the very rare diseases that can be treated almost exclusively by dietetics. For this reason alone, it could not escape being chosen as the subject of a Nestlé Nutrition Workshop.

At least in the case of some inborn errors, this is one of the extremely rare examples in which mother's milk is not the best food for a newborn, which means that more work needs to be done to develop optimal infant formulas for feeding such patients.

Interest in inborn errors peaked in the 1950s and 1960s. It was a time when technological progress allowed faster, easier, less expensive, and more accurate serum amino acid analysis; and the generalization of needle organ biopsies (liver, kidney, muscle, bone) made cellular exploration possible.

Now, at the beginning of the 1990s, there is renewed interest in the subject because of the increased possibilities for prenatal diagnosis and, if necessary, therapy. The fact that female patients are reaching the age of fecundity also raises new dietetic problems.

The subject is evolving rapidly, and this volume cannot give a definitive answer to every question. But, as our workshops are planned to allow ample time for detailed discussion, we hope this book will make an important contribution in this field.

PIERRE R. GUESRY, M.D.
Vice-President
Nestec Ltd, Vevey, Switzerland

Contents

Contributors

K. Bartlett
Department of Child Health
The Medical School
University of Newcastle-upon-Tyne
Framlington Place
Newcastle-upon-Tyne NE2 4HH, United
  Kingdom

Jean-Louis Dhondt
Centre Hospitalier Saint-Philibert
Laboratoire de Biochimie
115 Rue du Grand But
59462 Lomme, Cédex, France

Marinus Duran
University Children's Hospital
Het Wilhelmina Kinderziekenhuis
Nieuwe Gracht 137
NL-3512 LK Utrecht, The Netherlands

Ephrem Eggermont
Department of Pediatrics
Universitaire Ziekenhuizen Gasthuisberg
Herestraat 49
B-3000 Leuven, Belgium

Theodore Friedmann
Center for Molecular Biology and
Department of Pediatrics
University of California, San Diego
School of Medicine, M-034 CMG
La Jolla, California 92093, USA

Margit Hamosh
Department of Pediatrics and Physiology
  and Biophysics
Georgetown University Medical Center
3800 Reservoir Road NW
Washington DC, 20007-2197, USA

John R. Hobbs
Charing Cross and Westminster Medical
  School
Department of Chemical Immunology
17 Page Street
London SW1P 2AR, United Kingdom

John B. Holton
Department of Clinical Chemistry
Southmead General Hospital
Westbury-on-Trym
Bristol BS10 5NB, United Kingdom

Jaak Jaeken
Department of Pediatrics
Division of Metabolism and Nutrition
University Hospital Gasthuisberg
Herestraat 49
B-3000 Leuven, Belgium

André Kahn
Université Libre de Bruxelles
Clinique Pédiatrique
Hôpital Univesitaire des Enfants Reine
  Fabiola
Avenue JJ Crocq 15
1020 Brussels, Belgium

Stephen Krywawych
University College and Middlesex School
  of Medicine
Department of Medicine
The Rayne Institute
5 University Street
London WC1E 6JJ, United Kingdom

Guy P. Mannaerts
Department of Pharmacology
Katholieke Universiteit Leuven
Campus Gasthuisberg
B-3000 Leuven, Belgium

Alex P. Mowat
King's College School of Medicine and
  Dentistry
Department of Child Health
Variety Club Children's Hospital
Bessemer Road
London SE5 9PJ, United Kingdom

Michel Odièvre
Hôpital Antoine Béclère
Service de Pédiatrie
157 Rue de la Porte de Trivaux
92140 Clamart, France

Jean-Bernard Otte
Service de Chirurgie Pédiatrique
Générale & Abdominale
Université Catholique de Louvain
Cliniques Universitaires Saint-Luc
Avenue Hippocrate 10
1200 Brussels, Belgium

Charles R. Roe
Division of Pediatric Genetics and
* Metabolism*
Duke University Medical Center
Box 3028
Durham, North Carolina 27710, USA

Jean-Marie Saudubray
Département de Pédiatrie
Hôpital des Enfants Malades
149 Rue du Sèvres
75743 Paris, Cédex 15, France

Jürgen Schaub
Department of Pediatrics
University of Kiel
Schwanenweg 20
D-2300 Kiel 1, Federal Republic of
* Germany*

Georges Van den Berghe
Laboratory of Physiological Chemistry
International Institute of Cellular and
* Molecular Pathology*
Avenue Hippocrate 75
B-1200 Brussels, Belgium

François Van Hoof
Faculté de Médecine
Laboratoire de Chimie Physiologique
Université Catholique de Louvain
Avenue Hippocrate 75
1200 Brussels, Belgium

Henri L. Vis
Hôpital Universitaire des Enfants (HUDE)
15 Avenue JJ Crocq
1020 Brussels, Belgium

Ronald J. A. Wanders
Department of Pediatrics
University Hospital of Amsterdam
Meibergdreef 9
1105 AZ Amsterdam, The Netherlands

Invited Attendees

Kurt Baerlocher / *St. Gallen,*
* Switzerland*
B. Bhandari / *Udaipur, India*
Hans J. Böhles / *Frankfurt, Federal*
* Republic of Germany*
Johannes Brodehl / *Hannover,*
* Federal Republic of Germany*
Daniel Brasseur / *Brussels, Belgium*
Jean-Paul Buts / *Brussels, Belgium*
Paul Casaer / *Leuven, Belgium*
Lucien Corbeel / *Leuven, Belgium*
Linda de Meirleir / *Brussels, Belgium*
W. Th. Endres / *München, Federal*
* Republic of Germany*

Dr. Engohan / *Libreville, Gabon*
Philippe Gillis / *Hasselt, Belgium*
Philippe Goyens / *Brussels, Belgium*
Eric Harms / *Münster, Federal*
* Republic of Germany*
Jules G. Leroy / *Ghent, Belgium*
A. Jai Mohan / *Ipoh, Perak, Malaysia*
Musa Mohd. Nordin / *Seremban*
* N.S., Malaysia*
Albert Otten / *Giessen, Federal*
* Republic of Germany*
Etienne Sokal / *Brussels, Belgium*
Phienvit Tantibhedhyangkul /
* Bangkok, Thailand*

Esther Vamos / *Brussels, Belgium*
Jean-Pierre van Biervliet / *Bruge, Belgium*
Lionel van Maldergem / *Loverval, Belgium*
Alain Verloes / *Liège, Belgium*

Tso-Ren Wang / *Taipei, Taiwan, R.O.C.*
Udo Wendel / *Düsseldorf, Federal Republic of Germany*
Kurt Widhalm / *Vienna, Austria*

Nestlé Participants

Bianca Exl
Nestlé-Alete GmbH
Münich, Federal Republic of Germany

Karel De Block
Nestlé Belgilux
Brussels, Belgium

Cedric de Prelle
Nestlé Belgilux
Brussels, Belgium

Laila Dufour-Khouri
Nestec Ltd.
Vevey, Switzerland

Marie-José Mozin
Nestlé Belgilux
Brussels, Belgium

Nestlé Nutrition Workshop Series

Inborn Errors of Metabolism, edited by
J. Schaub, F. Van Hoof, and H. L. Vis.
Nestlé Nutrition Workshop Series, Vol. 24.
Nestec Ltd., Vevey/Raven Press, Ltd.,
New York © 1991.

Fatty Acid Oxidation: General Overview

Guy P. Mannaerts and Paul P. Van Veldhoven

*Department of Pharmacology, Faculty of Medicine, Katholieke Universiteit Leuven,
Campus Gasthuisberg, B-3000 Leuven, Belgium*

In 1949, Kennedy and Lehninger showed that fatty acids are β-oxidized in mitochondria. Twenty years later Cooper and Beevers found that glyoxysomes from
castor bean endosperm, organelles that belong to the peroxisome family, are also
capable of β-oxidizing fatty acids. In 1976, Lazarow and de Duve described the
presence of a fatty acyl-CoA oxidizing system in rat liver peroxisomes. Since then
it has become clear that in animal cells, mitochondria as well as peroxisomes can
β-oxidize fatty acids. In plant cells and eukaryotic microorganisms, peroxisomes are
the only site of β-oxidation. This overview will be limited to fatty acid oxidation in
animal cells. Substrates for β-oxidation include short (C4–C6), medium (C8–C12),
long (C14–C20), and very long chain (>C20) fatty acids, medium and long chain
dicarboxylic fatty acids, and the carboxy side chains of bile acid intermediates, prostaglandins and other eicosanoids, and xenobiotics. Long chain fatty acids are by far
the most abundant substrate. It should be emphasized that because of this abundance
they are the only substrate for β-oxidation that plays a major role in fuel homeostasis.

ACTIVATION OF FATTY ACIDS: UPTAKE BY MITOCHONDRIA AND PEROXISOMES

A prerequisite for β-oxidation is activation of the fatty acids to their CoA thioes-
ters. Long chain fatty acids are activated by long chain acyl-CoA synthetases present
in the mitochondrial outer membrane, peroxisomal membrane, and endosplasmic
reticulum (1). All three enzymes are most active toward fatty acids containing 10–
18 carbon atoms and appear to have identical or nearly identical molecular and catalytic properties.

The mitochondrial long chain acyl-CoA synthetase is present at the inner aspect
of the outer membrane (Fig. 1). Acyl-CoA esters cannot traverse the inner membrane. They are converted to carnitine esters (which are capable of crossing this
membrane) via a reaction catalyzed by carnitine palmitoyltransferase I. This enzyme
was believed to reside at the outer aspect of the inner membrane, but recent evidence
indicates that it is an outer membrane enzyme, the catalytic site of which faces the

1

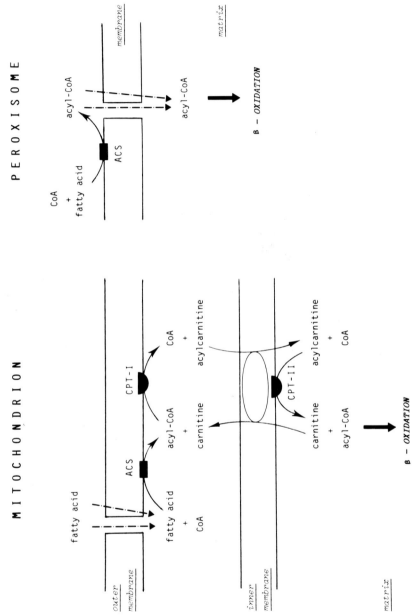

intermembrane space (2). The long chain acylcarnitines then diffuse through the inner membrane via a translocase that exchanges the acylcarnitine esters for intramitochondrial carnitine. At the matrical side of the inner membrane the acylcarnitine esters are reconverted to acyl-CoAs, a reaction catalyzed by carnitine palmitoyltransferase II. It is still a matter of debate whether carnitine palmitoyltransferase I and II are the same or different proteins.

Medium and short chain fatty acids can penetrate the mitochondria as the free acids and are activated mainly in the mitochondrial matrix. Very long chain fatty acids with a number of carbon atoms in excess of 20 are most probably not activated by mitochondria.

The peroxisomal long chain acyl-CoA synthetase is an integral membrane protein, the catalytic site of which faces the cytosol (Fig. 1). In a addition to this enzyme, peroxisomes (and endoplasmic reticulum) seem to possess an acyl-CoA synthetase specific for the activation of very long chain fatty acids (3). The acyl-CoA esters, formed at the outer aspect of the peroxisomal membrane, traverse the membrane without need for carnitine (4). When measured in homogenates or subcellular fractions, peroxisomal β-oxidation does not show latency, indicating that peroxisomes are readily permeable to acyl-CoA esters. The peroxisomal membrane contains a pore-forming protein (5). The diameter of the pore is large enough to allow the free diffusion of substrates, products, and cofactors of the peroxisomal enzymes. It is not known, however, whether long chain acyl-CoAs, which tend to partition in the lipid phase of membranes, also diffuse in the peroxisome via the hydrophilic pores or via some other mechanism.

Several substrates for β-oxidation, such as dicarboxylic fatty acids and the carboxy side chains of prostaglandins and of bile acid intermediates (di- and trihydroxycoprostanic acid), are not activated by mitochondria or by peroxisomes but solely by the endoplasmic reticulum. The enzymes that activate bile acid intermediates and dicarboxylic fatty acids are different from fatty acyl-CoA synthetase and are probably present only in liver (6,7).

MITOCHONDRIAL AND PEROXISOMAL β-OXIDATION

β-Oxidation of saturated fatty acids consists of four consecutive reactions (1,8, 9): a first reaction in which an acyl-CoA is oxidized to a 2-*trans*-enoyl-CoA, a second

---

FIG. 1. Long chain fatty acid entry in mitochondria and peroxisomes. Whether fatty acids traverse the mitochondrial outer membrane via the channel-forming protein (porin) or via some other mechanism is not known. At the inner aspect of the outer membrane the fatty acids are converted to acyl-CoAs and subsequently to acylcarnitines by the sequential action of long chain acyl-CoA synthetase (*ACS*) and carnitine palmitoyltransferase I (*CPT-I*), enzymes with their catalytic sites facing the intermembrane space. The acylcarnitines diffuse through the inner membrane via a carnitine:acylcarnitine exchange carrier. At the inner aspect of the inner membrane, carnitine palmitoyltransferase II (*CPT-II*) reconverts the acylcarnitines to acyl-CoAs. Peroxisomal long chain acyl-CoA synthetase (*ACS*) converts fatty acids to acyl-CoAs at the outer aspect of the membrane. The acyl-CoAs traverse the peroxisomal membrane without need for carnitine. It is not known whether the acyl-CoAs diffuse in the peroxisome via the channel-forming protein or via another mechanism.

one in which the 2-*trans*-enoyl-CoA is hydrated to L-3-hydroxyacyl-CoA, a third one in which L-3-hydroxyacyl-CoA is oxidized to 3-ketoacyl-CoA, and a fourth reaction in which 3-ketoacyl-CoA is cleaved in acetyl-CoA that is released and in acyl-CoA that is two carbon atoms shorter than the original molecule and which reenters the β-oxidation spiral (Fig. 2).

In mitochondria the first oxidation step is catalyzed by acyl-CoA dehydrogenase, a FAD-containing enzyme, which transfers its electron to another FAD-containing protein, namely electron-transferring flavoprotein. The latter protein donates its electrons to the respiratory chain. Mitochondria contain three separate acyl-CoA dehydrogenases, active toward long chain, medium chain, and short chain fatty acids, respectively.

The second reaction in mitochondrial β-oxidation is catalyzed by enoyl-CoA hydratase. There are two separate enoyl-CoA hydratases present in mitochondria: a short chain enoyl-CoA hydratase (crotonase) and a long chain enoyl-CoA hydratase. Although crotonase is not particularly active toward long chain enoyl-CoA, its total activity is so high in most tissues that it also seems to be responsible for the hydration of long chain enoyl-CoA.

The third step of mitochondrial β-oxidation is catalyzed by L-3-hydroxyacyl-CoA dehydrogenase, an enzyme that is dependent on NAD^+. There are two mitochondrial hydroxyacyl-CoA dehydrogenases: a soluble matrix enzyme that is active mainly toward short chain substrates, and a membrane-bound enzyme that is active mainly toward long chain substrates.

The last reaction of the β-oxidation cycle is catalyzed by thiolase. Mitochondria contain two thiolases: 3-ketoacyl-CoA thiolase, which is active toward molecules of various chain lengths, and acetoacetyl-CoA thiolase, which acts specifically on acetoacetyl-CoA. The former enzyme is involved in β-oxidation; the latter is thought to be involved in the synthesis (liver) and degradation (extrahepatic tissues) of ketone bodies. In the synthesis of ketone bodies the thiolase does not catalyze the cleavage of acetoacetyl-CoA but catalyzes the reverse reaction: the condensation of two acetyl-CoAs to acetoacetyl-CoA.

Peroxisomes (Fig. 2) degrade saturated fatty acids via a similar mechanism of β-oxidation which generates the same fatty acyl-CoA intermediates as described for mitochondria (1,8–10). Despite these similarities there are also important differences between the mitochondrial and peroxisomal systems (1,4,8,9). The first enzyme of the peroxisomal sequence is a FAD-containing oxidase, acyl-CoA oxidase, that transfers its electrons directly to molecular oxygen and thereby produces H_2O_2. Rat

———→

FIG. 2. The mitochondrial and peroxisomal β-oxidation system. β-Oxidation consists of four successive reactions. In mitochondria these reactions are catalyzed by acyl-CoA dehydrogenase (*1*), enoyl-CoA hydratase (*2*), L-3-hydroxyacyl-CoA dehydrogenase (*3*), and 3-ketoacyl-CoA thiolase (*4*). In peroxisomes the first reaction is catalyzed by acyl-CoA oxidase (*1*). The second and third reactions are catalyzed by a single bifunctional protein (enoyl-CoA hydratase/L-3-hydroxyacyl-CoA dehydrogenase) (*2,3*). The last reaction is catalyzed by peroxisomal 3-ketoacyl-CoA thiolase (*4*). ETF, electron-transferring flavoprotein.

Mitochondrial B-Oxidation

Peroxisomal B-Oxidation

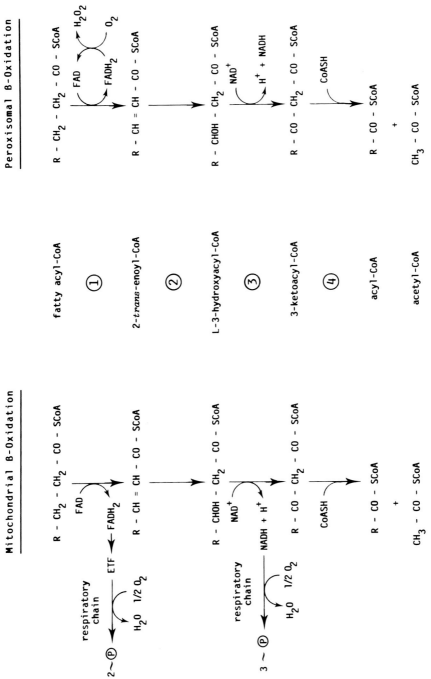

liver peroxisomes contain two fatty acyl-CoA oxidases with different isoelectric points. It is not known whether both enzymes are also present in extrahepatic tissues. In addition, liver peroxisomes contain trihydroxycoprostanoyl-CoA oxidase, an enzyme that oxidizes specifically the CoA derivatives of the bile acid intermediates di- and trihydroxycoprostanic acid (11). This enzyme is absent from extrahepatic tissues.

The second (hydration) and third (dehydrogenation) steps of peroxisomal β-oxidation are not catalyzed by two separate enzymes, as is the case in mitochondria, but by a single protein (enoyl-CoA hydratase/L-3-hydroxyacyl-CoA dehydrogenase), which is therefore often called bifunctional protein. The peroxisomal 3-ketoacyl-CoA thiolase, which catalyzes the last reaction of the cycle, is also different from its mitochondrial counterparts.

The oxidation of unsaturated fatty acids requires the presence of two auxiliary enzymes: Δ^3-*cis*-Δ^2-*trans*-enoyl-CoA isomerase and NADPH-dependent 2,4-dienoyl-CoA reductase (8,12). Isomerase and dienoyl-CoA reductase activities are found in mitochondria as well as in peroxisomes. The mitochondrial and peroxisomal enzymes appear to be distinct proteins. The presence of these auxiliary enzymes allows mitochondria and peroxisomes to oxidize polyunsaturated fatty acids.

Most naturally occurring unsaturated fatty acids contain cis double bonds. Fatty acids possessing double bonds extending from an odd-numbered carbon atom require only the isomerase as additional enzyme for their degradation. Oleic acid, for example, which is characterized by a 9-cis double bond, first undergoes three cycles of β-oxidation, which yield 3-*cis*-dodecenoyl-CoA. This intermediate is then isomerized by the isomerase to 2-*trans*-dodecenoyl-CoA, a normal enoyl-CoA intermediate of β-oxidation (Fig. 3).

Fatty acids with double bonds extending from an even-numbered carbon atom require both the dienoyl-CoA reductase and the isomerase. An example is linoleic acid, which possesses not only a 9-cis double bond such as oleic acid but also a 12-cis double bond. Linoleic acid is first degraded via three cycles of β-oxidation and isomerization to 2-*trans*,6-*cis*-dodecadienoyl-CoA. Completion of an additional β-oxidation cycle yields 4-*cis*-decenoyl-CoA, which is then oxidized in the first step of the next cycle to 2-*trans*,4-*cis*-decadienoyl-CoA. This compound is not further oxidized but is first reduced by 2,4-dienoyl-CoA reductase to 3-*trans*-decenoyl-CoA, and this in turn is isomerized to 2-*trans*-decenoyl-CoA, a normal intermediate of β-oxidation (Fig. 3).

In mitochondria, polyunsaturated fatty acids are oxidized exclusively via the dienoyl-CoA reductase/isomerase pathway. This pathway is also responsible for the major portion of polyunsatured fatty acid oxidation in peroxisomes (12). A minor alternative pathway, the description of which lies beyond the scope of this overview, may also exist in peroxisomes.

Partial hydrogenation of polyunsaturated fatty acids (e.g., during the production of margarines) creates trans double bonds. Trans polyunsaturated fatty acids are also degraded via the dienoyl-CoA reductase/isomerase pathway but at a slower rate.

The enzymes of mitochondrial and peroxisomal β-oxidation have been purified

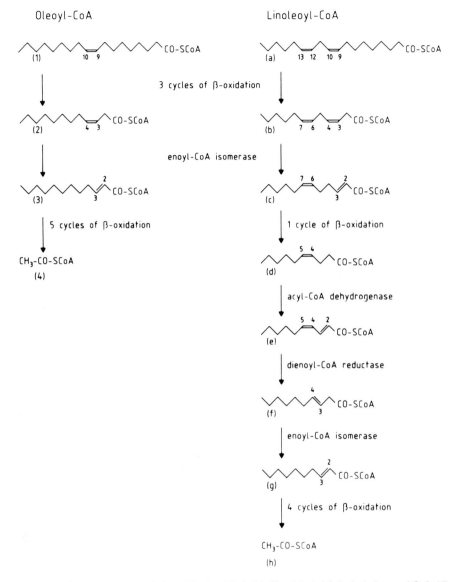

FIG. 3. β-Oxidation of oleoyl-CoA and linoleoyl-CoA. (*1*) Oleoyl-CoA; (*2*) 3-*cis*-dodecenoyl-CoA; (*3*) 2-*trans*-dodecenoyl-CoA; (*4*) acetyl-CoA; (*a*) linoleoyl-CoA; (*b*) 3-*cis*,6-*cis*-dodecadienoyl-CoA; (*c*) 2-*trans*,6-*cis*-dodecadienoyl-CoA; (*d*) 4-*cis*-decenoyl-CoA; (*e*) 2-*trans*,4-*cis*-decadienoyl-CoA; (*f*) 3-*trans*-decenoyl-CoA; (*g*) 2-*trans*-decenoyl-CoA; (*h*) acetyl-CoA.

and their molecular weight, subunit structure, and generally, their amino acid sequence are known (1,8,9). The β-oxidation enzymes are located in the mitochondrial and peroxisomal matrix. In mitochondria they are probably present as multienzyme complexes, in which the intermediates of β-oxidation are chaneled directly from one enzyme to the other without being released in the matrix (13). There are some indications that such multienzyme complexes also exist in peroxisomes.

Unlike mitochondrial β-oxidation, peroxisomal β-oxidation is not directly coupled to a respiratory chain and a phosphorylating system. Hence the energy that is released in the first oxidation step (H_2O_2 production) is completely lost as heat. The energy released in the third step of β-oxidation is conserved (NADH formation), so that from an energetic point of view peroxisomal β-oxidation is approximately half as efficient as mitochondrial oxidation (4).

The peroxisomal β-oxidation sequence is not active toward fatty acids with a chain length of less than eight carbon atoms (10). Thus, in contrast with mitochondrial β-oxidation, peroxisomal β-oxidation does not degrade fatty acyl-CoAs completely but acts as a chain-shortening system. This does not mean, however, that all acyl-CoAs entering peroxisomal β-oxidation are shortened to hexanoyl-CoA. There is evidence that in the intact cell peroxisomal β-oxidation does not normally go beyond two to three cycles. What stops further degradation in such instances remains unclear. Interestingly, peroxisomal β-oxidation goes to completion in plants and eukaryotic microorganisms where peroxisomes are the only site of β-oxidation (see above).

The product of mitochondrial β-oxidation, acetyl-CoA, condenses with oxaloacetate to form citrate, which enters the Krebs cycle. In liver, acetyl-CoA can also be converted to ketone bodies: acetoacetate and β-hydroxybutyrate (14). The ketone bodies leave the mitochondria and the hepatocytes and are an important source of metabolic fuel for extrahepatic tissues, especially in conditions such as starvation, where glucose is sparse. When hepatic fatty acid oxidation is high (e.g., starvation, diabetes; see below) most of the acetyl-CoA goes to ketone bodies. Low intramitochondrial levels of oxaloacetate, an intermediate that is also used for gluconeogenesis, or saturation of the Krebs cycle, may help to direct the acetyl units into the ketogenic pathway.

The fate of the products of peroxisomal β-oxidation (acetyl-CoA and shortened acyl-CoAs) is less clear. Peroxisomes lack the ketogenic and Krebs cycle enzymes and peroxisomal acetyl-CoA-consuming pathways remain to be discovered. The peroxisomal matrix contains carnitine octanoyltransferase. It is probable that this enzyme converts at least part of the acetyl-CoA and shortened acyl-CoAs to carnitine esters, which can then leave the peroxisomes and enter the mitochondria for further oxidation. It is not excluded that a portion of the acetyl-CoA escapes conversion and diffuses to the cytosol, where it might be used for biosynthetic purposes (e.g., cholesterol synthesis). In rat liver, the major portion of acetyl-CoA produced in peroxisomes seems to be hydrolyzed to acetate, which then diffuses into the circulation (15). Hepatic peroxisomes contain an acetyl-CoA hydrolase, which is perhaps responsible for this hydrolysis.

ROLE OF MITOCHONDRIAL AND PEROXISOMAL β-OXIDATION

Isolated mitochondria are capable of β-oxidizing short, medium, and long chain fatty acids, medium chain dicarboxylic fatty acids, and the carboxy side chains of prostaglandins and possibly of other arachidonic acid metabolites. Isolated peroxisomes can oxidize medium, long, and very long chain fatty acids; medium and long chain dicarboxylic acids; the carboxy side chains of xenobiotics, prostaglandins, and possibly other arachidonic acid metabolites; and the carboxy side chains of the bile acid intermediaters di- and trihydroxycoprostanic acid (liver peroxisomes).

The role of peroxisomal and mitochondrial β-oxidation *in vivo* and the contribution of each organelle to the *in vivo* oxidation of the above-mentioned substrates are not always clear. Evidently, short chain fatty acids such as butyrate are oxidized exclusively in mitochondria, since they are no substrate for peroxisomes (10). Mitochondria are also responsible for the major portion of the oxidation of medium and long chain fatty acids. The latter are by far the most abundant fatty acids in the organism and constitute a major source of metabolic fuel. Since mitochondrial β-oxidation conserves more energy than peroxisomal β-oxidation, it may seem logical that long chain fatty acids are oxidized preferentially in mitochondria. The contribution of mitochondria to palmitate or oleate oxidation in liver has been estimated at more than 90% (16). The contribution of mitochondria in extrahepatic tissues seems to be at least as high.

Very long chain fatty acids are predominantly, if not exclusively, oxidized by peroxisomes, perhaps because mitochondria do not have the ability to activate these fatty acids (3,17). The fatty acids are shortened in peroxisomes to long chain fatty acids, which in turn can be oxidized further by the mitochondria. Compared to long chain fatty acids, saturated very long chain fatty acids are only slowly oxidized by isolated peroxisomes. Very long chain polyunsaturated fatty acids are oxidized at rates comparable to those at which long chain fatty acids are oxidized (18). Although very long chain fatty acids form only an insignificant percentage of the overall fatty acids, a deficiency of peroxisomal β-oxidation leads to a deleterious accumulation of these poorly soluble compounds in various tissues, including the brain.

The contribution of mitochondria and peroxisomes to dicarboxylic fatty acid oxidation is controversial. Some authors favor an important role for peroxisomes (15, 19), whereas others oppose this view (20). Long chain dicarboxylic fatty acids are formed from long chain monocarboxylic fatty acids via ω-oxidation. Their production is increased under conditions of increased fatty acid supply (e.g., uncontrolled diabetes) or inhibition of mitochondrial fatty acid oxidation (e.g., enzyme deficiencies, inhibitors). Long chain dicarboxylic fatty acids are good substrates for isolated peroxisomes and apparently no substrate for isolated mitochondria—hence the opinion that peroxisomes shorten long chain dicarboxylic fatty acids to more polar medium chain dicarboxylic acids, which are then excreted. There is recent evidence from *in vivo* studies, however, that mitochondria also play a significant role in dicarboxylic fatty acid oxidation (20). In addition, the methods that have been used to measure long chain dicarboxylic fatty acid oxidation in isolated mitochondria were not always very sensitive. Since mitochondria are more numerous than peroxisomes in the cell, even low specific activity in mitochondria might suffice to yield a major mitochondrial contribution.

The same situation applies to the oxidation of the carboxy side chains of xenobiotics, formed via ω-oxidation of aliphatic side chains. The carboxy side chains of xenobiotics are good substrates for isolated peroxisomes and apparently poor substrates for isolated mitochondria (21). Here again, the detection methods were not very sensitive. As a result, it remains to be determined whether mitochondria or peroxisomes or both organelles play a significant role in the shortening of the side chains of xenobiotics. Chain shortening creates more polar metabolites that can more easily be excreted.

Prostaglandins (and other arachidonic acid metabolites) are excreted in the urine as dinor and tetranor metabolites whose side chains are, respectively, two and four carbon atoms shorter than those of the parent compounds, indicating that prostaglandins undergo β-oxidation before excretion. Isolated rat liver peroxisomes and mitochondria are capable of β-oxidizing prostaglandins, but the specific activity is severalfold higher in peroxisomes than in mitochondria (22). In whole liver homogenates, peroxisomes appear to oxidize the major portion of added prostaglandins, suggesting that peroxisomes play a dominant role in prostaglandin oxidation in the intact liver. Whether this is also the case in extrahepatic tissues remains to be seen.

The liver is the sole organ that can degrade cholesterol (Fig. 4). In a first series of reactions the steroid nucleus is altered (reduction of the double bond, hydroxylations) and one of the terminal methyl groups of the side chain is oxidized. The enzymes that catalyze these reactions are distributed among the endoplasmic reticulum, mitochondria, and cytosol and convert cholesterol to the C27 bile acids di- and trihydroxycoprostanic acid. The C27 bile acids are activated to their CoA esters in the endoplasmic reticulum (6) and subsequently β-oxidized in peroxisomes to chenodeoxycholoyl-CoA (derived from dihydroxycoprostanic acid) and choloyl-CoA (derived from trihydroxycoprostanic acid) (23). These CoA esters are then conjugated with taurine or glycine in peroxisomes and/or endoplasmic reticulum and the conjugates are excreted in the bile (24). Because the α-carbon atom of the C27 bile acids carries a methyl substitution, propionyl-CoA is released instead of acetyl-CoA. Fatty acyl-CoA oxidase is not active toward the C27 bile acids, but a separate oxidase, trihydroxycoprostanoyl-CoA oxidase, is responsible for the first step in the β-oxidation of bile acids (11). C27 bile acids are not a substrate for mitochondria.

α-OXIDATION OF PHYTANIC ACID

Phytanic acid is a 3,7,11,15-tetramethyl-substituted fatty acid with a chain length of 16 carbon atoms. The fatty acid, which is dietary in origin, is formed in various organisms from phytol, the fatty alcohol that is present in esterified form in chlorophyl. The methyl group at position 3 prevents the β-oxidation of phytanic acid. It is first degraded via α-oxidation (oxidative decarboxylation) to pristanic acid, the

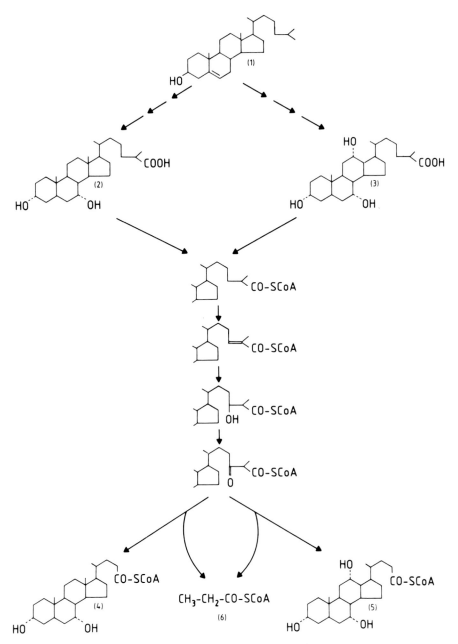

FIG. 4. Degradation of cholesterol. (*1*) Cholesterol; (*2*) dihydroxycoprostanic acid; (*3*) trihydroxy-coprostanic acid; (*4*) chenodeoxycholoyl-CoA; (*5*) choloyl-CoA; (*6*) propionyl-CoA.

chain length of which is one carbon atom shorter and which can now undergo β-oxidation. α-Oxidation consists most probably of a sequence of several reactions, the first of which may be a hydroxylation of position 2. Subcellular fractionation experiments with rat liver have provided evidence that α-oxidation is a mitochondrial process (25). Accumulation of phytanic acid in body fluids and tissues from patients with peroxisomal diseases suggests that in humans α-oxidation is a peroxisomal pathway (26).

REGULATION OF MITOCHONDRIAL AND PEROXISOMAL FATTY ACID OXIDATION

In liver, mitochondrial long chain fatty acid oxidation is regulated primarily by the nutritional state of the organism (14). In the fed state the liver synthesizes fatty acids from carbohydrate and the oxidation of fatty acids is low. On transition from the fed to the starved state the liver switches from fatty acid synthesis to fatty acid oxidation. Key factors in the regulation of hepatic fatty acid oxidation are the hepatic concentration of malonyl-CoA, the first intermediate committed to lipogenesis, and the fatty acid supply to the liver from the circulation. Both regulatory factors are controlled by the islet cell hormones insulin and glucagon. The high insulin and low glucagon levels in the fed state stimulate hepatic fatty acid synthesis. As a result, the concentration of malonyl-CoA increases. Malonyl-CoA is a potent inhibitor of carnitine palmitoyltransferase I (27), and its elevated concentration suppresses the entry of fatty acids in the mitochondria and, as a consequence, fatty acid oxidation (14). The newly synthesized fatty acids are now prevented from being oxidized and are directed toward triglyceride synthesis.

On transition to the starved state, glucagon levels increase and insulin levels decrease. The rates of fatty acid synthesis decline, as does the malonyl-CoA concentration. The suppression of fatty acid oxidation is thereby released (14). Under the influence of the altered hormonal balance, adipose tissue lipolysis is activated. This increases the fatty acid supply to the liver, which further enhances fatty acid oxidation. In addition, starvation causes modest increases in hepatic carnitine concentration and the activity of carnitine palmitoyltransferase I and a decrease in the affinity of the transferase for malonyl-CoA. As described above, a similar mechanism activates fatty acid oxidation in diabetes.

In starvation, hepatic fatty acid oxidation becomes a major source of metabolic energy, which can be used for gluconeogenesis. As explained earlier, most of the acetyl-CoA produced by mitochondrial β-oxidation is directed toward the synthesis of ketone bodies, which are released from the liver and serve as oxidizable substrates for extrahepatic tissues.

The regulation of mitochondrial long chain fatty acid oxidation in extrahepatic tissues is less clear. Extrahepatic carnitine palmitoyltransferase I is inhibited *in vitro* by malonyl-CoA and most extrahepatic tissues contain malonyl-CoA (28). Whether it plays a regulatory role in these tissues is not known. The increased supply of fatty acids from the circulation in starvation probably also stimulates extrahepatic fatty acid oxidation.

Peroxisomal fatty acid oxidation does not require carnitine, is not inhibited by malonyl-CoA, and does not seem to be regulated by feeding as opposed to starvation (4). The need for a regulatory mechanism for peroxisomal fatty acid oxidation seems to be less urgent, since peroxisomes oxidize only a small portion of the energetically important long chain fatty acids. Rather, peroxisomes seem to be engaged in the degradation and detoxification of those fatty acids (very long chain fatty acids, phytanic acid) or fatty acid derivatives (carboxy side chains of bile acid intermediates and perhaps of prostaglandins and xenobiotics) that do not play a significant role in fuel homeostasis. However, the activity and concentration of the hepatic peroxisomal β-oxidation enzymes increase two- to threefold when rodents are fed a high-fat diet, especially when the diet contains a large percentage of very long chain and/ or trans fatty acids (29). Smaller increases are observed in heart, kidney, and intestinal mucosa. The enzyme induction is accompanied by an increase in the number of peroxisomes. A 10-fold increase in hepatic peroxisome number and an even larger increase in the concentration and activity of the peroxisomal β-oxidation enzymes is seen when rodents are treated with certain plasticizers, herbicides, and hypolipidemic drugs of the fibrate type (30).

The mechanism of peroxisome induction remains unknown. Chronic peroxisome proliferation in rodent liver is accompanied by a dramatically increased incidence of liver cancer, which is a matter of serious concern to the industry and the regulatory authorities. It may sound reassuring, however, that until now there is no evidence for hepatic peroxisome proliferation and for an increased incidence of liver cancer in patients treated with these hypolipidemic fibrates.

REFERENCES

1. Hashimoto, T. Individual peroxisomal β-oxidation enzymes. *Ann NY Acad Sci* 1982;386:5–12.
2. Murthy MSR, Pande SV. Malonyl-CoA binding site and the overt carnitine palmitoyltransferase activity reside on the opposite sides of the outer mitochondrial membrane. *Proc Natl Acad Sci USA* 1987;84:378–82.
3. Singh H, Poulos A. Distinct long chain and very long chain fatty acyl-CoA synthetases in rat liver peroxisomes and microsomes. *Arch Biochem Biophys* 1988;266:486–95.
4. Mannaerts GP, Debeer LJ. Mitochondrial and peroxisomal β-oxidation of fatty acids in rat liver. *Ann NY Acad Sci* 1982;386:30–9.
5. Van Veldhoven PP, Just WW, Mannaerts GP. Permeability of the peroxisomal membrane to cofactors of β-oxidation. *J Biol Chem* 1987;262:4310–8.
6. Schepers L, Casteels M, Verheyden K et al. Subcellular distribution and characteristics of trihydroxycoprostanoyl-CoA synthetase in rat liver. *Biochem J* 1989;257:221–9.
7. Vamecq J, De Hoffmann E, Van Hoof F. The microsomal dicarboxylyl-CoA synthetase. *Biochem J* 1985;230:683–93.
8. Schulz H. Oxidation of fatty acids. In: Vance DE, Vance JE, eds. *Biochemistry of lipids and membranes.* Menlo Park: The Benjamin-Cummings Publishing Company, 1985;116–42.
9. Hashimoto T. Comparison of enzymes of lipid β-oxidation in peroxisomes and mitochondria. In: Fahimi HD, Sies H, eds. *Peroxisomes in biology and medicine* Berlin: Springer-Verlag, 1987;97–104.
10. Lazarow PB. Rat liver peroxisomes catalyze the β-oxidation of fatty acids. *J Biol Chem* 1978;253:1522–8.

11. Casteels M, Schepers L, Van Eldere J, Eyssen HJ, Mannaerts GP. Inhibition of 3α,7α,12α-trihydroxy-5β-cholestanoic acid oxidation and of bile acid secretion in rat liver by fatty acids. *J Biol Chem* 1988; 263:4654–61.
12. Schulz H, Kunau W-H. β-Oxidation of unsaturated fatty acids: a revised pathway. *Trends Biochem Sci* 1987;12:403–6.
13. Sumegi B, Srere PA. Binding of the enzymes of fatty acid β-oxidation and some related enzymes to pig heart inner mitochondrial membrane. *J Biol Chem* 1984;259:8748–52.
14. McGarry JD, Foster DW. Regulation of hepatic fatty acid oxidation and ketone body production. *Annu Rev Biochem* 1980;49:395–420.
15. Leighton F, Bergseth S, Rortveit T, Christiansen EN, Bremer J. Free acetate production by rat hepatocytes during peroxisomal fatty acid and dicarboxylic acid oxidation. *J Biol Chem* 1989;269:10347–50.
16. Mannaerts GP, Debeer LJ, Thomas J, De Schepper PJ. Mitochondrial and peroxisomal fatty acid oxidation in liver homogenates and isolated hepatocytes from control and clofibrate-treated rats. *J Biol Chem* 1979;254:4585–95.
17. Wanders RJA, van Roermund CWT, van Wijland MJA, et al. Studies on the peroxisomal oxidation of palmitate and lignocerate in rat liver. *Biochim Biophys Acta* 1987;919:21–5.
18. Hovik R, Osmundsen H. Peroxisomal β-oxidation of long chain fatty acids possessing different extents of unsaturation. *Biochem J* 1987;247:531–5.
19. Cerdan S, Künnecke B, Dolle A, Seelig J. *In situ* metabolism of 1,ω medium chain dicarboxylic acids in the liver of intact rats as detected by ^{13}C and ^{1}H NMR. *J Biol Chem* 1988;263,11664–74.
20. Draye JP, Veitch K, Vamecq J, Van Hoof F. Comparison of the metabolism of dodecanedioic acid *in vivo* in control, riboflavin-deficient and clofibrate-treated rats. *Eur J Biochem* 1988;178:183–9.
21. Yamada J, Ogawa S, Horie S, Watanabe T, Suga T. Participation of peroxisomes in the metabolism of xenobiotic acyl compounds: comparison between peroxisomal and mitochondrial β-oxidation of ω-phenyl fatty acids in rat liver. *Biochim Biophys Acta* 1987;921:292–301.
22. Schepers L, Casteels M, Vamecq J, Parmentier G, Van Veldhoven PP, Mannaerts GP. β-Oxidation of the carboxyl side chain of prostaglandin E$_2$ in rat liver peroxisomes and mitochondria. *J Biol Chem* 1988; 263:2724–31.
23. Pedersen JI, Kase BF, Prydz K, Björkhem I. Liver peroxisomes and bile acid formation. In: Fahimi HD, Sies H, eds. *Peroxisomes in biology and medicine*. Berlin: Springer-Verlag, 1987;67–77.
24. Kase BF, Björkhem I. Peroxisomal bile acid-CoA: amino-acid *N*-acyltransferase in rat liver. *J Biol Chem* 1989;264:9220–3.
25. Skjeldal OH, Stokke O. The subcellular localization of phytanic acid oxidase in rat liver. *Biochim Biophys Acta* 1987;921:38–42.
26. Wanders RJA, Heymans HSA, Schutgens RBH, Barth PG, Van den Bosch H, Tager JM. Peroxisomal disorders in neurology. *J Neurosci* 1988;88:1–39.
27. McGarry JD, Mannaerts GP, Foster DW. A possible role for malonyl-CoA in the regulation of hepatic fatty acid oxidation and ketogenesis. *J Clin Invest* 1977;60:265–70.
28. Scholte HR, Luyt-Houwen IEM, Dubelaar ML, Hülsmann WC. The source of malonyl-CoA in rat heart. The calcium paradox releases acetyl-CoA carboxylase and not propionyl-CoA carboxylase. *FEBS Lett* 1986;198:47–50.
29. Osmundsen H, Thomassen MS, Hiltunen JK, Berge RK. Physiological role of peroxisomal β-oxidation. In: Fahimi HD, Sies H, eds. *Peroxisomes in biology and medicine*. Berlin: Springer-Verlag, 1987;152–65.
30. Lock EA, Mitchell AM, Elcombe CR. Biochemical mechanisms of induction of hepatic peroxisome proliferation. *Annu Rev Pharmacol Toxicol* 1989;29:145–63.

DISCUSSION

Dr. Bartlett: You mentioned a number of differences between mitochondrial and peroxisomal β-oxidation. I would like to make a couple of comments. First, we have carried out some studies on the acyl-CoA intermediates of mitochondria and peroxisomal β-oxidation. There are some quite striking differences. In mitochondrial preparations oxidizing palmitate, during midpulse steady state conditions we could detect only C16, C14, and C12 intermediates, whereas in the peroxisomal system the complete range (C16 to C2) of intermediates was detected. The second point is that we detect all chain-length intermediates in the peroxisomal system, the implication being that peroxisomes are quite capable of β-oxidizing beyond C8. These are intact peroxisomes, not solubilized preparations.

Dr. Mannaerts: As far as short chain fatty acid oxidation is concerned, I think that other laboratories have also obtained evidence that peroxisomes can indeed oxidize short chain fatty acids. But the rate of oxidation seems to be very low. The reason might be that the K_m for short chain fatty acyl-CoA esters is high. This would mean that there may be some oxidation going on, but that the levels of the short chain intermediates would be high and perhaps easier to detect than the low levels of long chain intermediates, despite the fact that long chain fatty acid oxidation in peroxisomes is much more rapid than short chain fatty acid oxidation. However, I think that you are right that there is some short chain fatty acid oxidation in peroxisomes but that it is not very important compared to long chain fatty acid oxidation.

Dr. Bartlett: I would agree with that, but the point I really wanted to draw attention to was that there might be differences in organization. The implication of our study is that in the mitochondrial system, once palmitate is committed to oxidation it proceeds to completion, whereas this is not the case for peroxisomal β-oxidation.

Dr. Mannaerts: I think that one of the reasons is that the mitochondrial β-oxidation enzymes are probably organized in multienzyme complexes, in which the intermediates are channeled directly from one enzyme to the next one without being released in the surrounding medium. The system works perhaps less efficiently in peroxisomes.

Dr. Wanders: With regard to the comments about acyl-CoA oxidases, you stated that there were three of them: one specific for trihydroxycoprostanoyl-CoA and the other two reacting with fatty acyl-CoA esters. How do these findings relate to the finding by Hashimoto of having two messengers from one gene? The second question is: Did you look at the situation in human liver, where we know that clofibrate has no effect? Is there only one acyl-CoA oxidase there?

Dr. Mannaerts: This is very recent information. What we know is that in rat liver there is a trihydroxycoprostanoyl-CoA oxidase, which is not inducible and which specifically oxidizes the CoA esters of the bile acid intermediates, and that there are two fatty acyl-CoA oxidases, one that is inducible and one that is not. The two fatty acyl-CoA oxidases differ in isoelectric point and in subunit composition. As you know, the inducible enzyme consists mainly of components with molecular masses of approximately 50 and 20 kDa, which originate from the posttranslational cleavage of a 70-kDa component. The noninducible enzyme consists mainly of an uncleaved 70-kDa component. We don't know yet whether the two fatty acyl-CoA oxidases correspond to the two messengers recently discovered by the group of Osumi and Hashimoto, but we are planning to investigate this possibility in the near future. In human liver there seems to be only one fatty acyl-CoA oxidase, but as is the case for rat liver, there is also a separate trihydroxycoprostanoyl-CoA oxidase.

Dr. Wanders: The second question is relating to phytanic acid oxidation. It is not certain but probable that pristanic acid is oxidized in peroxisomes. The other thing that strikes me, at least, is the step at which phytanic acid is converted to pristanic acid. In every textbook it is stated that there is a sequence of three reactions, and I should like your comments on these. Professor Van Hoof has found that α-hydroxyacid oxidase B is capable of oxidizing the hydroxyphytanic acid to oxophytanic acid, but I have difficulty with these findings because this enzyme is in kidney only, whereas we know that in fibroblasts, for instance, or in liver, phytanic acid is efficiently degraded. So I wonder whether this whole sequence of reactions is indeed true. There is also another argument. If you look at the studies by Skjeldahl, Poll-Thé, and Saudubray on Refsum disease (1), they have done complementation analysis and have found that all the classical Refsum patients are in one complementation group, suggesting the likelihood that in all these patients the defect resides in one gene. If there were three enzymes, which could all cause Refsum disease, of course you would expect more than one complementation group. So my basic question is: What is your feeling about the phytanic acid degradation pathway, and might it not turn out that the whole metabolic pathway is wrong?

Dr. Mannaerts: I don't have very many ideas about α-oxidation, but I think there is still much to be discovered. If you look, for example, at the older publications regarding α-oxidation in brain, the data are always very hard to understand and very confusing. We have done some preliminary work on α-oxidation of phytanic acid and of the side chain of vitamin A in rat liver. We have the impression that you don't need mitochondria or peroxisomes but endoplasmic reticulum combined with the cytosolic fraction. So I don't know what to say about α-oxidation any more!

Dr. Van Hoof: It has been shown earlier that phytanic acid oxidation occurs in mitochondria, and defective oxidation corresponds to Refsum disease. We now know that some steps of α-oxidation of phytanate occur in peroxisomes and that deficiency of that function probably causes infantile Refsum disease (2). Here again, we see that fatty acid oxidation can occur in parallel in mitochondria and peroxisomes, and when we will discover the role of each organelle in each type of cell in the oxidation of phytanate, the problem of the etiology of the two Refsum diseases will become clear. May I ask Dr. Mannaerts to say a few words about β-oxidation and the evolution of species. Was not β-oxidation restricted mostly to peroxisomes before the appearance of mammals?

Dr. Mannaerts: Everybody now accepts or believes that in eukaryotic microorganisms and in plants peroxisomes are the only site of β-oxidation. Of course, for plants this has not been investigated in very many instances, but in those where it has, β-oxidation is in peroxisomes and not in mitochondria. This may not be absolute. Last week I saw a paper about algae, which apparently belong to the plant kingdom, and the authors claimed that they found peroxisomal as well as mitochondrial β-oxidation.

Dr. Van Hoof: The reason for evoking plants, which have a metabolism so different from that of mammals, is that they need peroxisomal β-oxidation at a specific stage of development: in the seeds. Seeds need to accumulate the largest possible food reserve in the least space. They do so by accumulating lipids, but at the time of germination, the plantlets will transform lipids into carbohydrates, thanks to specialized peroxisomes, the glyoxysomes. Mammalian peroxisomes lack the glyoxylate pathway and one might speculate that ancesters of mammals have lost the capacity of transforming lipids into carbohydrates, which has rendered more necessary the development of mitochondrial β-oxidation.

Dr. Hobbs: Just before World War II, the great Rudolf Schoenheimer studied atherosclerotic plaques and concluded that their biochemical evolution was compatible with the deposition of intravascular lipids within vascular endothelium up against the barrier of the elastic lamina. The phagocytes of the body attempt to remove them, but fail because they cannot metabolize the free cholesterol that crystallizes out, then generating the fibrosis and damage which underlies so much cardiovascular disease. I would like to ask if you think it is possible that when the cycle of the enzymes you are studying has been analyzed down to gene level, you might then be able to transfer the relevant enzymes into monocytes. Today, it is fairly easy to isolate monocytes from the peripheral blood of the patient and to grow these in tissue culture using recombinant monocyte stimulating factor (MSF). If at this stage you could insert the gene into the monocytes of the patient, they could then be returned to the patient and might clean out the atherosclerotic deposits. While such gene transfer clones might not last very long, the great advantage would be that the cells would be autologous and therefore nonantigenic, and of course the genes, being of normal human origin, should be able to generate a gene product that is not antigenic. It would therefore be possible to repeat such treatment at regular intervals in those patients who have a cholesterol overload. It could be a case of educating the patients' own monocytes and following up with refresher courses.

Dr. Friedman: I would like very much to be able to answer Dr. Hobbs's question. I don't have great experience with cholesterol metabolism, so I am not sure what the answer is. I think that such things are feasible, and many model systems and cell culture systems are available, so I don't think it is beyond the realm of possibility that these kinds of new functions can be supplied to cells. Of course, there are major questions about the longevity and stability of such a genetic reconstitution. But clearly it may be possible to carry out a gene transfer multiple times if one is dealing with circulating cells, and whether an organ other than the liver can function sufficiently well in reverse cholesterol transport is not a question that has been answered. There is too little information. But I would say the answer to your question in principle is: "Of course, let's get the genes and try."

Dr. Saudubray: Do you have any idea of the physiological significance of peroxisomal fatty acid oxidation in muscle? The general sense of my question is: Do you think it could be possible to find patients presenting with muscle symptoms due to peroxisomal fatty acid oxidation disorders?

Dr. Mannaerts: I don't know the exact role of peroxisomes in muscle. What I know is that peroxisomal β-oxidation in muscle is very low, as it is in the brain. An important portion of the very long chain fatty acids present in brain and perhaps also in muscle is probably oxidized locally in these tissues. Perhaps peroxisomes are also involved in the partial degradation of certain other lipid species that remain to be discovered or identified.

Dr. Duran: It was nice that you showed these auxiliary enzymes of unsaturated fatty acid oxidation, the dienoyl-CoA reductase and the enoyl-CoA isomerase. Could you predict if there would be clinical consequences for a deficiency of one of these enzymes? Would these patients present with hypoketotic hypoglycemia?

Dr. Mannaerts: A substantial portion of the fatty acids in the body are unsaturated fatty acids, so clinical consequences such as hypoglycemia might be a possibility. Perhaps Dr. Saudubray could answer this question.

Dr. Saudubray: It is only a guess, of course. One hypothesis would be that the clinical expression of such a defect would be largely dependent on the country where the patients live. In the south of France, for example, most fatty acids used for cooking are derived from olive oil, which is monounsaturated, whereas in Normandy or Britany, people mainly eat butter (saturated); so there is a large difference in the use of saturated and unsaturated fatty acids. It might be interesting to perform an epidemiological study of Reye's syndrome comparing the south of Europe or the United States, where people consume mainly polyunsaturated fatty acids, with other countries where butter or other saturated fatty acids are the main sources of fat. Another approach could be to measure systematically dienoyl-CoA reductase and isomerase in the liver of patients dying from Reye syndrome or other unexplained "hepatic encephalopathy."

Dr. Van Hoof: We could also have discussed the fate of medium and short chain fatty acids, which is different in the liver from that of long chain fatty acids. Indeed, fatty acids shorter than 12 carbons cross the mitochondrial membranes freely and are thus less actively driven to the mitochondrial β-oxidation. Part of them thus undergo ω-oxidation and form dicarboxylic acids. Excess of dicarboxylic acids could be harmful for our metabolism. I think that this will be discussed later by Dr. Hamosh.

REFERENCES

1. Poll-Thé BT, Skjeldal OH, Stokke O, et al. Phytanic acid alpha-oxidation and complementation analysis of classical Refsum and peroxisomal disorders. *Hum Genet* 1989;81:175–81.
2. Draye JP, Van Hoof F, de Hoffmann E, Vamecq J. Peroxisomal oxidation of L-2-hydroxyphytanic acid in rat kidney cortex. *Eur J Biochem* 1987;167:573–8.

Inborn Errors of Metabolism, edited by
J. Schaub, F. Van Hoof, and H. L. Vis.
Nestlé Nutrition Workshop Series, Vol. 24.
Nestec Ltd., Vevey/Raven Press, Ltd.,
New York © 1991.

Inherited Disorders of Mitochondrial β-Oxidation

K. Bartlett, A. Aynsley-Green, *J. V. Leonard, and
D. M. Turnbull

*Human Metabolism Research Centre, Departments of Child Health, Clinical Biochemistry and Neurology, Royal Victoria Infirmary, University of Newcastle upon Tyne, Newcastle upon Tyne, NE1 4LP; and the *Institute of Child Health, London, WC1N 1EH, United Kingdom*

Inherited abnormalities of mitochondrial oxidation of long chain fatty acids cause a number of clinical syndromes, including sudden infant death, Reye's syndrome, episodic hypoglycemia, and lipid storage myopathy. Since suberylglycinuria was first described in 1976, there has been a growing recognition that these inherited defects of the mitochondrial oxidation of fatty acids constitute an important group of disorders, some of which are treatable by simple dietary manipulation, such as the avoidance of starvation (1,2). Thus deficiencies of long chain acyl-CoA dehydrogenase (3,4), medium chain acyl-CoA dehydrogenase (5), short chain acyl-CoA dehydrogenase (6,7), ETF or ETF:QO [glutaric aciduria type II, multiple acyl-CoA dehydrogenase deficiency] (8), long chain 3-hydroxyacyl-CoA dehydrogenase (9), and acetoacetyl-CoA thiolase (10) have been described. Also of relevance to the present discussion, disorders of carnitine palmitoyltransferase (11) and of the Lynen cycle of ketogenesis (12,13) have been documented.

Mitochondrial β-oxidation of saturated acyl-CoA esters proceeds by a repeated cycle of four reactions: flavoprotein-linked dehydrogenation, hydration, NAD^+-linked dehydrogenation, and thiolysis. The three chain-length-specific acyl-CoA dehydrogenases (14) which catalyze the first dehydrogenation step are linked to the respiratory chain by the electron transfer flavoprotein (ETF) and ETF:ubiquinone oxidoreductase (ETF:QO) (Fig. 1). The second dehydrogenation step is catalyzed by two chain-length-specific NAD^+-dependent 3-hydroxyacyl-CoA dehydrogenases (15). There are two acyl-CoA hydratases (16) and two thiolases (17,18), which vary in their chain length specificity. These nine enzymes are required for the complete oxidation of long chain saturated acyl-CoAs. There are also auxillary systems for the transport of long chain fatty acids across the inner mitochondrial membrane and for the oxidation of polyunsaturated fatty acids. Carnitine palmitoyltransferase I is located on the inner face of the outer mitochondrial membrane and catalyzes the

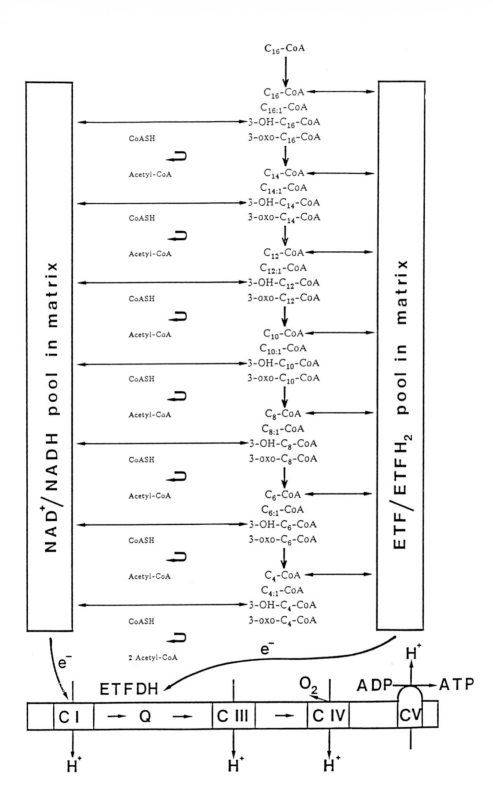

formation of long chain acylcarnitine from the corresponding long chain acyl-CoA, which can traverse the inner mitochondrial membrane in exchange for free carnitine via a specific translocase. The matrix acylcarnitine then becomes the substrate for carnitine palmitoyltransferase II to regenerate acyl-CoA. Two enzymes are required for the oxidation of polyunsaturated fatty acids: 2,4-dienoyl-CoA reductase and an isomerase (19,20).

The control of β-oxidation in the mitochondrial matrix occurs at several steps and depends on the redox state and the rate of recycling of CoA (Fig. 1; 21–24). The rate is lowered with reduced states since low $NAD^+/NADH$ ratios impair the activity of the hydroxyacyl-CoA dehydrogenase (25,26) and increase the formation of ETF_{sq}, which is a potent inhibitor of the acyl-CoA dehydrogenases (27). These changes affect the steady state concentrations of acyl-CoA intermediates, which in turn may change the control strength of other enzymes of the pathway as outlined in Fig. 1.

In liver mitochondria acetyl-CoA produced by each cycle of β-oxidation has four major routes of disposal: ketogenesis, oxidation by the citrate cycle, conversion to acetylcarnitine, or hydrolysis to acetate, and each of these reactions generates free CoA. During maximum flux through β-oxidation, up to 95% of the mitochondrial CoA pool is acylated (28) and thus the rate of recycling of CoA may partly control β-oxidation (29). Increased steady state concentrations of some acyl-CoA esters may also occur when one or more of the enzymes of β-oxidation is inhibited, as in hypoglycin poisoning (30) or where one or more of the enzymes of the pathway are absent.

In normal subjects under fasting conditions, lipolysis is stimulated and fatty acids are released into the circulation. Following their uptake by tissues, fatty acids are activated to acyl-CoA esters, which may be utilized for the formation of triacylglycerides or transported into the mitochondrial matrix for oxidation. The acetyl-CoA generated by β-oxidation may then be completely oxidized via the tricarboxylic acid cycle or utilized for ketogenesis. Circulating ketone bodies may then be oxidized by extrahepatic tissues, notably brain (31,32) and muscle (33,34). This system constitutes the Randle cycle and is the mechanism by which glucose utilization is spared

---

FIG. 1. β-Oxidation of hexadecanoate and its relation to the redox state of the mitochondrion. Each cycle of the mitochondrial β-oxidation of hexadecanoyl-CoA and all 27 intermediates is shown. The flow of electrons between 3-hydroxyacyl-CoA/3-oxoacyl-CoA esters and the $NAD^+/NADH$ pool, between the $NAD^+/NADH$ pool and the respiratory chain at the level of NADH dehydrogenase, between acyl-CoA/2-enoyl-CoA esters and the $ETF/ETFH_2$, between the $ETF/ETFH_2$ pool and the respiratory chain at the level of ETF:QO, and electron flow from NADH dehydrogenase and ETF:QO to O_2 along the respiratory chain is indicated by thin lines. Electron flow through NADH dehydrogenase and complexes III and IV of the respiratory chain to O_2 is associated with proton ejection from the matrix, and the proton gradient generated is used to drive the synthesis of ATP by complex V. The flux through the respiratory chain is controlled by the ATP/ADP ratio and is maximal in uncoupled mitochondria. Acetyl-CoA is converted to acetoacetate with recycling of CoA.

It can be seen that the flux through β-oxidation depends on the supply of hexadecanoyl-CoA (via CPT I/carnitine-acyl carnitine exchange carrier/CPT II not shown), the [acyl-CoA]/[CoA] ratio, and the redox states of the $NAD^+/NADH$ and $ETF/ETFH_2$ pools, which in turn depend on the rate of electron transport through the respiratory chain and are more oxidized when electron transport is fast.

for those tissues, such as brain, which have an obligatory requirement for glucose as a metabolic fuel (35). If fatty acid oxidation is impaired by one of the enzyme defects mentioned above, there are a number of metabolic consequences. The first effect is an impaired ability to withstand fasting, with rapid onset of hypoglycemia as glycogen reserves become depleted. Second, as lipolysis continues and the blood concentration of free fatty acids rises, the fatty acids entering the liver are either partially oxidized to a variety of abnormal metabolites or stored as triglyceride. Third, the impairment of mitochondrial β-oxidation appears to trigger the proliferation of hepatic peroxisomes (36), with resultant stimulation of peroxisomal β-oxidation and further production of chain-shortened intermediates. The abnormal metabolites generated by partial mitochondrial β-oxidation, peroxisomal β-oxidation, and a number of detoxification mechanisms are excreted and can be detected in urine (dicarboxylic acids, hydroxy acids, carnitine esters, and glycine conjugates) (37–40).

Thus β-oxidation defects cause major changes in whole body fuel economy, but changes that may only be apparent in response to metabolic stress such as fasting. We suggest that much of the argument regarding the presence or absence of putative pathognomic urinary metabolites (see, e.g., ref. 41), the usual mainstay of inborn error diagnosis, arises because the metabolic conditions under which specimens are collected are not defined with sufficient rigor. It is more logical to identify patients with impaired ketogenesis by monitoring the major metabolic fuels during a fast, and only then progressing to secondary investigations such as urine analysis and direct enzyme assay.

In many patients with inherited disorders of β-oxidation, hypoglycemia is the preeminent presenting feature. Hypoglycemia is one of the most common metabolic abnormalities in pediatric medicine. There are numerous causes and several different clinical manifestations, and its occurrence is often intermittent and unpredictable. These aspects, together with the involvement of several biochemical pathways in the maintenance of normoglycemia, has made the condition particularly difficult to investigate and manage. There have been few attempts to define a practical, logical approach to diagnosis. It is further complicated by the continued use of archaic terms such as "idiopathic hypoglycemia," "asymptomatic hypoglycemia," and "ketotic hypoglycemia."

Although the descriptive phrase "ketotic hypoglycemia" cannot be regarded as a final diagnosis, it is important to recognize whether children have hypoglycemia in the presence or absence of ketonemia or ketonuria. Ketotic hypoglycemia occurs when the falling glucose concentration results in mobilization of fatty acids from adipose tissue and generation of ketone bodies by fatty acid oxidation in the liver. Hypoglycemia without ketonuria or ketonemia has been regarded as pathognomic of hyperinsulinism in view of the anti-lipolytic effect of high circulating insulin concentrations.

It is now recognized that there exist a number of children in whom hypoglycemia is associated with unexpectedly low blood concentrations of ketone bodies due to impaired oxidation of fatty acids in the liver. This may be due to a primary defect in the enzymes of fatty acid oxidation or a secondary effect on mitochondrial fatty acid oxidation due to a defect elsewhere in intermediary metabolism.

This chapter documents an analysis of metabolic relationships in patients presenting with hypoglycemia associated with varying degrees of ketonemia, and from this we outline a practical, logical, and comprehensive approach to elucidate the underlying biochemical abnormality.

PATIENTS

Twenty-eight patients aged from 1 day to 4 years of age were referred for investigation of symptomatic hypoglycemia. Of the 28 patients, 13 were found on investigation to be suffering from hyperinsulinemic hypoglycemia, one child had fructose-1,6-diphosphatase deficiency, one child had glucose-6-phosphatase deficiency, and 13 had evidence of defects in the β-oxidation of fatty acids. Eight of these 13 patients were subsequently confirmed to have medium chain acyl-CoA dehydrogenase (MCAD) deficiency. In addition, results are presented from patients whose urine specimens and fibroblast cell lines were referred for analysis (cases 29–36).

METHODS

Clinical

In all children referred for investigation of spontaneous hypoglycemia a plastic cannula was inserted into a peripheral vein to allow the withdrawal of free-flowing venous blood samples. A small number of patients were studied by the withdrawal of a single blood sample at the time of an emergency admission to the hospital due to symptoms of spontaneous hypoglycemia. In all other cases, a starvation challenge was performed. The children were starved under careful clinical supervision and with hourly monitoring of blood glucose concentrations. There was an arbitrary limit on the maximum period of starvation allowed for each age group of children. Children during the first month after birth were subjected to a maximum period of starvation of 6 h. Infants between 1 and 3 months of age were starved to a maximum of 8 h; children 3 months to 1 year were starved for a maximum of 12 h. A maximum of 18 h of starvation was allowed for children between ages of 1 and 3 years, with a maximum limit of 24 h for children beyond this age. In all patients hypoglycemia occurred prior to these limits of starvation.

At the onset of symptoms or when the blood glucose concentration fell below 2.5 mmol/liter, a venous blood sample was obtained. An aliquot (0.5 ml) was immediately placed into 5 ml of ice-cold 5% (v/v) perchloric acid, and the remainder was used to prepare a plasma sample. In some of the older children a series of blood samples was drawn at 3-h intervals during the starvation procedure. The urine sample passed immediately after the episode of spontaneous or starvation-induced hypoglycemia was collected and deep frozen immediately.

The results of the metabolic investigations were compared with the profiles of circulating levels of intermediary metabolites in 46 normal children undergoing routine surgical procedures. The samples in these children were obtained immediately prior to the operation and the period of starvation was noted. The investigations performed on the patients and control children were approved by the Newcastle Joint Ethics Committee, and parental consent was obtained.

Measurement of Blood and Plasma Concentrations of Intermediary Metabolites, Insulin, and Carnitine

Whole blood concentrations of glucose, lactate, pyruvate, acetoacetate, 3-hydroxybutyrate, glycerol, and alanine were measured fluorometrically (42). Plasma free fatty acid concentrations were also measured by a spectrophotometric enzyme-linked assay using the Cobas Bio Fast Analyzer. Plasma insulin concentrations were measured by a double antibody radioimmunoassay (43). Plasma-free carnitine, short chain acylcarnitine, and long chain acylcarnitine were measured radioenzymatically (44).

Determination of Urinary Organic Acids and Acylcarnitine Concentrations

Urinary organic acid analysis was by gas chromatography–mass spectrometry. Acyl carnitines were analyzed by either reversed-phase high-performance thin layer chromatography or high-performance liquid chromatography (46,46).

Measurement of Fibroblast Acyl-CoA Dehydrogenase Activities

Acyl-CoA dehydrogenase activities were measured in cultured skin fibroblasts by the ETF-linked fluorometric method (47).

RESULTS

Interrelationships of Metabolic Fuels and Intermediary Metabolites

The concentrations of blood glucose, lactate, pyruvate, acetoacetate, hydroxybutyrate, glycerol, alanine, and free fatty acids in controls and patients are shown in Table 1. None of the control children were hypoglycemic under the conditions of preoperative starvation.

Thirteen patients could clearly be identified who had hypoglycemia with low concentrations of acetoacetate and hydroxybutyrate together with low concentrations of free fatty acids. All of these children had inappropriate concentrations of plasma insulin for the level of glycemia. One patient (case 14) had hypoglycemia accompanied by hyperlacticacidemia, hyperalaninemia, and hyperglycerolemia. This pa-

TABLE 1. *Blood intermediary metabolites, plasma non-esterified fatty acids and insulin*

Patient	lact	pyr	ala	β-OHB	AcAc	glu	NEFA	glyc	Insulin
Controls (fasted for 24 h; *n* = 19)									
Mean	1.26	0.11	0.20	1.98	0.74	3.6	1.58	0.16	
SD	0.56	0.07	0.06	1.38	0.56	0.60	0.39	0.04	<1.0
Hyperinsulinemics: patients 1–13									
Mean	1.07	0.09	0.24	0.29	0.14	2.5	0.58	0.13	9.8
SD	0.53	0.04	0.08	0.47	0.17	0.9	0.45	0.11	7.6
Fructose-1,6-diphosphatase deficiency									
14	8.77	0.32	0.60	0.28	0.09	2.6	0.91	0.74	nd
Glucose-6-phosphatase deficiency									
15	5.61	0.30	0.50	0.04	0.01	2.3	1.30	0.18	1.5
Medium chain acyl-CoA dehydrogenase deficiency									
16	1.45	0.09	0.16	0.67	0.50	2.7	2.58	0.32	<1.0
17	1.90	0.14	0.16	0.28	0.18	1.9	2.99	0.43	<1.0
18	0.85	0.05	0.14	0.01	0.01	2.6	1.93	0.09	<1.0
19	1.25	nd	nd	0.40	nd	2.2	2.21	nd	nd
20	1.00	nd	nd	0.40	nd	3.9	1.86	nd	nd
21	1.66	nd	nd	0.42	nd	1.9	2.46	nd	<1.5
22	0.85	nd	nd	0.39	nd	2.3	1.90	nd	nd
23	0.96	nd	nd	0.62	nd	2.8	nd	nd	nd
Probable β-oxidation defects									
24	1.05	0.11	0.10	0.54	0.44	15.0*	1.83	0.08	nd
25	1.26	nd	nd	0.10	nd	1.8	3.09	nd	nd
26	1.43	nd	nd	0.10	nd	1.8	2.06	nd	nd
27	1.35	0.11	0.17	0.21	0.10	1.8	2.88	0.28	nd
28	6.92	0.32	0.40	0.27	0.09	1.4	2.28	0.30	nd

tient was shown subsequently to have a deficiency of fructose-1,6-diphosphatase. Case 15 had hypoglycemia with hyperlacticacidemia and low concentrations of ketone bodies. Measurement of glucose-6-phosphatase in her liver biopsy demonstrated that she had glycogen storage disease type 1B. The remaining children had hypoglycemia with normal concentrations of lactate, pyruvate, alanine, and glycerol, and elevated levels of free fatty acids but low concentrations of blood ketone bodies. This finding strongly suggested a defect in the oxidation of fatty acids in the liver.

While these findings provide some clues for further investigation of patients, considerably more information can be obtained by relating the concentration of blood glucose to that of plasma insulin and from the relationship between the concentrations of ketone bodies and fatty acids to blood glucose concentration. Another interrelationship of great clinical value is between plasma free fatty acid concentrations and the concentrations of total ketone bodies (acetoacetate plus 3-hydroxybutyrate). Figure 2 demonstrates a linear relationship with 95% confidence limits between these two variables as derived from the data from normal children. With increasing levels of free fatty acids there is a direct increase in the concentration of ketone bodies.

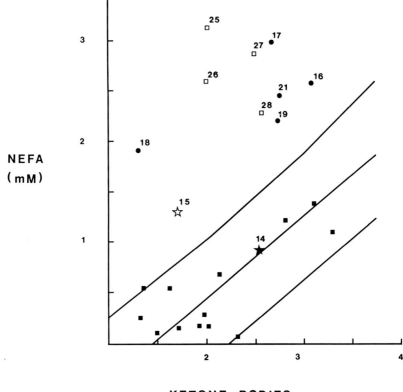

KETONE BODIES
log umol/l

FIG. 2. Relationship of plasma NEFA concentrations to blood ketone body concentrations in controls (the line of best fit and the 95% confidence limits determined by Deming's method are as indicated), patients with medium chain acyl-CoA dehydrogenase deficiency (●), glycogen storage disease type 1B (☆), fructose-1,6-diphosphatase deficiency (★), patients with probable β-oxidation disorders (□), and hyperinsulinemic patients (■). The case numbers are as shown in Table 1.

The relationship of children with hyperinsulinism falls within the 95% confidence limits. Thus, although these children had an inappropriately low concentration of ketone bodies for the level of glycemia, the relationship with free fatty acids was appropriate. The hypoketonemia was therefore due to a failure of free fatty acid release as a result of the antilipolytic effect of insulin on adipose cells.

The child with fructose-1,6-diphosphatase deficiency had an appropriate level of ketone bodies for the degree of free fatty acidemia. However, the child with glycogen storage disease type 1B clearly had an inappropriately low level of ketone bodies for the degree of free fatty acidemia, suggesting a secondary effect on fatty acid oxidation. The children with suspected and proven defects of β-oxidation had high

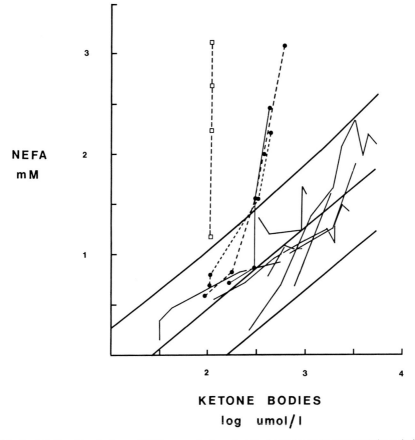

FIG. 3. Relationship of plasma NEFA concentrations to blood ketone body concentrations during the course of fasting in controls (solid lines, no symbols), patients with proven medium chain acyl-CoA dehydrogenase deficiency (●), and a patient with a probable β-oxidation disorder (□).

concentrations of free fatty acids but inappropriately low concentrations of ketone bodies for that degree of lipolysis.

Figure 3 shows the sequential change in the relationship during the progression of the starvation provocation test between free fatty acids and ketone bodies in five children with medium chain acyl-CoA dehydrogenase deficiency. It is clear that while the relationship is normal at the onset of the starvation, with increasing starvation-induced stress the relationship rapidly becomes abnormal.

Concentrations of Carnitine and Acylcarnitines in Plasma

The results of the assays of plasma carnitine, short chain acylcarnitine, long chain acylcarnitine, and percentage acylated carnitine in patients, adult controls, and nor-

TABLE 2. *Fasting plasma concentrations of free carnitine, short chain acylcarnitine, long chain acylcarnitine, and percentage carnitine acylated*

	Carnitine	Short chain acylcarnitine	Long chain acylcarnitine	% Acylated
Adults ($n = 30$)				
Mean	32.8	6.2	3.2	23
SD	6.3	2.3	0.7	5
Normal children (aged <5 years) ($n = 11$)				
Mean	26.2	17.2	3.1	44
SD	7.7	5.9	0.8	9
Hyperinsulinemic patients ($n = 8$)				
Mean	24.2	7.5	2.9	32
SD	12.4	2.7	1.5	12
Medium chain acyl-CoA dehydrogenase-deficient patients ($n = 7$)				
Mean	11.4	13.4	2.8	58
SD	5.9	7.4	1.1	12
Patients with probable β-oxidation disorders				
Case				
24	7.1	7.2	1.5	55
25	2.7	0.0	3.2	54
26	4.3	0.0	5.1	54
27	6.4	3.8	4.8	57
28	34.9	21.7	7.1	55

mal children during ketosis are shown in Table 2. Patients with hyperinsulinism, fructose-1,6-diphosphatase deficiency, and glycogen storage disease type 1B did not demonstrate any abnormality in carnitine metabolism. However, patients with MCAD deficiency had an abnormally high short chain acylcarnitine concentration and a low free carnitine concentration. In two patients with probable defects of β-oxidation there was a total absence of short chain acylcarnitine, which is suggestive of a defect in long chain fatty acid oxidation. The total absence of plasma short chain acylcarnitine is abnormal; taken in conjunction with the hypoketonemic hypoglycemic hyper-fatty-acidemia, it is suggestive of a disorder of long chain acyl-CoA metabolism.

Urinary Dicarboxylic Acids and Acylcarnitines

Patients with proven MCAD deficiency excreted dicarboxylic acids, suberylglycine, and octanoylcarnitine when hypoglycemic. However, case 17, who presented in the neonatal period, did not excrete suberylglycine at presentation, but did so when fasted at 7 months of age. One patient, case 24, who had normal MCAD activity, also excreted the dicarboxylic acids suberylglycine, and octanoylcarnitine, and as can be seen from the results presented in Table 1, clearly had hypoketotic,

TABLE 3. *Acylcarnitines excreted by patients with proven and suspected medium chain acyl-CoA dehydrogenase deficiency*

	C6	C8	C10	
	μmol·mmol^{-1} creatinine			Suberylglycine[a]
16[b]	53.4	239.6	6.8	+ve
17[b] (neonatal)	10.9	75.2	0	−ve
17[b] (infantile)	6.1	120.5	0	+ve
22[b]	14.8	44.1	1.3	nd
23[c]	10.1	101.6	2.4	nd
24[d]	0	42.1	0	+ve
29[b]	2.9	16.1	0	+ve
33[b]	8.8	14.7	8.6	+ve
34[c]	280.7	1004.0	27.6	+ve
35[c]	1.5	232.1	0	nd
36[c]	0	73.0	2.4	+ve

[a] nd, not determined.
[b] Proven medium chain acyl-CoA dehydrogenase-deficient patient.
[c] Suspected medium chain acyl-CoA dehydrogenase-deficient patients.
[d] Proven normal acyl-CoA dehydrogenases.

hyper-fatty-acidemic hypoglycemia. The results of urinary acylcarnitine analysis from patients with proven and suspected medium chain acyl-CoA dehydrogenase deficiency are presented in Table 3. Some typical HPLC chromatograms of urinary acylcarnitines are shown in Fig. 4.

Fibroblast Acyl-CoA Dehydrogenase Activities

The activities of short, medium, and long chain acyl-CoA dehydrogenases are shown in Table 4.

DISCUSSION

The cause of hypoglycemia cannot be determined by the measurement of blood glucose concentration alone. It is essential to examine blood glucose levels in relation to the concentrations of other major metabolic fuels, intermediary metabolites, and metabolic hormones at the time of hypoglycemia. This diagnostic strategy is not always used, and many of these children have experienced recurrent episodes of severe hypoglycemia, with an unacceptable delay in establishing an appropriate diagnosis due to measurement of blood glucose alone. Our data support our contention that it is important to obtain a blood and a urine sample at the time of hypoglycemia, either during a spontaneous attack or during a supervised fast.

We suggest the following protocol for the investigation of children with hypoglycemia:

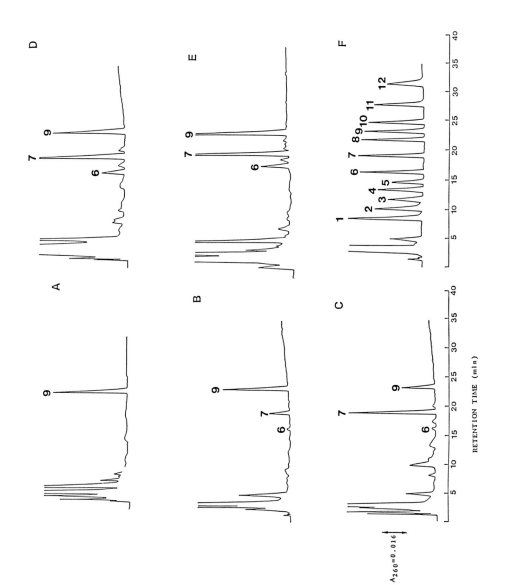

D

A

E

B

F

C

RETENTION TIME (min)

$A_{260} = 0.016$

TABLE 4. *Fibroblast acyl-CoA dehydrogenase activities*[a]

Patient	SCAD	MCAD	LCAC
16	0.24	0.10	1.11
17	0.04	0	0.32
19	0.24	0.16	1.34
22	0.25	0.13	1.37
29	0.03	0	0.79
30	0.12	0.05	0.78
31	0.16	0.19	1.10
32	0.17	0.08	1.45
24	0.13	0.63	0.75
26	0.24	0.94	1.52
Controls ($n = 18$)			
Mean	0.22	0.95	1.42
SD	0.10	0.17	0.21

[a] Units: nmol ETF reduced·min^{-1}·mg protein^{-1}

Stage 1 is the recognition that the child's symptoms could be explained on the basis of hypoglycemia.

Stage 2 is obtaining a blood and urine sample at the time of spontaneous hypoglycemia to measure the blood concentrations of intermediary metabolites, free fatty acids and hormones, and urinary organic acids and acylcarnitines.

Stage 3 is the determination of all metabolic fuels, metabolites, and hormones during the course of a starvation provocation test.

Since hypoglycemic episodes may be intermittent, we have introduced a starvation provocation test to stress the counterregulatory metabolic and endocrine systems. Over 100 formal starvation tests have now been performed on children of different ages, and within the strict time limits for maximum periods of starvation as outlined above, no adverse sequelae have been documented. However, it is essential to recognize that prolonged starvation could be dangerous for a child with a defect of β-oxidation in view of the elevation of free fatty acid concentrations that can occur under these circumstances. Our approach is to pay meticulous attention to the clinical condition of the child during the starvation, with an indwelling venous canula *in situ* for the withdrawal of the blood sample and for the immediate correction of hypoglycemia or a deteriorating circumstance by intravenous glucose.

FIG. 4. HPLC analysis of urinary acylcarnitines (46). **A:** A normal ketotic child. **B:** case 17 aged 48 h. **C:** case 17 aged 7 months following a starvation provocation test. **D:** case 16. **E:** case 22. **F:** standard mixture of acylcarnitines containing (*1*) carnitine, (*2*) acetylcarnitine, (*3*) propionylcarnitine, (*4*) butyrylcarnitine, (*5*) 2-methylbutyrylcarnitine, (*6*) hexanoylcarnitine, (*7*) octanoylcarnitine, (*8*) decanoylcarnitine, (*9*) undecanoylcarnitine (internal standard), (*10*) dodecanoylcarnitine, (*11*) tetradecanoylcarnitine, (*12*) hexadecanoylcarnitine.

The etiology and management of hyperinsulinemic states due to dysregulation of the islets of Langerhans have been described previously (48,49). It is evident from our series of patients that this cause of hypoketotic hypoglycemia is associated with the lowest concentrations of ketone bodies; in some cases both hydroxybutyrate and acetoacetate are virtually undetectable. This hypoketonemia is associated with low concentrations of free fatty acids, although the relationship between the two substrates is within the normal range. Recognition of this relationship should alert the clinician to the possibility of hyperinsulinism and the patient should then be investigated as outlined previously (49).

The relationship of free fatty acids to total ketone bodies is highly informative. All patients with enzyme-proven medium chain acyl-CoA hydrogenase deficiency have demonstrated an abnormal relationship as indicated in Fig. 2. Confirmation that this abnormal ratio is due to MCAD deficiency is shown by the measurement of abnormal concentrations of plasma carnitine and its derivatives, and by the demonstration of the excretion of abnormal urine constituents.

However, as is evident from our data, there remains a group of children who demonstrate an abnormally low concentration of ketone bodies for the degree of free fatty acidemia, implying impaired ketogenesis, yet who do not excrete abnormal constituents in their urine. Moreover, some children who do demonstrate abnormal urinary constituents with an abnormal fatty acid/ketone body ratio do not have abnormal activity of MCAD on enzyme analysis of tissue culture samples. These children presumably have defects of the other enzymes of fatty acid oxidation, and further investigations are in progress. Some children with impaired β-oxidation are able to generate ketone body concentrations in the blood but the concentration is inappropriately low for the level of free fatty acids.

We conclude that it is too simplistic to classify children with hypoglycemia into "ketotic" and "hypoketotic" categories. There is a spectrum of relationship which can only be assessed by the direct relationship shown in Figs. 2 and 3. Determination of the concentration of metabolic fuels, intermediates, and hormones during fasting is extremely valuable in the diagnosis of these children.

Finally, it is emphasized that some children may have a secondary impairment of fatty acid oxidation as a result of a primary enzyme defect elsewhere. This is exemplified by the observation that a child with glycogen storage disease type 1B also has an abnormal relationship between free fatty acids and ketone bodies. However, another disorder of gluconeogenesis, fructose-1,6-diphosphatase deficiency, although also characterized by an abnormal elevation of blood lactate levels, was not associated with the secondary disturbance of ketogenesis. Secondary effects on β-oxidation are further illustrated by the data presented in Fig. 5. This shows the acyl CoA intermediates generated by the incubation of [U-^{14}C]palmitate with isolated skeletal muscle mitochondria from a patient with a lipid storage myopathy due to a deficiency of complex I of the respiratory chain. Thus an impaired ability to oxidize NADH results in a slowing of β-oxidation flux (Fig. 6), the accumulation of hexadec-2-enoyl-CoA, tetradec-2-enoyl-CoA, and 3-hydroxyhexadecanoyl-CoA, and lowered production of acetyl-CoA. These observations provide a mechanism for the lipid

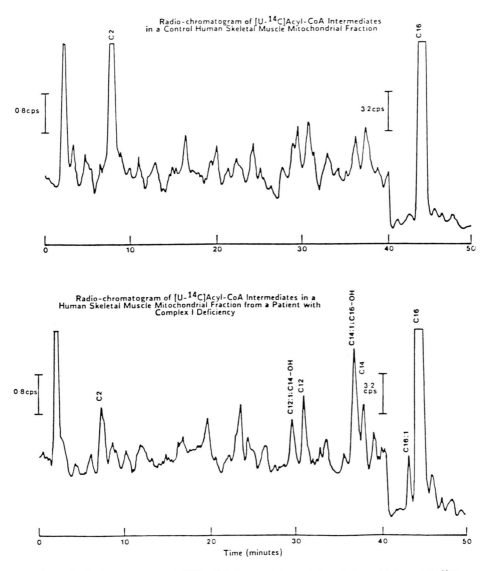

FIG. 5. Radiochromatograms of [¹⁴C]acyl-CoA ester intermediates of the oxidation of [U-¹⁴C]-hexadecanoate by skeletal muscle mitochondria from a patient with a deficiency of complex I of the respiratory chain and controls. Analysis was by reversed-phase HPLC with on-line photodiode array and radiochemical detection as described previously (50). The identity of hexadec-2-enoyl-CoA (C16:1) was confirmed by its characteristic UV absorbance spectrum. Tetradec-2-enoyl-CoA (C14:1) and 3-hydroxyhexadecanoyl-CoA (C16-OH) coelute.

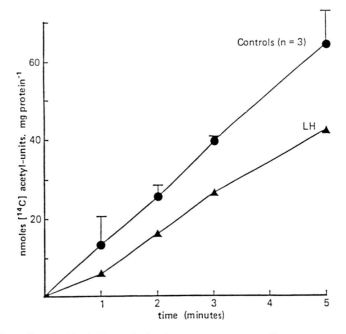

FIG. 6. Generation of acid-soluble metabolites from the oxidation of [U-^{14}C]hexadecanoate by skeletal muscle mitochondrial fractions from a patient with deficiency of complex I of the respiratory chain (<2% of controls) and three controls. Mitochondrial fractions (0.55–4.4 mg protein) were incubated with 60 nmol of [U-^{14}C]hexadecanoate and acid-soluble radioactivity determined at the indicated times. The rates of oxidation were: patient (▲) 9.9 nmol·min^{-1}·mg protein^{-1}; controls (●) (mean ± SD) 15.0 ± 1.9 nmol·min^{-1}·mg protein^{-1}.

storage observed in this patient. This clearly illustrates the intimate relationship between β-oxidation flux and mitochondrial redox state depicted in Fig. 1.

REFERENCES

1. Vianey-Liaud C, Divry P, Gregersen N, Matthieu M. The inborn errors of mitochondrial fatty acid oxidation. *J Inher Metabol Dis* 1987;10(Suppl 1):159–98.
2. Turnbull DM, Shepherd I, Aynsley-Green A. Inherited defects of mitochondrial fatty acid oxidation. *Biochem Soc Trans* 1988;16:424–7.
3. Hale DE, Coates PM, Stanley CA, Lortner JA, Hall CL. Long-chain acyl-CoA dehydrogenase deficiency. *Pediatr Res* 1983;17:290A.
4. Hale DE, Batshaw ML, Coates PM, et al. Long-chain acyl-CoA dehydrogenase deficiency: an inherited cause of non-ketotic hypoglycaemia. *Pediatr Res* 1985;19:666–71.
5. Stanley CA, Hale DE, Coates PM, et al. Medium-chain acyl-CoA dehydrogenase deficiency in children with non-ketotic hypoglycaemia and low carnitine levels. *Pediatr Res* 1983;17:877–84.
6. Turnbull DM, Bartlett K, Stevens DL, et al. Short-chain acyl-CoA dehydrogenase deficiency associated with a lipid-storage myopathy and secondary carnitine deficiency. *N Engl J Med* 1984;311:1232–6.
7. Amendt BA, Rhead WJ. The multiple acyl-coenzymeA dehydrogenation disorders, glutaric aciduria type II and ethylmalonic-adipic aciduria. *J Clin Invest* 1986;78:205–13.
8. Frerman FE, Goodman SI. Deficiency of electron transfer flavoprotein or electron transfer flavopro-

tein:ubiquinone oxidoreductase in glutaric acidaenia type II fibroblasts. *Proc Natl Acad Sci USA* 1985; 82:4517–20.

9. Wanders RJA, Duran M, Ijlst L, et al. Sudden infant death and long-chain 3-hydroxyacyl-CoA dehydrogenase. *Lancet* 1989;ii:52–3.

10. Middleton B, Bartlett K. The synthesis and characterization of 2-methylacetoacetyl-coenzyme A and its use in the identification of the site of the defect in 2-methylacetoacetic and 2-methyl-3-hydroxybutyric aciduria. *Clin Chim Acta* 1983;128:291–305.

11. Bougneres PF, Saudubray JM, Marsac C, Bernard O, Odievre M, Girard J. Fasting hypoglycaemia resulting from hepatic carnitine palmitoyl transferase deficiency. *J Pediatr* 1981;98:742–6.

12. Faull K, Bolton P, Halpern B, et al. Patient with defect of leucine metabolism. *N Engl J Med* 1976; 294:1013.

13. Leonard JV, Seakins JWT, Griffin NK. β-Hydroxy-β-methylglutaric aciduria presenting as Reye's syndrome. *Lancet* 1979;i:680.

14. Ikeda Y, Dabrowski C, Tanaka K. Separation and properties of five distinct acyl-CoA dehydrogenases from rat liver mitochondria. Identification of a new 2-methyl branched chain acyl-CoA dehydrogenase. *J Biol Chem* 1983;258:1066–76.

15. El Fakhri M, Middleton B. The existence of an inner-membrane-bound, long acyl-chain specific 3-hydroxyacyl-CoA dehydrogenase in mammalian mitochondria. *Biochim Biophys Acta* 1982;713:270–9.

16. Fong JC, Schulz H. Purification and properties of pig heart crotonase and the presence of short-chain and long-chain enoyl-CoA hydratases in pig and guinea pig tissues. *J Biol Chem* 1977;252:542–7.

17. Middleton B. The acetoacetyl-CoA thiolases of rat brain and their relative activities during post-natal development. *Biochem J* 1973;132:717–30.

18. Staack H, Binstock JF, Schulz H. Purification and properties of a pig heart thiolase with broad chain-length specificity and a comparison of thiolases from pig heart and *Escherichia coli*. *J Biol Chem* 1978; 253:1827–31.

19. Kunau W-H, Dommes P. Degradation of unsaturated fatty acids. *Eur J Biochem* 1978;91:533–44.

20. Schulz H, Kunau W-H. Beta-oxidation of unsaturated fatty acids: a revised pathway. *Trends Biochem Sci* 1987;12:403–6.

21. Lopes-Cardozo M, Van Den Bergh SG. Ketogenesis in isolated rat liver mitochondria. I. Relationship with the citric acid cycle and with the mitochondrial energy state. *Biochim Biophys Acta* 1972;283:1–15.

22. Lopes-Cardozo M, Van Den Bergh SG. Ketogenesis in isolated rat liver mitochondria. II. Factors affecting the rate of β-oxidation. *Biochim Biophys Acta* 1974;357:43–52.

23. Lopes-Cardozo M, Van Den Bergh SG. Ketogenesis in isolated rat liver mitochondria. III. Relationship with the rate of β-oxidation. *Biochim Biophys Acta* 1974;357:53–62.

24. Schultz H. Fatty acid oxidation. In: Vance DE, Vance JE, eds. *Biochemistry of lipids and membranes*. Menlo Park, CA: The Benjamin-Cummings Publishing Company, 1985;116–42.

25. Bremer J, Wojtczak AB. Factors controlling the rate of fatty acid β-oxidation in rat liver mitochondria. *Biochim Biophys Acta* 1972;280:515–30.

26. Latipää PM, Karki TT, Hiltunen JK, Hassinen IE. Regulation of palmitoylcarnitine oxidation in isolated rat liver mitochondria. Role of the redox state of NAD(H). *Biochim Biophys Acta* 1986;875:293–300.

27. Beckmann JD, Frerman FE. Reaction of electron transfer flavoprotein with electron transfer flavoprotein-ubiquinone oxidoreductase. *Biochemistry* 1985;24:3922–5.

28. Garland PB, Shepherd D, Yates DW. Steady state concentrations of coenzyme A, acetyl-coenzyme A and long-chain acyl-coenzyme A in rat liver mitochondria oxidizing palmitate. *Biochem J* 1965;97:587–94.

29. Billington D, Osmundsen H, Sherratt HSA. Mechanism of the metabolic disturbances caused by hypoglycin and by pent-4-enoic acid *in vitro* studies. *Biochem Pharmacol* 1979;27:2879–85.

30. Sherratt HSA. Hypoglycin, the infamous toxin of the Jamaican Ackee fruit. *Trends Pharmacol Sci* 1986; 7:186–91.

31. Owen QE, Morgan AP, Kemp HG, Sullivan JM, Herrera MG, Cahill GF Jr. Brain metabolism during fasting. *J Clin Invest* 1967;46:1589–95.

32. Hawkins RA, Williamson DH, Krebs HA. Ketone body utilisation by adult and suckling rat brain *in vitro*. *Biochem J* 1971;122:13–18.

33. Williamson JR, Krebs HA. Acetoacetate as the fuel of repiration in the perfused rat heart. *Biochem J* 1961;80:540–7.

34. Page MA, Krebs HA, Williamson DH. Activities of enzymes of ketone-body utilisation in brain and other tissues of suckling rats. *Biochem J* 1971;121:49–53.

35. McIlwain H, Bachelard HS. Metabolism of the brain *in situ*. In: *Biochemistry and the central nervous sytem*, 5th ed. London: Churchill Livingstone, 1985;7–29.
36. Lake BD, Clayton PT, Leonard JV, Bhuiyan AKMJ, Bartlett K, Aynsley-Green A. Ultrastructure of liver in inherited disorders of fat oxidation. *Lancet* 1987;i:382–3.
37. Duran M, Mitchell G, De Klerk JB. Octanoic acidemia and octanoyl-carnitine excretion with dicarboxylic aciduria due to defective oxidation of medium-chain fatty acids. *J Pediatr* 1985;107:397–404.
38. Roe CR, Millington DS, Maltby DA, Bohan TP, Kahler SG, Chalmers RA. Diagnostic and therapeutic implications of medium-chain acyl-CoA dehydrogenase deficiency. *Pediatr Res* 1985;19:459–65.
39. Divry P, David M, Gregersen N, et al. Dicarboxylic aciduria due to medium-chain acyl-CoA dehydrogenase defect. A cause of hypoglycaemia in childhood. *Acta Pediatr Scand* 1983;72:943–8.
40. Gregersen N, Lauritzen R, Rasmussen K. Suberylglycine excretion in the urine from a patient with dicarboxylic aciduria. *Clin Chim Acta* 1976;70:417–25.
41. Rinaldo P, O'Shea JJ, Coates PM, Hale DE, Stanley CA, Tanaka K. Medium-chain acyl-CoA dehydrogenase deficiency. Diagnosis by stable isotope dilution measurement of urinary *n*-hexanoylglycine and 3-phenylpropionylglycine. *N Engl J Med* 1988;319:1308–13.
42. Harrison J, Hodson AW, Skillen AW, Stappenbeck R, Agius L, Alberti KGMM. Blood glucose, lactate, pyruvate, glycerol, 3-hydroxybutyrate and acetoacetate measurements in man using a fast centrifugal analyser with a fluorimetric attachment. *J Clin Chem Clin Biochem* 1988;26:141–6.
43. Soeldner JS, Slone D. Critical variables in the radioimmunoassay of serum insulin using the double antibody technique. *Diabetes* 1965;14:771–9.
44. Bhuiyan AKMJ, Bartlett K, Sherratt HSA, Agius L. Effects of ciprofibrate and 2-[5-(4-chloro-phenyl)pentyl]oxirane-2-carboxylate (POCA) on the distribution of carnitine and CoA and their acyl esters and on enzyme activities in rats. *Biochem J* 1988;253:337–43.
45. Bhuiyan AKMJ, Watmough NJ, Turnbull DM, Aynsley-Green A, Leonard JV, Bartlett K. A new simple screening method for the diagnosis of medium-chain acyl-CoA dehydrogenase deficiency. *Clin Chim Acta* 1989;165:39–44.
46. Bhuiyan AKMJ, Bartlett K. Reverse-phase high performance liquid chhromatographic analysis of short-, medium-, and long-chain acylcarnitines in urine and plasma. *Biochem Soc Trans* 1988;16:796–7.
47. Frerman FE, Goodman SI. Fluorimetric assay of acyl-CoA dehydrogenase in normal and mutant human fibroblasts. *Biochem Med* 1985;33:38–44.
48. Soltesz G, Aynsley-Green A. Hyperinsulinism in infancy and childhood. In: *Advances in internal medicine pediatrics*. Berlin: Springer-Verlag 1984;151–202.
49. Aynsley-Green A, Soltesz G. Hypoglycemia due to hyperinsulinism. In: *Current reviews in paediatrics 1; Hypoglycaemia in infancy and childhood*. London: Churchill Livingstone 1985;54–102.
50. Watmough NJ, Turnbull DM, Sherratt HSA, Bartlett K. Measurement of the acyl-CoA intermediates of β-oxidation by h.p.l.c. with on-line radiochemical and photodiode array detection. *Biochem J* 1989; 262:261–9.

DISCUSSION

Dr. Wanders: One of the problems, as Professor Van Hoof says, with regard to the mitochondrial β-oxidation defects is that it is difficult to identify them if you look at organic acids in urine. You suggest doing starvation provocation tests, but perhaps there is another possibility and I should like to have your ideas about it. Mitochondrial β-oxidation is expressed in leukocytes and blood platelets. We have been working on this aspect for several months, and what we do now, in our hospital at least, is to take blood for isolation of leukocytes and platelets from any patient with hypoketotic hypoglycemia to study octanoate β-oxidation and palmitate β-oxidation, looking at CO_2 production and acid-soluble material. In this group of disorders particularly, in which you should intervene with diet treatment as soon as possible, it is of utmost importance to know straight away whether or not there is a mitochondrial β-oxidation defect. Hence in this case enzyme analysis should not be at the end of the investigations but rather should be one of the first things to do. What is your view on this?

Dr. Bartlett: I agree. I think we have a problem here: If you measure a specific enzyme and you find it is normal, you may then conclude that you are not dealing with a β-oxidation defect.

This is obviously a dangerous assumption. There are two possible solutions. You can either devise a method to measure the flux of the whole process, for example by measurement of total acid soluble radioactivity derived from radiolabeled substrates, or measure all the enzymes of β-oxidation directly. The latter course would be a major undertaking.

Dr. Wanders: But the first is very easy to do. To look at octanoate β-oxidation and palmitate β-oxidation is simple. I would like to make a strong plea for overall β-oxidation testing in leukocytes or platelets.

Dr. Bartlett: We have tried to devise a radiochemical method for the measurement of β-oxidation flux, although we have not yet applied it to routine screening. I should explain that the conventional way to approach this problem is to incubate fibroblasts or leukocytes with [1-^{14}C]-labeled substrates, for example [1-^{14}C]octanoate and [1-^{14}C]palmitate, and to measure $^{14}CO_2$. The logic is that if octanoate oxidation is normal and palmitate oxidation is impaired, a long chain disorder is indicated. The problem with this technique is that it is difficult to obtain reliable assays, probably because CO_2 is quantitatively a minor product in these tissues. We would like to have a reliable single method to measure β-oxidation flux. We have tried using universally labeled substrates and measuring CO_2 production and acid-soluble radioactivity. To date we have obtained rather poor discrimination between affected and nonaffected cell lines. Whether or not there is still a place for CO_2 release assays I am not sure.

Dr. Van Hoof: One of the difficulties in the interpretation of results obtained with 1[^{14}C]-labeled fatty acids is that $^{14}CO_2$ production can result both from α- and β-oxidations. I think that Dr. Saudubray has some experience with the use of radiolabeled fatty acids in the diagnosis of mitochondrial β-oxidation defects.

Dr. Saudubray: I have a comment and a question. The comment is about fatty acid oxidation in fresh isolated lymphocytes. To me it is a very convenient method: very rapid and reliable for screening most fatty acid oxidation disorders, but not all. I should like to emphasize the value of performing an *in vivo* oral loading test with polyunsaturated long chain fatty acids. This procedure is very reliable and very safe; you can perform the test after an overnight fast of 10 to 12 h, with 1.5 g per kilogram of polyunsaturated sunflower oil. Blood ketones are measured at 0, 1.2, and 3 h after the load. We have used this test successfully in every fatty acid oxidation disorder we have investigated, including PCTI, PCTII, long chain, medium chain, and generalized fatty acid oxidation disorders, and also 3-hydroxyacyl-CoA-dehydrogenase deficiency. In addition, we identified four patients with this loading test who had a clinical and metabolic pattern very suggestive of long chain fatty acid disorders (hypoketotic hypoglycemia, Reye-like encephalopathy), but without any defect identified *in vitro* in lymphocytes or "film blasts." These four patients presented with a complete absence of increase of blood ketones after the loading test with the polyunsaturated long chain fatty acids. There was no abnormal plasma carnitine level, no abnormal organic acids in the urine, and fatty acid oxidation was completely normal in fibroblasts and lymphocytes. We are now planning to carry out *in vitro* fatty acid oxidation experiments in liver biopsy specimens. Because these patients suggest the possibility of fatty acid oxidation defects restricted to the liver, it seems to me at the moment that the best system for screening such patients is the long chain fatty acid loading test.

Dr. Bartlett: We certainly considered that possibility when we started our studies. We came to the conclusion that as a general principle, once one has administered something to a patient it is impossible to remove it if something goes wrong. We concluded that the safest course was a fasting provocation test, because it is straightforward to abort the test by the administration of glucose. So although I take the point that it is possible to stress β-oxidation by the administration of a fat load, we have no direct experience.

Dr. Endres: I think that fasting is a relatively dangerous procedure for young babies or infants.

As a pediatrician I have some difficulty in deciding what is the most suitable screening test for defects in β-oxidation in children with near-miss sudden infant death syndrome. Tanaka proposed that one should just take a random sample of urine and use a stable isotope dilution technique for gas chromatography–mass spectrometry (GC-MS). What is your experience with this method, since the loading with phenylpropionic acid proposed by Seakins and co-workers can be used only for the diagnosis of MCAD deficiency? What do you think about this special technique for GC-MS?

Dr. Bartlett: I believe you are referring to a paper by Rinaldo et al. (1) which describes a stable isotope dilution assay for glycine conjugates in urine. They measured hexanoylglycine, phenylpropionylglycine, and suberylglycine and reported that they could detect abnormal concentrations of some of these during periods of remission: in other words, under normoglycemic conditions. The only problem with this approach is that the technique requires gas chromatography–mass spectrometry, and the stable isotopically labeled internal standards are not commercially available. I cannot say from my own experience whether the technique is reliable, although I am sure Dr. Roe has something to say about the alternatives.

Dr. Roe: That is an interesting point. I think the use of phenylpropionate loading, as Professor Endres indicated, would seem to be relatively restricted to MCAD patients. So it is a rather focused approach, almost like doing an enzyme assay selectively. On the other hand, it should be recognized that phenylpropionyl glycine is not seen in newborns because it is a metabolite produced by established bacterial flora. I would agree with Professor Endres that one should avoid fasting young infants when looking for β-oxidation disorders.

Dr. Bartlett: We have now performed over 200 fasting stress tests, including tests of patients with subsequently proven β-oxidation disorders. In none have we experienced any untoward clinical sequelae. However, it is important to emphasize that these were always carried out under close clinical supervision and that fasts were always terminated within the limits indicated.

Dr. Roe: The Hopkins group lost one child in the course of the fasting, and another child in Denmark was lost.

Dr. Eggermont: In the newborn, ketonuria is very rare. Can you comment on the metabolism of ketone bodies in the newborn and the infant?

Dr. Bartlett: Ketone bodies are a major substrate for brain in the newborn period. There are, of course, some important dietary transitions in early life, from a largely carbohydrate-based economy during fetal life to a high-fat diet in the neonatal period and a further transition to a mixed diet at weaning. Thus in the newborn period it is really not surprising that ketone bodies are extensively utilized, both as metabolic fuels and as lipogenic precursors in the brain.

Dr. Holton: Screening for MCAD has been recommended, particularly in siblings of SIDS patients. It is suggested that the urine metabolites could be picked up during the first couple of days of life, and some groups are doing this in large numbers. Do you think that this is reliable?

Dr. Bartlett: If you assume that about 2–3% of SIDS cases are caused by medium chain acyl-CoA dehydrogenase deficiency, although the precise proportion is still open to debate, and further that it is an autosomal condition, then in order to obtain statistically significant results, large numbers of siblings of SIDS would have to be screened. There is a more serious problem with screening siblings of SIDS. It is accepted that the excretion of informative abnormal metabolites is critically dependent on the metabolic milieu at the time the urine is collected. If conventional gas chromatographic methods are used rather than the stable isotope/GCMS method described by Rinaldo et al. (1), I am not convinced that even if MCAD were present, it would be detected by analysis of random urines, that is, without some form of metabolic stress.

Dr. Duran: I would like to comment on the neonatal urine screening of sibling case of the SIDS. We had the opportunity to study two siblings of proven MCAD-deficient patients in the first week of life and we did not find any abnormal metabolites then. What we then did was a phenoylpropionate loading test 2 months later and we found that the result of that loading test was positive. We are content with this loading test because it cannot only pick up the MCAD deficiency but probably also other defects. For example, we showed that we could pick up long chain 3-hydroxyacyl-CoA-dehydrogenase deficiency.

Dr. Hobbs: I realize that your particular assay at the moment requires a large number of cells, but it is possible these days to produce them in culture. There does tend to be a dogma that it is almost impossible to insert extraneous enzymes into mitochondria, but if you were to grow the fibroblasts of a deficient patient and then add the cells or plasma from a normal subject, the hypothesis could be tested. If, indeed, the normal cells were able to deliver the deficient enzyme into mitochondria of the patient's cells, you would have a clear indication of future possible treatments.

Dr. Bartlett: Most polypeptide precursors of mitochondrial proteins have a peptide leader sequence that both targets them to the corret intracellular compartment and allows them to traverse the inner mitochondrial membrane. This leader sequence is removed to allow generation of active enzyme. I did not show the data, but we have studied a patient whom we find difficult to explain. She presented with hypoketotic, hyper-fatty acidemic hypoglycemia and excreted the metabolites characteristic of medium chain acyl-CoA dehydrogenase deficiency. However, we found normal activity as measured in homogenates of cultured skin fibroblasts. We were puzzled by this until it was pointed out that a mutation in the leader sequence could account for these findings. It is possible that an accumulated precursor peptide could undergo maturation to active enzyme following homogenization. I agree that it may be possible to study enzyme replacement therapy for mitochondrial disorders by such a technique, but I think it would be necessary to use the precursor peptide.

Dr. Krywawych: In those cases where you see dicarboxylic acids, is it only saturated dicarboxylic acids or are unsaturated acids also present? If there are unsaturated dicarboxylic acids, do you think that this is simply a reflection of dietary intake of unsaturated acids, or do you think that this may be used as an indicator of a more specific enzyme lesion in β-oxidation?

Dr. Bartlett: We do see C10 unsaturated dicarboxylic acids. I have always assumed that these are generated from polyunsaturated fatty acids which are dietary in origin.

Dr. Saudubray: I have a question on the 3-hydroxybutyrate–acetoacetate ratio and lactate biorate ratio in the blood. Have you checked these ratios in fatty acid oxidation defects?

Dr. Bartlett: The 3-hydroxybutyrate/acetoacetate and lactate/pyruvate ratios were normal, as were the lactate concentrations in medium chain acyl-CoA dehydrogenase deficiency. However, we have observed raised lactate concentrations in three cases of long chain 3-hydroxyacyl-CoA dehydrogenase deficiency.

Dr. Saudubray: We could expect to find lowered ratios. The fatty acid oxidation defect should lower the production of NADH and FADH in mitochondria, resulting in secondary lowering of lactate.

Dr. Bartlett: I would not anticipate an altered mitochondrial redox state simply because of impaired β-oxidation. There are, after all, plenty of other oxidizable substrates, at least under normoglycemic conditions.

Dr. Krywawych: You have said that control of β-oxidation occurs at the CPT1 stage. Presumably, the carnitine concentration can influence the rate of β-oxidation, as carnitine is a substrate for the CPT1 enzyme. Does the carnitine status, reflected in the plasma carnitine concentrations, alter the plot of plasma concentrations of fatty acids against ketone bodies in

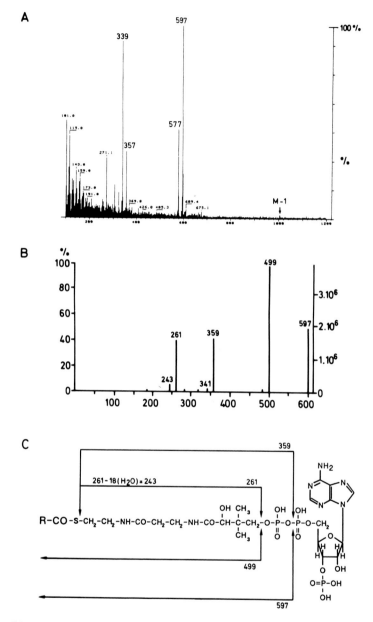

FIG. 1. Triple-quadrupole mass spectrometric detection of palmitoyl-CoA. In the simple FAB-MS spectrum the molecular ion (M-1) is almost undetectable (**A**). The most intense signal corresponding to a negative ion with a mass of 597 results from the loss of adenosine 3′- and 5′-bisphosphate. Daughter fragments of this 597 ion displayed in (**B**) are typical. Three among them with masses of 243, 261, and 359 are common to all CoA esters; the other two (499 and 597) vary with the length of the fatty acid, as explained on the formula of a coenzyme A ester, in (**C**).

normal subjects? Can carnitine deficiency, which may be secondary to some other problem, produce a condition that appears to be a block in β-oxidation?

Dr. Bartlett: Early reports of what were thought to be cases of primary systemic carnitine deficiency have been shown to be, I think without exception, secondary to β-oxidation disorders. As far as I am aware, there have been very few substantiated cases of inherited primary carnitine deficiency.

Dr. Van Hoof: Important progress in the diagnosis of disorders of mitochondrial β-oxidation has resulted from the development of tandem mass spectrometry. Acylcarnitine in blood and urine reflect the accumulation of acyl-CoA esters in the mitochondrial matrix. I would like to show you that acyl-CoA can be directly analyzed with a tandem mass spectrometer. Figure 1, obtained with the collaboration of S. Ponchaut, as well as E. de Hoffmann from the Department of Mass Spectrometry of the University of Louvain (Louvain-la-Neuve), shows that specific fragments are formed by fast atom bombardment, which allow one to recognize the CoA esters. The upper part of the figure (A) displays a positive ion scan of deionized palmitoyl-CoA dissolved in a mixture of glycerol and 1% glycolic acid. The molecular ion is barely detectable at a mass of 1004, but there is an intense fragment at mass 597. The daughter scan of this fragment submitted to collision with xenon atoms (B) reveals interesting fragments, some (at mass 499) containing the fatty acid and some (at mass 243, 261, 359) which are common to all CoA derivatives. An explanation of each of these fragments is given in the inferior part of the figure (C).

Dr. Bartlett: We have done a similar sort of thing with FAB-MS and intact CoA esters. We have been able to carry out FAB-MS analysis of the complete series of saturated C4–C16 mono-CoA esters of dicarboxylic acids. It also works well for the carnitine esters, of course.

REFERENCE

1. Rinaldo P, O'Shea JJ, Coates PM, Hale DE, Stanley CA, Tanaka K. Medium chain acyl-CoA dehydrogenase deficiency: diagnosis by stable isotope dilution measurement of urinary *n*-hexanoylglycine and 3-phenylpropionylglycine. *N Engl J Med* 1988;319:1308–13.

Inborn Errors of Metabolism, edited by
J. Schaub, F. Van Hoof, and H. L. Vis.
Nestlé Nutrition Workshop Series, Vol. 24.
Nestec Ltd., Vevey/Raven Press, Ltd.,
New York © 1991.

Disorders of Peroxisomal Fatty Acid β-Oxidation

Ronald J. A. Wanders, Carlo W. T. van Roermund,
Ruud B. H. Schutgens, and *Joseph M. Tager

*Department of Pediatrics, University Hospital of Amsterdam, Meibergdreef 9, 1105 AZ Amsterdam; *Department of Biochemistry, E. C. Slater Institute, University of Amsterdam, Meibergdreef 15, 1105 AZ Amsterdam, The Netherlands*

The functional significance of a second fatty acid β-oxidizing system localized in peroxisomes has remained obscure for some time. In recent years, however, much has been learned about the physiological importance of the peroxisomal β-oxidation system. The recognition of a group of inherited diseases in humans associated with a dysfunction in one or more steps involved in peroxisomal β-oxidation stresses the importance of this β-oxidation system.

As discussed in detail elsewhere (1), peroxisomes are now known to be involved in the β-oxidative chain shortening of a distinct set of compounds. In case of some of these compounds, notably very long chain fatty acids (VLCFA) and the bile acid intermediates di- and trihydroxycholestanoic acid (DHCA and THCA), oxidation takes place virtually exclusively in peroxisomes, whereas in other cases (long chain fatty acids, mono- and polyunsaturated fatty acids, prostaglandins, dicarboxylic acids), both mitochondria and peroxisomes contribute to their β-oxidation.

ENZYMES INVOLVED IN THE PEROXISOMAL β-OXIDATION OF VERY LONG CHAIN FATTY ACIDS AND DI- AND TRIHYDROXYCHOLESTANOIC ACIDS

β-Oxidation of Very Long Chain Fatty Acids

As discussed in more detail elsewhere (1,2) the peroxisomal enzymes involved in fatty acid β-oxidation are different from their mitochondrial counterparts, except for the long chain fatty acyl-CoA synthetase. This enzyme, present on the cytosolic site of the peroxisomal membrane (3), is identical to the enzyme present in the mito-

---

Corresponding author: RJA Wanders.

chondrial outer membrane and the membrane of the endoplasmic reticulum (4). Recently, it has become clear that there is a separate acyl-CoA synthetase involved in the activation of very long chain fatty acids. This enzyme activity is present in peroxisomes and endoplasmic reticulum but not in mitochondria (5,6). That the enzyme is, indeed, different from the long chain fatty acyl-CoA synthetase, is concluded from their different subcellular localization (5,6), kinetic properties (7), competition experiments (5), their behavior toward various detergents (8), immunological studies (9), and the findings in X-linked adrenoleukodystrophy (see below). Following their activation, the very long chain fatty acyl-CoA esters are subsequently β-oxidized via the concerted action of acyl-CoA oxidase, bifunctional protein with enoyl-CoA hydratase and L-3-hydroxyacyl-CoA dehydrogenase activity, and peroxisomal thiolase.

β-Oxidation of Di- and Trihydroxycholestanoic Acid

Recent studies by the groups of Mannaerts and Pedersen, respectively, have shed new light on the pathway of di- and trihydroxycholestanoic acid oxidation in peroxisomes. First, activation of trihydroxycholestanoic acid does not occur in peroxisomes but instead is catalyzed by a specific activating enzyme present in the endoplasmic reticulum (10,11). Furthermore, it is now clear that the first step in the subsequent β-oxidation of the THCA-CoA ester is carried out by a distinct trihydroxycholestanoyl-CoA oxidase (12,13). The findings in some of the disorders of peroxisomal β-oxidation (see below) suggest that, at least in humans, subsequent oxidation of the unsaturated Δ^{24}-THCA-CoA is catalyzed by the same enzymes as those involved in the oxidation of α,β-unsaturated VLCFA-CoA esters (i.e., bifunctional protein and peroxisomal thiolase; see Fig. 1).

INBORN ERRORS OF PEROXISOMAL β-OXIDATION

The inborn errors of peroxisomal β-oxidation known today are listed in Table 1. These include diseases in which peroxisomal β-oxidation is impaired due to a deficiency of all peroxisomal β-oxidation enzyme proteins resulting from the (virtual) absence of peroxisomes (group A), diseases in which peroxisomal β-oxidation is impaired due to the loss of multiple peroxisomal β-oxidation enzyme activities (group B), and diseases in which a single peroxisomal β-oxidation enzyme activity is lost (group C). In the latter two groups, morphologically distinguishable peroxisomes are present in normal amounts. The characteristics of these disorders are described below.

The Peroxisome Deficiency Disorders

The clinical and biochemical characteristics of this group of disorders have recently been described in detail (14,15) and will only be summarized briefly here, especially

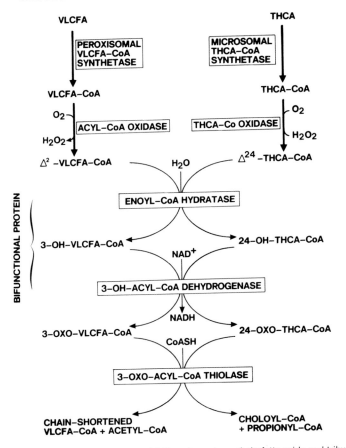

FIG. 1. The activation and subsequent β-oxidation of very long chain fatty acids and trihydroxycholestanoic acid in peroxisomes.

since these disorders cannot be taken to be true disorders of peroxisomal β-oxidation. The prototype of the group of peroxisome deficiency disorders, alternatively named disorders of peroxisome biogenesis (15), is the cerebro-hepato-renal syndrome of Zellweger. In patients suffering from the classical form of Zellweger syndrome there are multiple abnormalities, including craniofacial, neurological, ocular, hepatological, renal, skeletal, and other aberrations [see (14,15) for details].

Morphologically distinguishable peroxisomes are also (virtually) absent in neonatal adrenoleukodystrophy, infantile Refsum disease, and the four cases of hyperpipecolic acidemia described in the literature. Without going into detail, it can be concluded that disorders of group A are overlapping syndromes, the clinical course being mildest in patients suffering from infantile Refsum disease (16).

The (virtual) absence of peroxisomes in these patients is associated with a generalized loss of peroxisomal functions, including peroxisomal fatty acid β-oxidation. Indeed, immunoblotting experiments have shown that the three peroxisomal β-ox-

TABLE 1. *Inborn errors of peroxisomal β-oxidation*

Peroxisomal disorder	Peroxisomal β-oxidation defect
A. *Peroxisomes absent, generalized dysfunction*	
Cerebro-hepato-renal (Zellweger) syndrome	Generalized
Neonatal adrenoleukodystrophy	Generalized
Infantile Refsum disease	Generalized
Hyperpipecolic acidemia	Generalized
B. *Peroxisomes present, multiple defects*	
"Zellweger-like" syndrome	Multiple defects (acyl-CoA oxidase, bifunctional protein, and peroxisomal thiolase)
C. *Peroxisomes present, single defect*	
X-linked adrenoleukodystrophy	Peroxisomal very long chain acyl-CoA synthetase
Acyl-CoA oxidase deficiency (pseudo-NALD)	Acyl-CoA oxidase
Peroxisomal thiolase deficiency (pseudo-ZS)	Peroxisomal thiolase
Bifunctional protein deficiency	Bifunctional protein

idation enzyme proteins (acyl-CoA oxidase, bifunctional protein, and peroxisomal thiolase) are strongly deficient in Zellweger patients as well as in other patients in whom there is a major deficiency of peroxisomes (see ref. 1 for references). This explains the strong impairment in the oxidation of very long chain fatty acids such as tetracosanoic acid (24:0) and hexacosanoic acid (26:0), as first described by Singh and co-workers (17). Oxidation of palmitate and stearate was found to proceed normally in these cells in accordance with the view that oxidation of these fatty acids occurs primarily in mitochondria. The deficiency of bifunctional protein and peroxisomal thiolase also explains the impairment in THCA-CoA β-oxidation (18,19) in Zellweger patients, leading to their accumulation in plasma and other body fluids. Recent studies have shown that the oxidation of other fatty acids is also impaired in patients lacking peroxisomes. Indeed, Christensen and co-workers (20,21) recently reported that the oxidation of erucic acid [C22:1 (*n*-9)] and adrenic acid [C22:4 (*n*-6)] is deficient in fibroblasts from Zellweger (20) and neonatal adrenoleukodystrophy patients, whereas the oxidation of linolenic acid [18:3 (*n*-3)], arachidonic acid [20:4 (*n*-6)], and eicosapentaenoic acid [C20:5 (*n*-3)] was found to proceed normally (21). In a recent study by Street et al. (22) oxidation of tetracosatetraenoic acid [C24:4 (*n*-6)] was also found to be deficient in Zellweger patients (see ref. 1).

Abnormalities in plasma and other body fluids of Zellweger patients are not restricted to very long chain fatty acids and bile acid intermediates, but also include various medium and long chain dicarboxylic acids. Although not related to peroxisomal β-oxidation directly, it is interesting to note that Martinez (23) recently reported remarkable abnormalities in the content of some polyunsaturated fatty acids, notably C22:6 (*n*-3) and C22:5 (*n*-6), in tissues from a Zellweger infant.

Disorders of Peroxisomal β-Oxidation Characterized by the Multiple Loss of Peroxisomal β-Oxidation Enzyme Activities

The only peroxisomal disorder known to belong to this category is "Zellweger-like syndrome," so far described in two patients (24,25). In these patients, who had a clinical presentation indistinguishable from Zellweger syndrome, the three peroxisomal β-oxidation enzyme proteins were found to be deficient upon immunoblotting. Furthermore, the activity of the peroxisomal enzyme acyl-CoA:dihydroxyacetonephosphate acyltransferase was found to be deficient in accordance with a deficiency of plasmalogens. Morphological studies, however, revealed the normal presence of peroxisomes.

Disorders of Peroxisomal β-Oxidation Associated with a Deficiency of Only One Peroxisomal β-Oxidation Enzyme Activity

X-Linked Adrenoleukodystrophy (Adreno-testiculo-leuko-myelo-neuropathic Complex)

The presentation of adrenoleukodystrophy (ALD) in its classical form is that of a boy who develops normally for the first years of life and then presents with signs of central nervous system involvement as manifested in behavioral abnormalities, visual and auditory disturbances, abnormal gait, loss of school performances, and other derangements (see refs. 26 and 27 for reviews). Studies in the 1970s have established that there is an accumulation of very long chain fatty acids in tissues as well as in fibroblasts and plasma of ALD patients. The discovery of a biochemical marker for ALD has enabled Moser and co-workers to study the phenotype of ALD, which they have shown to vary enormously, not only between families but also within the same pedigree (26).

Recent studies have identified the enzyme defect in ALD. A key finding in this respect was the observation by Hashmi et al. (28), who reported that the oxidation of lignoceroyl-CoA was unimpaired in ALD fibroblasts in contrast to the oxidation of lignoceric acid itself. Studies by Singh and co-workers (29) and ourselves (30) have shown that the defect in ALD is indeed at the level of a deficient activity of the peroxisomal enzyme which activates very long chain fatty acids to their CoA esters. In microsomes, however, a normal VLCFA-CoA synthetase activity was found (29,30). This suggests that the two VLCFA-CoA synthetases have different functions in the cell and that the VLCFA-CoA ester synthesized at the site of the endoplasmic reticulum is not available for β-oxidation in the peroxisome. This situation closely resembles the situation in the yeast *Candida lipolytica* (31). Interestingly, Lazo et al. (31) recently suggested that the inability of the microsomal VLCFA-CoA synthetase to generate VLCFA-CoA esters for β-oxidation in the peroxisome is due to the hydrolysis of VLCFA-CoA esters by acyl-CoA hydrolases present in the cytosol.

Acyl-CoA Oxidase Deficiency (Pseudo-neonatal Adrenoleukodystrophy)

This condition has only been described in two patients within the same family (32). Both patients presented with early seizures, muscle hypotonia, progressive hearing loss, and visual impairment. There was psychomotor retardation but no facial dysmorphia. These and other clinical findings led to the diagnosis of neonatal ALD. Peroxisomes were found to be normally present, however. Subsequent immuno-blotting studies revealed a deficiency of acyl-CoA oxidase (32). This was associated with elevated plasma VLCFA levels, whereas the bile acid intermediates were normal, which is in line with the recent findings of a separate THCA-CoA oxidase (12, 13).

Bifunctional Protein Deficiency

Recently, Watkins et al. (33) identified the first case of bifunctional protein deficiency in a patient who showed a variety of clinical abnormalities resembling those found in Zellweger syndrome and neonatal ALD. There was no dysmorphia, however. The patient remained hypotonic and showed no developmental progress. Interestingly, a brain biopsy at 6 weeks of age revealed polymicrogyria. Morphologically distinguishable peroxisomes were found to be normally present in this patient. In plasma accumulation of VLCFAs and bile acid intermediates was found. Bifunctional protein was subsequently found to be deficient upon immunoblotting. We have recently identified a second patient with this disorder (see below).

Peroxisomal 3-Oxoacyl-CoA Thiolase Deficiency (Pseudo-Zellweger Syndrome)

In 1986, Goldfischer et al. (34) described a patient with all the clinical and pathological features of Zellweger syndrome, including facial dysmorphia, hypotonia at birth, and neuronal heterotopia. Abnormal VLCFA and bile acid intermediates levels were found in plasma. Subsequent studies revealed the presence of hepatic peroxisomes in normal amounts. Furthermore, plasmalogen biosynthesis was found to proceed normally. The defect in this patient turned out to be at the level of peroxisomal 3-oxoacyl CoA thiolase (35).

Unidentified Disorders of Peroxisomal β-Oxidation

In recent years several patients with a defect in peroxisomal β-oxidation of unknown etiology have been described (see ref. 1 for a review). In one of these patients we have recently found that the defective VLCFA β-oxidation is due to a deficient activity of bifunctional protein. Interestingly, the protein itself was found to be normally present upon immunoblotting, which suggests that the mutation affects the active site of the enzyme without resulting in reduced enzyme protein levels.

DIAGNOSIS OF INBORN ERRORS OF PEROXISOMAL β-OXIDATION

It is clear from the data described above (see also Table 2) that there is accumulation of very long chain fatty acids in all disorders of peroxisomal β-oxidation known so far, which allows identification by means of gas chromatographic analysis of plasma VLCFAs. If, indeed, VLCFAs are found to accumulate in plasma from a particular patient, additional analyses in plasma (bile acid intermediates, pipecolic acid, phytanic acid), platelets (activity measurements of DHAPAT), and fibroblasts (plasmalogen biosynthesis, VLCFA β-oxidation, phytanic acid oxidation, and particle-bound catalase) will have to be done to find out whether the impairment in peroxisomal VLCFA β-oxidation is the result of a deficiency of peroxisomes (as in group A) or due to the loss of multiple (group B) or single (group C) β-oxidation enzyme activities (see ref. 1 for details).

TABLE 2. *Biochemical characteristics of the inborn errors of peroxisomal β-oxidation*

Parameter measured	Peroxisome deficiency disorders	Zellweger-like syndrome	X-linked ALD	Pseudo-Zellweger syndrome	Pseudo-neonatal ALD	Bifunctional protein deficiency
Metabolites in body fluids						
Very long chain fatty acids	Elevated	Elevated	Elevated	Elevated	Elevated	Elevated
Bile acid intermediates	Elevated	Elevated	Normal	Elevated	Normal	Elevated
Pipecolic acid	Elevated[a]	Normal	Normal	Normal	Normal	Normal
Phytanic acid	Elevated[a]	Normal	Normal	Normal	Normal	Normal
Plasmalogen synthesis						
DHAPAT	Deficient	Deficient	Normal	Normal	Normal	Normal
Alkyl DHAP synthase	Deficient		Normal	Normal	Normal	Normal
De novo synthesis	Impaired	Impaired	Normal	Normal	Normal	Normal
Peroxisomes						
Hepatic peroxisomes	(Virtually) absent	Present	Present	Present	Present	Present
Particle-bound catalase (% of total)	<5	n.d.	>65	>65	>65	>65
Peroxisomal β-oxidation						
Activity with C26:0	Deficient	Deficient	Deficient	Deficient	Deficient	Deficient
Enzyme proteins						
Acyl-CoA oxidase	Deficient	Deficient	Normal	Normal	Deficient	Normal
Bifunctional protein	Deficient	Deficient	Normal	Normal	Normal	Deficient
Peroxisomal thiolase	Deficient	Deficient	Normal	Deficient	Normal	Normal

[a] Age dependent.
n.d., not done.

PRENATAL DIAGNOSIS

Prenatal diagnosis is possible in any of the inborn errors of peroxisomal β-oxidation known today (see ref. 1 for a review). This can be done in the first trimester of pregnancy via analyses in chorionic biopsy material or cultured chorionic villous fibroblasts.

PATHOGENIC ASPECTS

Although our knowledge regarding disorders of peroxisomal β-oxidation is of rather recent date, it is clear that they are all devastating diseases with severe neurological involvement. If we restrict the discussion to the true disorders of peroxisomal β-oxidation (i.e., group C), the available information suggests that the severity of the disease is related to the exact site of the enzymic defect. Indeed, the deficiency of peroxisomal thiolase is associated with a clinical phenotype indistinguishable from the Zellweger syndrome, whereas a deficiency of acyl-CoA oxidase is associated with a much milder phenotype (32). This is even more so if X-linked adrenoleukodystrophy is concerned. A possible explanation for this relationship is that a deficiency of peroxisomal VLCFA-CoA synthetase or peroxisomal thiolase affects VLCFA β-oxidation to the same extent but affects the peroxisomal β-oxidation of other compounds differently. Indeed, peroxisomal VLCFA-CoA synthetase is probably involved in activation of very long chain fatty acids only, whereas peroxisomal thiolase is not only involved in VLCFA β-oxidation, but also in the β-oxidation of THCA-CoA and (most likely) mono- and polyunsaturated fatty acyl-CoA esters, prostaglandin CoA-esters, and other compounds yet to be identified. The same probably applies to acyl-CoA oxidase, which is not only involved in VLCFA β-oxidation but also in the β-oxidation of other compounds, such as prostaglandin CoA-esters (but not THCA-CoA).

With regard to the relationship between biochemical abnormalities on the one hand and clinical and pathological aberrations on the other, little is known even in the case of X-linked ALD, in which the accumulation of VLCFAs is the only known abnormality. Recent studies by Whitcomb et al. (36) suggest that very long chain fatty acids are toxic to the cell, changing the microviscosity of the membrane and subsequently its biological properties. This was concluded from experiments with adrenocortical cells which showed a decreased rate of ACTH-induced cortisol production upon addition of hexacosanoic acid. Interestingly, Meyer et al. (37) reported that leukocytes from ALD patients lack detectable ACTH-binding sites.

One of the most striking neuropathological abnormalities in Zellweger patients is the greatly disturbed neuronal migration. This disordered migration leads to unique cytoarchitectonic abnormalities which involve the cerebral hemispheres, the cerebellum, and the inferior olivary complex (26). In the cerebral hemispheres, neurons that are destined to migrate to outer cortical layers remain scattered within the inner cortical layers. The finding that a deficiency of peroxisomal thiolase leads to the same abnormalities (34) suggests a direct causal relationship between the disturbance in neuronal migration and the deficiency of peroxisomal thiolase, although there is no information on the exact mechanism. According to this rationale, the deficiency of plasmalogens is not of major pathogenic significance in this respect.

THERAPY IN DISORDERS OF PEROXISOMAL β-OXIDATION

In 1986, Rizzo et al. (38) discovered that addition of oleic acid to the culture medium of ALD fibroblasts leads to a drastic reduction in C26:0 levels. Since very long chain fatty acids originate primarily from endogenous fatty acids via chain elongation, it was suggested that oleic acid exerted its effect via competition at the level of chain elongation. These findings inspired Rizzo et al. (39) and Moser et al. (40) to try to reduce very long chain fatty acids in patients via a combined approach consisting of the use of a diet low in VLCFAs together with the administration of a glycerol trioleate oil. This combined approach would reduce exogenous as well as endogenous sources of the VLCFA burden in ALD. The results obtained so far indicate that plasma C26:0 levels in ALD patients can be reduced significantly via this regimen (39,40). However, clinical and neurological evaluation revealed little or no improvement. Along the same lines both Moser and Rizzo have instituted a new therapy involving the use of erucate rather than oleate. Preliminary results show that plasma C26:0 levels normalize almost completely. Whether or not this will be beneficial to ALD patients is studied intensively at this moment.

ACKNOWLEDGMENTS

Supported by grants from the Netherlands Fund for Medical Health Foundation (MEDIGON) and the Princess Beatrix Fund (The Hague, The Netherlands). Simone Majoor is gratefully acknowledged for preparation of the manuscript.

REFERENCES

1. Wanders RJA, van Roermund CWT, Schutgens RBH, et al. The inborn errors of peroxisomal β-oxidation. *J Inher Metab Dis* 1990;13:4–36.
2. Mannaerts GP, Van Veldhoven PP. Fatty acid oxidation: general overview, chapter in this volume.
3. Mannaerts GP, Van Veldhoven P, Van Broekhoven A, Van de Broek G, De Beer LJ. Evidence that peroxisomal acyl-CoA synthetase is located at the cytoplasmic site of the peroxisomal membrane. *Biochem J* 1982;204:17–23.
4. Miyazawa S, Hashimoto T, Yokota S. Identity of long-chain acyl coenzyme A synthetase of microsomes, mitochondria, and peroxisomes in rat liver. *J Biochem* 1985;98:723–33.
5. Wanders RJA, van Roermund CWT, van Wijland MJA, et al. Peroxisomal fatty acid β-oxidation in relation to the accumulation of very long chain fatty acids in peroxisomal disorders. *J Clin Invest* 1987; 80:1778–83.
6. Singh H, Derwas N, Poulos A. Very long chain fatty acid β-oxidation by rat liver mitochondria and peroxisomes. *Arch Biochem Biophys* 1987;359:382–90.
7. Bhusnan A, Singh RP, Singh I. Characterization of rat brain microsomal acyl-coenzyme A ligase: different

enzymes for the synthesis of palmitoyl-CoA and lignoceroyl-CoA. *Arch Biochem Biophys* 1986;246:374–80.

8. Singh H, Poulos A. Distinct long chain and very long chain fatty acyl-CoA synthetases in rat liver peroxisomes and microsomes. *Arch Biochem Biophys* 1988;266:486–95.

9. Singh I, Bhusnan A, Relan NK, Hashimoto T. Peroxisomal lignoceroyl-CoA ligase: an immunological study. *Biochim Biophys Acta* 1989;963:509–14.

10. Schepers L, Casteels M, Verheyden K, et al. Subcellular distribution and characteristics of trihydroxy-coprostanoyl-CoA synthetase. *Biochem J* 1989;257:221–9.

11. Prydz K, Kase BF, Björkhem I, Pedersen JI. Subcellular localization of 3α,7α-dihydroxy-and 3α,7α, 12α-trihydroxy-5β-cholestanoyl-coenzyme A ligase(s) in rat liver. *J Lipid Res* 1988;29:997–1004.

12. Casteels M, Schepers L, Van Eldere J, Eyssen H, Mannaerts GP. Inhibition of 3α, 7α, 12α-trihydroxy-5β-cholestanoic acid oxidation and of bile acid secretion in rat liver by fatty acids. *J Biol Chem* 1988; 263:4654–61.

13. Pederson JI, Hvattum E, Flatabo T, Björkhem I. Clofibrate does not induce peroxisomal 3α, 7α,12α-trihydroxy-5β-cholestanoyl coenzyme A oxidation in rat liver: evidence that this reaction is catalyzed by an enzyme system different from that of peroxisomal acyl-CoA oxidation. *Biochem Int* 1988; 17:163–9.

14. Wanders RJA, Heymans HSA, Schutgens RBH, Barth PG, van den Bosch H, Tager JM. Peroxisomal disorders in neurology. *J Neurol Sci* 1988;88:1–39.

15. Lazarow PB, Moser HW. Disorders of peroxisome biogenesis. In: Scriver CR, Beaudet AL, Sly WS, Valle D, eds. *The metabolic basis of inherited disorders*. New York: McGraw-Hill, 1989:1497–509.

16. Poll-Thé BT, Saudubray JM, Ogier HAM, et al. Infantile Refsum disease: an inherited peroxisomal disorder; comparison with Zellweger syndrome and neonatal adrenoleukodystrophy. *Eur J Pediatr* 1987; 146:477–83.

17. Singh I, Moser AB, Goldfischer S, Moser HW. Lignoceric acid is oxidized in the peroxisome: implications for the Zellweger cerebro-hepato-renal syndrome and adrenoleukodystrophy. *Proc Natl Acad Sci USA* 1984;81:4203–7.

18. Kase BF, Björkhem I, Haga P, Pedersen JI. Defective peroxisomal cleavage of the C27-steroid side chain in the cerebro-hepato-renal syndrome of Zellweger. *J Clin Invest* 1985;75:427–35.

19. Casteels M, van Roermund CWT, Schepers L, et al. Deficient oxidation of trihydroxycoprostanoic acid in liver homogenates from patients with peroxisomal diseases. *J Inher Metab Dis* 1989;12:415–22.

20. Christensen E, Hagve T-A, Christopherson BO. The Zellweger syndrome: deficient chain-shortening of erucic acid (22:1 (*n*-9)) and adrenic acid (22:4 (*n*-6)) in cultured skin fibroblasts. *Biochim Biophys Acta* 1988;959:95–9.

21. Christensen E, Gronn M, Hagve T-A, Kase BF, Christopherson BO. Adrenoleukodystrophy: the chain shortening of erucic acid (C22:1 (*n*-9)) and adrenic acid (C22:4 (*n*-6)) is deficient in neonatal adrenoleukodystrophy and normal in X-linked adrenoleukodystrophy fibroblasts. *Biochim Biophys Acta* 1989; 1002:79–83.

22. Street JM, Johnson DW, Singh H, Pouls A. Metabolism of saturated and polyunsaturated fatty acids by normal and Zellweger syndrome skin fibroblasts. *Biochem J* 1989;260:647–55.

23. Martinez M. Polyunsaturated fatty acid changes suggesting a new enzymatic defect in Zellweger syndrome. *Lipids* 1989;24:261–5.

24. Suzuki Y, Shimozawa N, Orii T, et al. Zellweger-like syndrome with detectable hepatic peroxisomes: a variant form of peroxisomal disorder. *J Pediatr* 1988;113:841–5.

25. Paturneau-Jouas M, Taillard F, Gansmuller A, et al. Clinical, biochemical, pathological "Zellweger-like" disorder with morphological normal peroxisomes. In: Salvayre R, Douste-Blazy L, Gatt S, eds. *Lipid storage disorders: biological and medical aspects*. NATO ASI series. *Life Sci* 1988;150:805–9.

26. Moser HW. Adrenoleukodystrophy: from bedside to molecular biology. *J Child Neurol* 1987;2:140–50.

27. Powers JM. Adreno-leukodystrophy. *Clin Neuropathol* 1985;4:191–9.

28. Hashmi M, Stanley W, Singh I. Lignoceroyl-CoASA ligase: enzyme defect in fatty acid β-oxidation systems in X-linked childhood adrenoleukodystrophy. *FEBS Lett* 1986;196:347–50.

29. Lazo O, Contreras M, Hashmi M, Stanley W, Irazu C, Singh I. Peroxisomal lignoceroyl-CoA ligase deficiency in childhood adrenoleukodystrophy and adrenomyeloneuropathy. *Proc Natl Acad Sci USA* 1988;85:7647–51.

30. Wanders RJA, van Roermund CWT, van Wijland MJA, et al. Direct demonstration that the deficient oxidation of very long chain fatty acids in X-linked adrenoleukodystrophy is due to an impaired ability of peroxisomes to activate very long chain fatty acids. *Biochem Biophys Res Commun* 1988; 153:618–24.

31. Lazo O, Contreras M, Bhusnan A, Stanley W, Singh I. Adrenoleukodystrophy: impaired oxidation of fatty acids due to peroxisomal lignoceroyl-CoA ligase deficiency. *Arch Biochem Biophys* 1989;270: 722–8.
32. Poll-Thé BT, Roels F, Ogier, H, et al. A new peroxisomal disorder with enlarged peroxisomes and a specific deficiency of acyl-CoA oxidase (pseudoneonatal adrenoleukodystrophy). *Am J Hum Genet* 1988; 42:422–34.
33. Watkins PA, Chen WW, Harris CJ, et al. Peroxisomal bifunctional enzyme deficiency. *J Clin Invest* 1989;83:771–7.
34. Goldfischer S, Collins H, Rapin I, et al. Pseudo-Zellweger syndrome: deficiencies in several peroxisomal oxidative activities. *J Pediatr* 1986;108:25–32.
35. Schram AW, Goldfischer S, van Roermund CWT, et al. Human peroxisomal 3-oxoacyl-coenzyme A thiolase deficiency. *Proc Natl Acad Sci USA* 1987;84:2494–7.
36. Whitcomb RW, Linehan WM, Knazek RA. Effects of long-chain saturated fatty acids on membrane microviscosity and adrenocorticotropin responsiveness of human adrenocortical cells in vitro. *J Clin Invest* 1988;81:185–8.
37. Meyer WJ, Smith EM, Richards GE, Greger NG, Brosnan PG, Keenan BS. ACTH receptor defect in adrenoleukodystrophy (abstract). *Pediatr Res* 1987;21:465A.
38. Rizzo WB, Watkins PA, Phillips MW, Cranin D, Campbell B, Avigan J. Adrenoleukodystrophy: oleic acid lowers fibroblast C22–26 fatty acids. *Neurology* 1986;26:357–61.
39. Rizzo WB, Phillips MW, Damman AL, et al. Adrenoleukodystrophy: dietary oleic acid lowers hexacosanoate levels. *Ann Neurol* 1987;21:232–9.
40. Moser AE, Borel J, Odone A, et al. A new dietary therapy for adrenoleukodystrophy: biochemical and preliminary clinical results in 36 patients. *Ann Neurol* 1987;21:240–9.

DISCUSSION

Dr. Van Hoof: Detection of a specific defect of the peroxisomal β-oxidation of fatty acids can be difficult. Demonstration of the presence of an enzyme using specific antibodies does not imply that this enzyme is active *in vivo*. If biochemical techniques are used, one has to cope with the existence of isoenzymes, most of them present in mitochondria. Distinction between acyl-CoA dehydrogenase and acyl-CoA oxidase is easy because only the latter forms H_2O_2. But what with the peroxisomal bifunctional protein and thiolase?

Dr. Wanders: In general, that is true. It is very difficult but not impossible. We have developed a technique with which you can fractionate fibroblasts in mitochondria and in peroxisomes. You can then assay bifunctional protein and peroxisomal thiolase in the peroxisomes and in fact that was the way in which we discovered the patients with an isolated enoyl-CoA hydratase and 3-hydroxyacyl-CoA dehydrogenase deficiency. You can also use antibodies to selectively immunoprecipitate enzyme proteins, for example bifunctional protein or the peroxisomal thiolase, and you can assay the enzymic activity of these proteins on the Sepharose beads to which the proteins are now attached. So it is difficult but it is not impossible (1).

Dr. Duran: It looks so easy if you just say that very long chain fatty acids are increased. Could you be a bit more specific? What do we need? Do we need the ratio C26 to C22? Do we need absolute concentrations? Do we need the unsaturated C26? What about the bifunctional protein deficiency? Do we see increased unsaturated or hydroxy acids?

Dr. Wanders: Basically, for most disorders of peroxisomal β-oxidation it is very simple. It is simple because both the absolute amount of C26:0 and the ratio are greatly increased in the patient's plasma: they are four times higher than the normal values. The biggest problem is, of course, X-linked adrenoleukodystrophy, which is sometimes very hard to detect. In this case we do two things. We look at the C26:0 level itself, and also the C26:0/C22:0 ratio. Sometimes the ratio is in the high normal range, but the C26:0 level exceeds the normal range and in those cases in which only one of the two results is abnormal, we proceed to investigate fibroblasts in which we can measure C26:0 β-oxidation as well as the C26:0 levels and the C26/C22 ratio. We have only missed one case of X-linked adrenoleukodystrophy by looking at very low chain fatty acids in plasma. So saying that it is simple is an overstatement, but at least the results look much more unequivocal than in case of the mitochondrial β-oxidation disorders. We have adopted the procedure of Moser and co-workers (2) which is a very good procedure, but I know that other people use other methods and then it might be more problematic. For example, with different assay methods there may be great difficulty in discriminating between controls and X-linked adrenoleukodystrophy patients.

Bile acid intermediates are elevated in those peroxisomal disorders of β-oxidation in which either bifunctional protein or the peroxisomal thiolase is deficient, simply because the pathways of very long chain fatty acid oxidation and bile acid intermediate oxidation converge at the level of bifunctional protein. Only in case of acyl-CoA oxidase deficiency and X-linked adrenoleukodystrophy are the bile acid intermediates normal, as in Dr. Saudubray's patients. To summarize, we always perform these measurements because they contribute to the diagnosis and we can immediately say the defect is at the level of acyl-CoA oxidase, or at the level of bifunctional protein or peroxisomal thiolase.

Dr. Leroy: I have two questions. In infantile or juvenile adrenoleukodystrophy, as well as in adult adrenomyeloneuropathy, the functional deficiency of peroxisomal fatty-acyl-CoA synthetase has been demonstrated. There is no apparent enzymatic difference between these two types of patients. It is my experience and that of others that in children the adrenal symptoms may precede the neurological symptoms, and vice versa. Is there any way of explaining this kind of variability? My second question is the following. Did I hear correctly from Dr. Mannaerts that the peroxisomal very long chain fatty acid CoA synthetase is a peroxisomal membrane enzyme? Do we already know anything of the distribution of that enzyme within the peroxisomal membrane? Can differences in distribution be the explanation of the fascinating but disturbing fact of clinical differences between males in the same pedigree? One type has a devastating neurological disorder from early childhood and the other type of male patient can, at least for some time, lead a reasonably normal life and have children.

Dr. Wanders: It is most difficult to understand the relationship between a biochemical abnormality and the clinical and pathological presentation of a patient. The second part of the question is less difficult than the first, in that we know that this enzyme (i.e., very long chain acyl-CoA synthetase, VLCFA-CoA synthetase) is most probably located at the peroxisomal membrane. Recent experiments that we have done suggest that the enzyme sticks to the cytosolic site of the peroxisome, like palmitoyl-CoA synthetase, as shown by Professor Mannaerts, but I doubt whether this actually gives a clue to the variation between X-linked ALD as you see it in young boys and AMN patients. With regard to the first part of the question concerning the ACTH receptors, I have no information about studies that have been done in ALD as compared to AMN patients.

Dr. Hobbs: How about detecting the carriers? Have you any experience on hair follicles, for example? Have you any test sensitive enough to work on single hair follicles?

Dr. Wanders: I must rely on the data from Moser again because he has the greatest experience in this field. According to his information, you can do carrier detection by looking at very long chain fatty acids in plasma and in fibroblasts. You should combine the two because carrier detection in plasma is very difficult, and is successful in only 85% of cases. You can increase this percentage by doing additional assays in fibroblasts and of course there is now the DNA analysis where you can detect carriers using the ST14 probe.

Dr. Saudubray: The two most intriguing categories of patients with peroxisomal disorders are undoubtedly chondrodysplasia puntata and the so-called Zellweger-like syndrome. You did not speak about chondrodysplasia punctata because it was outside the scope of your topic. Could you give some additional information on phytanic acid oxidation in both these disorders, and also comment on the two enzymes necessary for the synthesis of plasmalogens? You spoke about the first enzyme, dihydroxyacetonephosphate acyltransferase, but what about the other enzyme?

Dr. Wanders: First I did not speak about rhizomelic chondrodysplasia punctata because it is not a β-oxidation disorder, but it is interesting, of course. In this disease there is a deficiency of the two enzymes involved in plasmalogen biosynthesis, DHAPAT (dihydroxyacetonephosphate acyltransferase) and alkyl dihydroxyacetonephosphate synthase. Furthermore, this disorder is characterized by a deficient activity of phytanic acid oxidation, and next to that there is an abnormality in the peroxisomal thiolase. As to the other question with regard to phytanic acid oxidation in all the β-oxidation disorders: we know that in acyl-CoA oxidase deficiency, bifunctional protein deficiency, and thiolase deficiency, phytanic acid oxidation is normal. We have found, however, that pristanic acid is increased in all these cases. We have just started these studies, but it looks at if phytanic acid breakdown to pristanic acid is normal, but that subsequent oxidation of pristanic acid is deficient. This might contribute, of course, to the pathogenesis of these disorders.

Dr. Hobbs: Xenobiotic toxicity shows an idiosyncratic susceptibility. Has anyone studied peroxisomal carriers or defects in victims of the condition?

Dr. Van Hoof: We know that more than 100 cytochromes P450 and P448 exist. Genetic differences in these multiple isoenzymes might contribute to the heterogeneity in the individual response to xenobiotics. Some of these cytochromes are needed for the formation of dicarboxylic acids, which will later be β-oxidized, mainly in peroxisomes. May I remind you of the observation made by Van den Branden et al. (3). Rats receiving high amounts of phytol in their diet accumulate very long chain fatty acids in their tissues. Phytol is the precursor of phytanate. Part of it is oxidized in peroxisomes and the action of β-oxidation enzymes is required for this. It is likely that very long chain fatty acid accumulation can result from a competition between substrates of the peroxisomal β-oxidation. The same competition is expected to occur in conditions in which high amounts of dicarboxylic acids are formed [e.g., in subjects receiving medium chain triglycerides (MCT)]. One of the conclusions that should be drawn from this is that phytol-, phytanic acid- or MCT-containing foods should be avoided hours or days before collecting blood for the search of heterozygotes for X-linked adrenoleukodystrophy.

Dr. Krywawych: I come back to the point you have just raised. We have looked at the tissues from a patient with a dicarboxylic aciduria which we suspect was due to a lesion in the oxidation of long chain fatty acids and found an accumulation of very long chain fatty acids present only in cardiac tissue.

Dr. Hobbs: I am intrigued by the difference between "brown fat" persons and others. I would like to ask both Dr. Wanders and Dr. Mannaerts whether anybody has studied either peroxisomal function or malonyl-CoA functions to explore such differences.

Dr. Mannaerts: There have been some studies on mitochondria and peroxisomes in brown adipose tissue, mainly from the laboratory of Barbara Cannon in Sweden. Brown adipose tissue contains peroxisomes, which are inducible in rodents. Most of the thermogenesis is mitochondrial, however, and peroxisomes contribute to an only minor degree.

Dr. Van Hoof: I agree. We failed to demonstrate a significant activity of acyl-CoA oxidase in brown fat, and there is good evidence that mitochondria are responsible for the thermogenesis, which is important in newborns.

Dr. Mannaerts: At the beginning at least, the idea of peroxisomes being involved in thermogenesis was attractive, since the energy that is released during the first step of peroxisomal β-oxidation is completely lost as heat. That was the main reason why people thought about the role of peroxisomes in terms of thermogenesis. The regulatory role of malonyl-CoA I think has been proven only for liver and not for extrahepatic tissues. Malonyl-CoA is present in extrahepatic tissues, and it inhibits extrahepatic carnitine palmitoyltransferase I *in vitro*, but it is not known whether its concentration fluctuates, or fluctuates in the right direction. There is some indication that it might have a regulatory role in the heart.

REFERENCES

1. Wanders RJA, van Roermund CWT, Schelen A, et al. A bifunctional protein with deficient enzymic activity: identification of a new peroxisomal disorder using novel methods to measure the peroxisomal β-oxidation enzyme activities. *J Inher Metab Dis* 1990;13:375–9.
2. Moser HW, Moser AB, Kawamura N, et al. *Ann Neurol* 1980;7:542–9.
3. Van den Branden C, Vamecq J, Wÿbo I, Roels F. Phytol and peroxisome proliferation. *Pediatr Res* 1986; 20:411–5.

Inborn Errors of Metabolism, edited by
J. Schaub, F. Van Hoof, and H. L. Vis.
Nestlé Nutrition Workshop Series, Vol. 24.
Nestec Ltd., Vevey/Raven Press, Ltd.,
New York © 1991.

Carnitine and the Organic Acidurias

Charles R. Roe, David S. Millington, S. G. Kahler, N. Kodo,
and D. L. Norwood

*Division of Pediatric Genetics and Metabolism, Duke University Medical Center,
Durham, North Carolina 27710, USA*

The earliest observation of a deficiency of carnitine associated with an inherited metabolic disorder was with 5,10-methylene tetrahydrofolate reductase deficiency (1). A survey of carnitine status in patients with organic acidurias revealed an apparent secondary deficiency in all except maple syrup urine disease (2). There is considerable diagnostic value in the identification of acylcarnitine profiles for the recognition of organic acidurias. Furthermore, some of these disorders are effectively treated by supplemental carnitine therapy. The diagnostic and therapeutic applications of L-carnitine will be reviewed.

CARNITINE AS A DIAGNOSTIC TOOL

The development of fast atom bombardment–mass spectrometry (FAB-MS) facilitated the detection and analysis of specific acylcarnitines in urine (3). In particular, it enabled the recognition of new acylcarnitines, whose structures were subsequently investigated by auxiliary techniques (4). It was discovered that patients with inherited disorders of branched-chain amino acid and fatty acid catabolism excrete disease-specific acylcarnitines that reflect abnormal acylcoenzyme A (CoA) species accumulating at or near the site of the metabolic block (5). In situations where one would not expect unusual acyl-CoA thioester accumulation, as in maple syrup urine disease (MSUD) or phenylketonuria (PKU), for example, no unusual acylcarnitines are detected. In addition, the acylcarnitines were much more easily detected after loading patients with L-carnitine, which enhances the excretion of the abnormal, diagnostic species in patients with metabolic disorders.

In some cases, a single major, diagnostic acylcarnitine is predominant, facilitating the diagnosis, as exemplified by isovalerylcarnitine in isovaleric acidemia (6) and propionylcarnitine in propionic acidemia (7). In fat catabolism disorders, including medium chain acyl-CoA dehydrogenase deficiency and multiple acyl-CoA dehydrogenase deficiency (MADD), a specific pattern of acylcarnitines is excreted and the diagnosis cannot be reliably made on the basis of detection of any single species.

These acylcarnitine patterns are of considerable diagnostic utility because unlike branched-chain amino acid disorders, where the defects are expressed by a persistent and grossly abnormal organic aciduria, the levels of diagnostic organic acids vary considerably with clinical state (8). In our experience, the differential diagnosis of fatty acid catabolism disorders is greatly improved by including both GC-MS analysis of organic acids and FAB-MS analysis of acylcarnitines.

In an older child, or an infant not breast-fed, a significant carnitine deficiency can develop in MCAD deficiency, making the FAB-MS profile unclear or uninterpretable. The safe and simple expedient of collecting urine after an oral carnitine load of 100 mg/kg enhances the diagnostic acylcarnitine profile and removes ambiguity (9). This is illustrated in Fig. 1, which compares the FAB-MS results obtained on an affected presymptomatic boy aged 3½ years, whose first clinical symptoms did not occur until 7 years of age. The profile in Fig. 1A is uninterpretable, owing to chemical interference and low acylcarnitine concentration, but after the load (Fig. 1B) the characteristic pattern of MCAD deficiency (9) is clearly observed.

When a child with MCAD deficiency was given a bolus of [methyl-$^2H_3$]L-carnitine, a stable-isotope-labeled form of carnitine, each of the diagnostic signals was accompanied by a "satellite" with a mass increment of +3 (Fig. 1C). Analogous results were obtained in a patient with propionic acidemia (11). This result is very significant for several reasons. It shows that exogenous carnitine equilibrates rapidly with the endogenous acyl-CoA pool and the percentage incorporation of labeled carnitine in each acylcarnitine is similar (Fig. 1C), indicating the general specificity of the carnitine acyltransferases to form short and medium chain length acylcarnitines *in vivo*. It also demonstrates a simple, definitive method of confirming the identities of acylcarnitine signals observed in the FAB-MS spectrum. This woud be especially important in the identification of hitherto unknown acylcarnitines. The labeling experiments also confirm the existence of a general pathway for detoxification in several of the organic acidurias. Carnitine produces rapid transport of potentially toxic acyl groups out of the cell as acylcarnitines, which are then excreted as nontoxic metabolites. This is the biochemical rationale for L-carnitine therapy in these diseases.

Standard FAB-MS is limited to detection of acylcarnitines in urine when their individual concentrations exceed about 50 nmol/ml (4). The detection limit is a function of the chemical noise due in the biological matrix, which is variable. The absolute signal strength of acylcarnitines is also affected by the relative concentration of other surface-active components, including alkali metal cations. The successful detection of acylcarnitines at low concentration in urine, liver tissue (12), and blood plasma by FAB-MS has been possible in some cases, but only after extensive sample purification. Consequently, a more selective routine method was developed recently in our laboratory using a triple quadrupole—an example of a tandem mass spectrometer that incorporates two stages of mass analysis (MS/MS) in a single instrument. As with other combined techniques, such as GC/MS and LC/MS, MS/MS offers the potential for improving specificity and enabling the direct analysis of mixtures (13). This technique is particularly well suited to FAB-MS, since the appli-

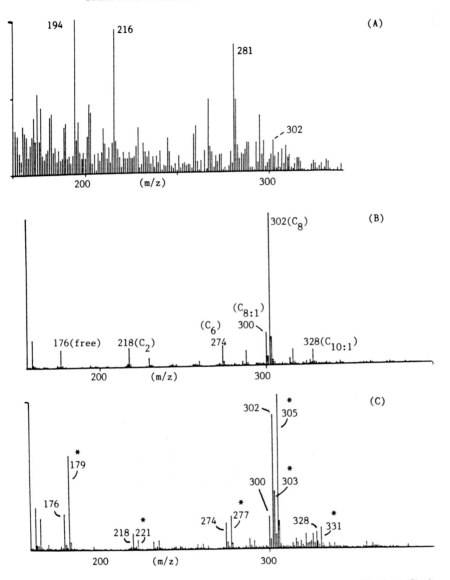

FIG. 1. MCAD deficiency FAB-MS profiles (**A**) untreated patient (**B**) after carnitine load (**C**) after [methyl $^2H_3$]carnitine load showing incorporation of the label (*) into the acylcarnitines. From Roe CR, et al. (10).

cability of on-line chromatographic separation is very limited at present. The added specificity achieved by FAB-MS/MS has facilitated its application to the quantitative analysis of individual acylcarnitines in urine, plasma, and tissue using isotope dilution assay (14).

The FAB mass spectra of acylcarnitine methyl esters and the daughter ion spectra of the M^+ ions generated by tandem MS show a prominent common fragment at m/z 99 (5,14). This ion is derived from the loss of both the acyl moiety, as the corresponding acid, and the quaternary ammonium function as trimethylamine. The structure of this highly characteristic fragment can be formally represented as $^+CH_2$—CH=CH—CO_2CH_3 and represents the "backbone" of the acylcarnitine molecule. Isotopically labeled forms, having ^2H or ^{13}C in either the acyl or trimethylamino group, also exhibit the m/z 99 fragment. Because the precursors of m/z 99 are predominantly acylcarnitine molecular cations, the new scan function, when applied to a biological sample, generates a metabolic "profile" of acylcarnitines in the sample (14,15).

The most immediately obvious difference between acylcarnitine profiles obtained by FAB-MS/MS and those performed by the standard FAB-MS (5) procedure is a large reduction in the chemical "noise." This results from the increased selectivity (specificity) of the analytical procedure, which has improved the detection limit for individual acylcarnitine methyl esters in urine from 50 nmol/ml to better than 1 nmol/ml (14). It is possible to observe diagnostic acylcarnitine signals in urine samples even from neonatal MCAD-deficient patients (with carnitine deficiency) that were completely masked by chemical interference using the older method. When the availability of free carnitine is compromised, however, low levels of unusual acylcarnitine species, including dicarboxylic acylcarnitines, have been observed. Furthermore, the probability of interference from "background" ions or from compounds other than acylcarnitines is high in these cases. For these reasons, the interpretation of acylcarnitine profiles from urine is more straightforward and reliable when the patient is in a carnitine-sufficient state. This is assured if the sample is collected after the administration of a bolus of L-carnitine or if the patient is breast-fed or receiving carnitine supplement.

Most of the even-mass ions above m/z 200 in the m/z 99 precursor ion spectra of urine samples are derived from acylcarnitines. This is based on the profiles of patients with well-defined metabolic defects whose diagnostic acylcarnitines have been previously characterized and reported (3,8,16). Thus, as observed in these earlier studies (5), the normal profile (Fig. 2A) is dominated by acetylcarnitine (M^+ = 218), with lesser amounts of C3, C4, C5, and C8:1 (M^+ = 300) acylcarnitines. In isovaleric acidemia (IVA), isovalerylcarnitine (M^+ = 260, Fig. 2B) is the dominant species (6), and in propionic acidemia (PA), propionylcarnitine (M^+ = 232, Fig. 2C) is the major acylcarnitine (7). In methylmalonic aciduria (MMA), the profile of which is not shown here, propionylcarnitine is also very prominent and is accompanied by a prominent signal for acetylcarnitine (3). In many cases, a signal corresponding to methylmalonylcarnitine (m/z 290) is also observed. Similarly, the profiles of glutaric aciduria type I (glutaryl-CoA dehydrogenase deficiency GAI, Fig. 2D), 3-ketothio-

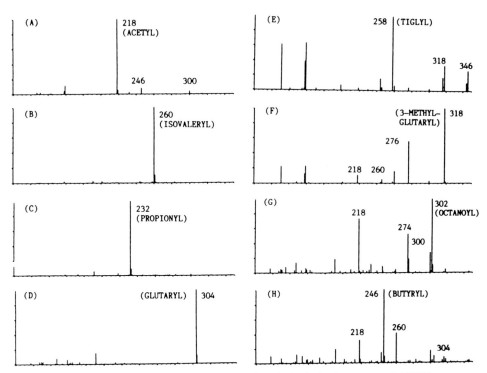

FIG. 2. Acylcarnitine profiles obtained by FAB-MS/MS analysis of urine from a normal child (**A**) compared with those (**B–H**) with metabolic diseases (see the text for details). From Roe CR, et al. (10).

lase deficiency (KT, Fig. 2E), and 3-hydroxy-3-methylglutaryl-CoA lyase deficiency (HMG, Fig. 2F) revealed the expected dominant molecular cations corresponding to glutarylcarnitine (m/z 304), tiglylcarnitine (m/z 258), and 3-methylglutarylcarnitine (m/z 318), respectively (16,17). The two remaining profiles are from patients with disorders of fatty acid catabolism. The profile in Fig. 2G is from a patient with medium chain acyl-CoA dehydrogenase (MCAD) deficiency and is characterized by the M^+ ions of medium chain acylcarnitines (8,9): hexanoyl (m/z 274), octanoyl (m/z 302), octenoyl (m/z 300), and decenoyl (m/z 328). In Fig. 2H a patient with multiple acyl-CoA dehydrogenase deficiency (MADD) is presented, showing increased excretion of butyrylcarnitine (M^+ = m/z 246) plus C5, C6, and C8 acylcarnitines.

These patients, with the exception of the one with KT, were receiving carnitine supplements when the urine collections were made. In patients with IVA, PA, MMA, and GAI, the profiles appear to be very clean even without carnitine supplement.

Using the "precursors of m/z 99" scan, individual acylcarnitines can be detected in blood plasma at concentrations of less than 0.5 nmol/ml (14). This compares with typical physiological concentrations for total acylcarnitines of 6–10 nmol/ml, which can increase two- or threefold in patients with metabolic disease (2).

The ability to detect acylcarnitines in blood is very important since it enables

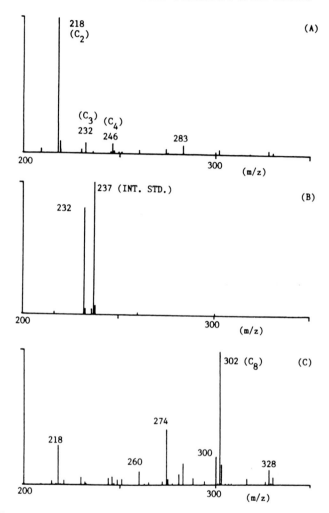

FIG. 3. Plasma acylcarnitine profiles by FAB-MS/MS (**A**) normal child (**B**) child with propionic acidemia (**C**) postmortem blood from SIDS case. From Roe CR, et al. (10).

recognition and diagnosis of inherited metabolic diseases after death. The overall
composition of blood is much less variable than that of urine, and the range of
acylcarnitine concentration is much narrower. Furthermore, the pattern of acylcarnitines in blood appears to be a better reflection of the status in tissue than that of
urine. Initial results with blood have been very encouraging. For example, diagnostic
profiles representative of the metabolic diseases summarized in Fig. 2 have been
achieved, and in general, appear to be similar to the urine profiles after carnitine
supplement. In Fig. 3 the profile of a metabolically normal child (Fig. 3A) is compared
with that of a postmortem specimen from a carnitine-supplemented child with PA
(Fig. 3B) and of another postmortem sample from a previously undiagnosed and

asymptomatic child that succumbed to "sudden infant death" (Fig. 3C). The classical profile of MCAD deficiency is evident from this profile. Clearly, such deaths could be avoided by neonatal screening of blood. An authentic "PKU card" which had been stored 6 months at room temperature was obtained from a patient later confirmed as MCAD deficiency. Although the recovery of acylcarnitines from the blood spots may deteriorate with age, the characteristic profile of MCAD deficiency was still detectable after 6 months. PKU cards from other organic acidurias stored in the freezer for 2 years still revealed the diagnostic profiles. It has already been demonstrated (14,15) that rapid sequential analysis of samples by FAB-MS/MS is feasible using a continuous liquid introduction system. A study has begun at Duke to determine the feasibility of large-scale neonatal screening.

Tissue samples have generally posed the biggest problem for the application of FAB-MS. Even after extensive cleanup, the acylcarnitine-enriched fractions are very complex matrices. The best success has been obtained with muscle, where the acylcarnitine concentrations are relatively high. Acetylcarnitine and butyrylcarnitine were detected and quantified by high-resolution FAB-MS (3) in muscle from normal mice and from a mutant strain with short chain acyl-CoA dehydrogenase deficiency (18). With the FAB-MS/MS technique individual acylcarnitines are detectable down to concentrations of 1 nmol/g wet weight in liver tissue (14), for example.

A number of liver samples from patients with known defects, including MCAD and PA, have subsequently been analyzed and revealed clear diagnostic profiles. Postmortem liver is therefore another useful material for the recognition of metabolic diseases by FAB-MS/MS. The liver must be deep-frozen soon after excision to preserve the integrity of the acylcarnitines. Tissue that has been preserved in formalin is unsuitable.

CARNITINE THERAPY

Early experience with carnitine loading in PA (7), MMA (19), and IVA (6) provided valuable biochemical clues to the potential therapeutic value of carnitine supplementation in these disorders. The dynamic biochemical effects of an oral carnitine challenge in a patient with isovaleric acidemia are illustrated in Fig. 4. Isotope-dilution assays showed a rapid increase in isovalerylcarnitine (IVC) excretion and a corresponding decrease in isovalerylglycine (IVG) excretion. This demonstrates effective competition for isovaleryl-CoA by carnitine. The increase in benzoylglycine (hippurate) excretion concomitant with the changes in IVG and IVC concentration strongly indicates that the formation of IVC is largely intramitochondrial, since the liberated CoASH would be available for formation of benzoyl-CoA and hence hippurate, an exclusively intramitochondrial event.

Most of the organic acidurias are characterized by a "secondary" carnitine deficiency (2). In some instances the inability to conserve carnitine at the renal level offers a reasonable explanation (20). In several of these disorders, however, the total quantities of free carnitine and acylcarnitines excreted per kilogram of body weight

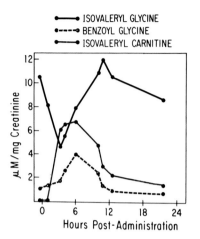

FIG. 4. Biochemical effects of a bolus of L-carnitine in isovaleric acidemia. From Roe CR, et al. (10).

per 24 h are markedlly below normal. Untreated patients with IVA (6) and MCAD deficiency (8,9), for example, have a marked reduction in plasma free carnitine associated with decreased excretion of total carnitine. Renal loss, therefore, is not an adequate explanation for their deficiency state. The integrity of carnitine biosynthesis or uptake by tissue may be compromised in these disorders.

In PA and MMA it is not unusual to observe relatively normal levels of total carnitine in the plasma and normal quantities excreted in the urine. However, the bulk of the carnitine is esterified, predominantly as propionylcarnitine. It is perhaps appropriate to describe this not as a true "deficiency" state, but rather as a relative insufficiency of carnitine to meet metabolic needs. Oral supplementation with L-carnitine results in increased excretion of propionylcarnitine and elevation of the free carnitine fraction, supporting the concept that additional carnitine is needed to handle the large quantities of propionyl-CoA being produced.

Despite widespread acceptance of the concept of carnitine deficiency or insufficiency and the compelling biochemical evidence for the detoxification pathway of carnitine conjugation, there is considerable controversy about the general use of L-carnitine as a therapeutic agent in the organic acidurias. This is surprising in view of the acceptance of glycine therapy in isovaleric acidemia (21), the purpose of which is solely to enhance the removal of a toxic metabolite. Carnitine supplementation in PA, MMA, and IVA is analogous, and in the latter case at least, has the bonus of correcting a known deficiency. In MCAD deficiency, carnitine supplementation would also seem to be justified on the basis of correcting a true deficiency state and for conjugation and excretion of medium chain acyl-CoA derivatives, especially octanoyl-CoA. Chronic oral carnitine supplementation of numerous patients with organic acidurias referred to Duke Medical Center has been taking place with close observation for up to 8 years. The range of disorders treated includes PA, IVA, MMA, HMG lyase, 3-ketothiolase deficiency (KT), MCAD deficiency, and MADD. Typical daily oral doses are 200 mg/kg for PA and MMA and 100 mg/kg for the others. It should be noted that only about 15% of the oral dose is absorbed, and the daily dose is divided into four portions, owing to the speed of the biochemical response.

These experiences may be summarized as follows. In all cases, with the exception of MCAD deficiency, parents report increased interaction with and awareness of the environment and at least a subjective overall clinical improvement. The degree of compliance has been very high. The patients with IVA, KT, HMG, and MADD have experienced no further hospitalizations while on carnitine supplement. In IVA, carnitine supplementation was used *instead* of glycine. When carnitine supplementation was discontinued for lengthy periods in certain patients with IVA, KT, and MADD, serious deterioration requiring hospitalization did occur.

Carnitine supplementation in PA, MMA, and MCAD has not eliminated recurrent illness, but it has reduced the severity of the illnesses and reduced the number of hospitalizations, especially in PA. Only one of seven treated MCAD patients has had recurrent illnesses. Although four have had chickenpox, they did not require hospitalization. Because the clinical course is so variable in this disorder, it is difficult to determine the significance of these observations. However, there are compelling reasons to support chronic carnitine therapy for MCAD deficiency. A high proportion (~30%) of deaths attributable to the disease occur with the first episode of illness. We believe that "systemic" carnitine deficiency in an untreated child would seriously limit mobilization of sufficient carnitine to conjugate the rapidly accumulating and potentially fatal medium chain fatty acyl-CoA compounds during such an episode. Chronic and acute carnitine supplementation should protect against this. Observations in a family with four affected children, two of whom had died reportedly with a Reye-like episode and sudden infant death syndrome (9) before a diagnosis was made, tend to support these concepts. The data shown in Fig. 5 are from one

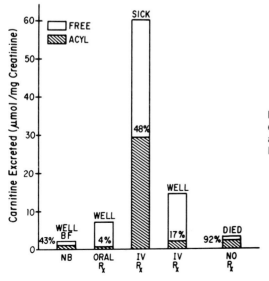

FIG. 5. Carnitine supplementation and excretion in MCAD deficiency during acute illness and when clinically well. From Roe CR, et al. (10).

of the survivors and one of the deceased children, in whom MCAD deficiency was diagnosed after death. MCAD was diagnosed at Duke in the surviving sibling at 2 months of age and prior to clinical symptoms by analysis of organic acids and acyl-carnitines. The diagnosis was subsequently confirmed by enzyme assay in cultured fibroblasts. Before initiating carnitine therapy, this patient, who was breast-fed at the time, excreted 2 µmol/mg creatinine total carnitine, of which 43% was acylated. Quantitative analysis by isotope-dilution FAB-MS (3) showed that octanoylcarnitine exceeded the acetylcarnitine concentration in this urine by a factor of 3. When receiving oral L-carnitine supplement at 100 mg/kg·day but asymptomatic, the typical output of total carnitine was 7 µmol/mg creatinine, of which 0.5 µmol was acylated. During a severe clinical episode, she was given intravenous carnitine (30 mg/kg bolus followed by 30 mg/kg over the next 24 h) and recovered rapidly with regained sensorium within 5 h. The total carnitine excreted during the intravenous therapy was 61 µmol/mg creatinine, 48% of which was acylated. Octanoylcarnitine and acetylcarnitine concentrations were 13 and 16 µmol/mg, respectively. A repeat of the same intravenous carnitine regimen when the patient was clinically well revealed much lower acylcarnitine as a percentage of the total with octanoylcarnitine representing about 25% of the acylated fraction. Analysis of postmortem urine from the deceased, untreated sibling revealed a total carnitine excretion of only 3 µmol/mg, of which about 90% was acylated (Fig. 5).

We infer from these data that untreated MCAD-deficient patients are at increased risk owing to their inability to mobilize carnitine during clinical episodes. By maintaining a steady intake, some additional reserve of carnitine is available for detoxification during the onset of illness. The use of intravenous carnitine during acute illnesses has been conducted under our supervision with excellent clinical results in patients with MCAD, MADD, IVA, and PA. Patients typically recover within a few hours, compared with 1–3 days when intravenous glucose alone is employed acutely.

SUMMARY

The detection of acylcarnitines by FAB-MS in human physiological fluids has added another valuable diagnostic tool for the recognition of specific metabolic diseases. The newly developed technique of FAB-MS/MS, which embodies the principles of tandem mass spectrometry, affords a quantum leap in specificity, enabling the detection and quantification of acylcarnitines in concentrations well within the physiological ranges in urine, blood, and tissue. The therapeutic use of L-carnitine appears to offer protection against the harmful consequences of catabolism. A reduction in the number of clinical episodes requiring hospitalization has been observed in most cases. When such occurrences have necessitated intravenous fluids, the addition of L-carnitine to the intravenous infusate has led to dramatic reduction in recovery times. It has also been shown that there is no discernible toxicity associated with carnitine therapy, even under high-dose intravenous conditions.

ACKNOWLEDGMENTS

These studies were supported by FDA Orphaned Products Division Grant FD-R-000177, Food and Drug Administration, Washington, DC; NIH Grant HD-22704, and HD-24908, National Institutes of Health, Bethesda, Maryland, and the RR-30 General Clinical Research Centers Program Division of Research Resources, National Institutes of Health, Bethesda, Maryland. The expert assistance of Diane Gale and Denise Kenyon is gratefully acknowledged.

REFERENCES

1. Allen RJ, Wong P, Rathenberg SP, Dimauro S, Headington JT. Progressive neonatal leukoencephalomyopathy due to absent methylenetetrahydrofolate reductase, responsive to treatment. *Ann Neurol* 1980; 8:211.
2. Chalmers RA, Roe CR, Stacey TE, Hoppel CL. Urinary excretion of L-carnitine and acylcarnitines by patients with disorders of organic acid metabolism: evidence for secondary insufficiency of L-carnitine. *Pediatr Res* 1984;18:1325–8.
3. Millington DS, Roe CR, Maltby DA. Application of high resolution fast atom bombardment and constant *B/E* ratio linked scanning to the identification and analysis of acylcarnitines in metabolic disease. *Biomed Mass Spectrom* 1984;11:236–41.
4. Millington DS. New methods for the analysis of acylcarnitines and acyl-CoA compounds. In: Gaskell SJ, ed. *Mass spectrometry in biomedical research.* Chichester, UK: John Wiley & Sons, 1986;97–114.
5. Roe CR, Millington DS, Maltby DA. Diagnostic and therapeutic implications of acylcarnitine profiling in organic acidurias associated with carnitine insufficiency. In: Borum PR, ed. *Clinical aspects of human carnitine deficiency.* Elmsford, NY: Pergamon Press, 1986;97–107.
6. Roe CR, Millington DS, Maltby DA, Kahler SG, Bohan TP. L-Carnitine therapy in isovaleric acidemia. *J Clin Invest* 1984;74:2290–5.
7. Roe CR, Millington DS, Maltby DA, Bohan TP, Hoppel CL. L-Carnitine enhances excretion of propionyl coenzyme A as propionylcarnitine in propionic acidemia. *J Clin Invest* 1984;73:1785–8.
8. Roe CR, Millington DS, Maltby DA, Bohan TP, Kahler SG, Chalmers RA. Diagnostic and therapeutic implications of medium-chain acylcarnitines in medium-chain acyl-CoA dehydrogenase deficiency. *Pediatr Res* 1985;19:459–66.
9. Roe CR, Millington DS, Maltby DA, Kinnebrew P. Recognition of medium-chain acyl-CoA dehydrogenase deficiency in asymptomatic siblings of children dying of sudden infant death or Reye-like syndromes. *J Pediatr* 1986;108:13–8.
10. Roe CR, et al. Carnitine homeostasis in the organic acidurias. In: Coates PM, Tanaka K, eds. *Fatty acid oxidation: clinical, biochemical, and molecular aspects. Prog Clin Biol Res* 1989;321.
11. Millington DS, Maltby DA, Gale D, Roe CR. Synthesis and human applications of stable isotope-labelled L-carnitine. In: Baillie TA, Jones R, eds. *Synthesis and applications of isotopically labelled compounds 1988.* Amsterdam: Elsevier, 1988.
12. Roe CR, Millington DS, Maltby DA, Wellman RB. Post-mortem recognition of inherited metabolic disorders from specific acylcarnitines in tissue in cases of sudden infant death. *Lancet* 1987;1:512.
13. Yost RA, Enke CG. Tandem quadrupole mass spectrometry. In: McLafferty FW, ed. *Tandem mass spectrometry.* New York: John Wiley & Sons, 1987;175–95.
14. Millington DS, Norwood DL, Kodo N, Roe CR, Inoue F. Application of fast atom bombardment with tandem mass spectrometry and liquid chromatography/mass spectrometry to the analysis of acylcarnitine in human urine, blood and tissue. *Anal Biochem* 1989;180:331–9.
15. Norwood DL, Kodo N, Millington DS. Application of continuous-flow liquid chromatography/fast atom bombardment mass spectrometry to the analysis of diagnostic acylcarnitines in human urine. *Rapid Commun Mass Spectrom* 1988;2:269–72.
16. Millington DS, Roe CR, Maltby DA. Characterization of new diagnostic acylcarnitines in patients with β-ketothiolase deficiency and glutaric aciduria type 1 using mass spectrometry. *Biomed Environm Mass Spectrom* 1987;14:711–6.

17. Roe CR, Millington DS, Maltby DA. Identification of 3-methylglutaryl-carnitine. A new diagnostic metabolite of 3-hydroxy-3-methylglutaryl-coenzyme-A lyase deficiency. *J Clin Invest* 1986;77:1391–4.
18. Wood PA, Amendt BA, Rhead WJ, Millington DS, Inoue F, Armstrong D. Short-chain acyl-coenzyme A dehydrogenase deficiency in mice. *Pediatr Res* 1989;25:38–43.
19. Roe CR, Hoppel CL, Stacey TE, Chalmers RA, Tracey BM, Millington DS. Metabolic response to carnitine in methylmalonic aciduria. An effective strategy for elimination of propionyl groups. *Arch Dis Child* 1983;58:916–20.
20. Bernardini I, Rizzo WB, Dalakas M, Bernar J, Gahl WA. Plasma and muscle free carnitine deficiency due to renal Fanconi syndrome. *J Clin Invest* 1985;75:1124–30.
21. Yudkoff M, Cohn RM, Ruschak R, Rothman R, Segal S. Therapeutic effects of glycine in isovaleric acidemia. *Pediatr Res* 1976;10:25–9.

DISCUSSION

Dr. Wendel: What carnitine doses do you recommend for the long-term treatment of an organic aciduria like β-ketothiolase deficiency?

Dr. Roe: We all have so little experience with large populations that it is hard to know exactly what would be the best level. Our β-ketothiolase patients have been treated with 100 mg/kg·day in four divided doses and that seemed to be sufficient. HMG and MCAD patients were given 50 mg/kg·day and propionics and methylmalonics 200 mg and higher. The dose is given every day since it is not possible to predict when crises will occur.

Dr. Van Hoof: With Professor E. de Hoffmann's Finnigan-MAT TSQ 70 tandem mass spectrometer, we avoided the methylation step and obtained equally good results in the detection of carnitine esters. The advantage of this is that one can escape the alkaline step of methylation, during which methanolysis of carnitine esters is expected to occur. Another point: You did not mention the danger of using valproate in children suffering from these disorders.

Dr. Roe: Two cases (one an MCAD and the other a multiple acyl-CoA dehydrogenase deficiency) received valproate and both went immediately into coma. It is clearly contraindicated in these disorders.

Dr. Van Hoof: The use of valproate might be the cause of several episodes of Reye's syndrome. Valproate is probably not the only culprit. The use of mosquito repellent has also been mentioned in the literature. These hazards, however, are expected to occur only in persons in whom mitochondrial β-oxidation is at the lower normal limit.

Dr. Roe: That is a very good comment. I would like to make two responses. In the biochemical literature it has been suggested that carnitine could enhance the branched-chain ketoacid decarboxylase, which would tend to suggest that it might produce a greater turnover of amino acids precursors. The same question has been raised in relation to the fatty acid pathway (i.e., that high-dose carnitine might enhance lipolysis). We have done this study on branched chain disorders and in the fat disorders, giving 100 mg carnitine per kilogram daily. It is clear that neither in propionic acidemia nor in the MCADs is there any enhancement of endogenous turnover as measured by the quantitative excretion of the acylcarnitine, nor any change in dicarboxylic acids. So I think that from a toxicity point of view it is good to know this. Referring to valproate, I think you are absolutely right. We are only beginning to understand what the contraindications would be in a number of these disorders. Tom Baillie, who is in Seattle, Washington with Dr. René Lévy, is very interested in the interactions of valproate in the inborn errors. This is one of the things we have worked on together recently and we have rationalized the origin of the intermediates that have been identified in valproate therapy.

Dr. Leroy: How sensible or how relevant is it to talk about normal carnitine levels? Can the hypothesis of carnitine deficiency be maintained in the case of myogenic hypotonia? Do we know really what normal serum levels of carnitine mean? Too few control data in children from infancy to late childhood are available. Do carnitine levels in plasma or muscle mean anything at all, and if so, how will they be useful? Can you please comment?

Dr. Roe: That is an excellent question. I get very concerned when I encounter situations where someone has measured the total carnitine and says it is normal. We don't rely on "normal" values at all. We do plasma carnitine by radioenzymatic assay and also by the FAB technique with internal standards that are reliable for quantification. The species of acylcarnitine is more important than the total carnitine value. We frequently refer to ratios, (e.g., the acylcarnitine to free carnitine ratio), but those of us who do these tests know how rapidly they change in disease. But I think you have a valid point in doing carnitine measurements on the plasma of a child with hypotonia. It is a good starting point because there may be a secondary deficiency state. I would move just as quickly to the other studies, even if the carnitine levels were normal.

Dr. Bartlett: I agree with that statement. We have spent a lot of time and effort devising reliable assays of free carnitine, short chain acylcarnitine and long chain acylcarnitine. Our long chain acylcarnitine method relies on internal standardization with palmitoyl[methyl-^{3}H]carnitine and is accurate and reproducible. However, it has become clear to us that in most instances the data generated are no more than confirmatory. The situation is particularly complicated during ketosis, when a high percentage of acylated carnitine is observed. This is largely due to short chain acylcarnitine, which can reach plasma concentrations in excess of 20 μmol/liter. This is nearly all acetylcarnitine and reflects a normal physiological resonse to fasting. However, in the absence of chromatographic analysis it would be very easy to confuse this normal physiological response with the pathological response, due, for example, to high octanoylcarnitine in medium chain acyl-CoA dehydrogenase deficiency. Under extreme conditions we could probably distinguish the two situations, but I would certainly not like to rely on analysis of carnitine and acylcarnitine alone.

Dr. Otten: Is there a defect of carnitine uptake into the cells? And if this is the case, does it make sense to supplement these patients with carnitine, and do you know the metabolic outcome? In patients with rickets with cardiomyopathy and low carnitine values, there is a high urinary carnitine output. When you supplement with carnitine there is a slight improvement in the cardiomyopathy.

Dr. Roe: Charles Stanley has definitely demonstrated the carnitine transport defect in terms of uptake, which I think is extremely interesting. In the cardiomyopathy area, we have had a similar experience. We have seen two types, one like the one you are talking about with excessive carnitine loss and others where there is really not an excessive carnitine loss, but there is a response to carnitine. I do not know the mechanism, but cardiomyopathy has improved with carnitine supplementation without any major dietary alteration. If one looks at the carnitine data, one can see that in MCAD and isovaleric acidemia, for example, the patients are actually excreting only a small fraction of the carnitine, maybe 10%, that normal children excrete in a 24-h period. These data suggest that the earlier work on the integrity of carnitine biosynthesis in "systemic carnitine deficiency" needs to be re-explored. There is probably some secondary problem in the biosynthetic pathway that may account for the so-called secondary carnitine deficiency producing a true deficiency state.

Dr. Saudubray: A very severe secondary carnitine deficiency is also observed in glutaric aciduria type I due to glutaryl-CoA dehydrogenase deficiency. We investigated three patients and found free and total carnitine plasma levels close to zero (around 1 μmol/liter). I guess these very low levels were not explained through enhanced urinary losses of glutaryl carnitine.

Of course, there was some glutaryl carnitine in the urine but only a small amount. So why are the carnitine levels so low in glutaric aciduria type I? What is your experience?

Dr. Roe: It is exactly the same as yours. There is an extraordinary deficiency that is not accounted for by enhanced excretion. We synthesized a CD3 carnitine for intravenous use, and we have shown that there is an inhibition of carnitine production in MCAD patients.

Dr. Mowat: This is a simple clinical question. When cases of MCAD present in the emergency room we do not usually know the diagnosis. Are there any conditions, for example Reye's syndrome, in which you think that carnitine might be dangerous if given as emergency treatment in this acute clinical presentation? I wonder also if the same would apply to the other clinical situations: for example, a child presenting with hypotonia, apnea, and bradycardia.

Dr. Roe: From our studies with high-dose intravenous carnitine and high-dose acetyl carnitine with stable isotope labels, there is absolutely no evidence of any toxicity at doses which would be far greater than one would employ in an acute emergency therapy situation. Intravenous carnitine has no obvious toxicity. I think its intravenous benefits need more documentation by other investigators. It could be an extraordinarily valuable emergency medication.

Inborn Errors of Metabolism, edited by
J. Schaub, F. Van Hoof, and H. L. Vis.
Nestlé Nutrition Workshop Series, Vol. 24.
Nestec Ltd., Vevey/Raven Press, Ltd.,
New York © 1991.

Sudden Infant Death Syndrome, as First Expression of a Metabolic Disorder

E. Rebuffat, M. Sottiaux, P. Goyens, D. Blum, E. Vamos,
G. Van Vliet, D. Hasaerts, P. Steenhout, *L. Demeirler,
and A. Kahn

*Pediatrics Clinic, Children's University Hospital Reine Fabiola, Free University of
Brussels, Avenue J J Crocq 15, 1020 Brussels; and *the V.U.B., Brussels, Belgium*

INTRODUCTION AND DEFINITIONS

Sudden Infant Death Syndrome

Sudden infant death syndrome (SIDS) is the sudden death of a young child which is unexpected, given the child's history, and for which no explanation can be found despite postmortem examination (1). The need for a complete postmortem investigation is shown by the fact that in up to 15% of the autopsies, an explanation for the death can be found (1). In 5% of the cases, a "fatty liver" is found, revealing a possible prior metabolic disorder (2). The prevalence of SIDS is between one and three deaths per 1,000 live births. In Belgium, the SIDS rate is 1.72 per 1,000, and represents one third of all deaths occurring between the age of 1 month and 1 year, by far the most frequent cause of death in the postnatal period.

Apparent Life-Threatening Event

Pediatricians have been asked by anxious parents to care for an infant who has survived an apparent life-threatening event (ALTE). The child was found unresponsive, pale or cyanotic, and apparently not breathing. The accident occurred unexpectedly, and only prompt intervention by one of the parents revived the child. The initial episodes appear to occur during periods of sleep, waking, or feeding, and are most commonly described as some combination of apnea, color change (usually cyanosis or pallor, occasionally erythema), marked change in muscle tone (usually limpness, but in rare cases rigidity), and choking or gagging. In most cases observers reported the episode as being potentially life threatening, and in some cases they stated that the child had actually died (1,2). There is epidemiological evidence that some of the infants studied after an ALTE might have survived a potential SIDS episode (3,4).

Metabolic Abnormalities, Sudden Infant Death Syndrome, and Apparent Life-Threatening Events

The possible role played in SIDS by inherited metabolic diseases could be illustrated by some epidemiological characteristics of these deaths, such as the tripled death rate in families with a SIDS case, or the frequent observation of gastrointestinal infections or fasting in the days preceding a SIDS event (1,4,5). Fasting could have enhanced the occurrence of metabolic crises related to acylcoenzyme A dehydrogenase deficiency. The inherited metabolic disorder is associated with life-threatening episodes of hypoketotic hypoglycemia, accompanied by dicarboxylic aciduria, and steatosis in various tissues. The clinical findings are similar to those of Reye's syndrome with fulminant hepatic encephalopathy following a minor illness with diarrhea and/or vomiting (8). Subtle clinical symptoms, as seen in some future SIDS or ALTE victims, are also compatible with an underlying metabolic problem, such as the observation of recurrent episodes of "fatigue" during feeds, muscular hyptonia, or excessive sweating during sleep (1,5).

As early as 1976, an unrecognized but specific disease was suspected in a small number of the SIDS cases in which a diffuse fatty change was found in the liver (2). Since 1984, several cases of "sudden Reye-like deaths" and SIDS have been attributed to defects of free fatty acid metabolism or to a systemic carnitine deficiency (7–12). Deaths have also been related to nesidioblastosis-induced hypoglycemia, or to a deficiency of pyruvate dehydrogenase (13), thiamine (14), or biotinidase (15). It was estimated that up to 1 of 10 SIDS cases could be attributed to inherent errors of metabolism, and that at least 31 metabolic defects could be potential candidates for SIDS (16).

RETROSPECTIVE ANALYSIS OF APPARENT LIFE-THREATENING EVENTS RELATED TO METABOLIC ABNORMALITIES

Retrospective Analysis of Data

We have reviewed the available data on the 844 infants admitted between 1977 and 1984 after having survived an apparent life-threatening event (ALTE). The mean age was 9 weeks (range 1 to 52 weeks). After a systematic clinical investigation was conducted to rule out possible causes for the event, a medical or surgical cause was found in 563 infants (67%). In decreasing order of frequency, the main abnormalities were digestive (47%), neurological (30%), and respiratory problems (10%). Impaired breathing regulation during sleep was found in about a third of the infants (3,6). In five infants a metabolic cause was found (0.6% of all ALTE cases, or 0.9% of the "explained" ALTE cases) (3).

Results

The results are shown in Table 1.

Infant 1. The child with Leigh's syndrome was a 9-week old girl admitted 5 days

TABLE 1. *ALTE infants with metabolic abnormalities: retrospective study (1977–1984)*

Number of infants studied	844
Number of patients with a metabolic disorder	5
Sex (M/F)	2/3
Gestational age (weeks)	38.8 ± 1.0
Legal age (weeks)	8.8 ± 1.7
Diagnosis:	
(1) Subacute necrotic encephalopathy (Leigh)	1
(2) Menkes' syndrome	1
(3) "Reye's syndrome"	1
(4) NEFA oxydation deficiency (?)	1
(5) Fructosemia	1

after an upper airway infection. She was found limp, pale, and with irregular shallow breathing. On admission she was in a coma and hypothermic. She had severe metabolic acidosis, with normal aciduria. She died 15 days later, and the diagnosis was confirmed by the postmortem.

Infant 2. A 3-month-old boy was found in a state of respiratory arrest and metabolic acidemia. His rectal temperature was 39°C, his hair was sparse, and he had palmar hyperkeratosis. The diagnosis of Menkes' syndrome was supported by the finding of pili torti, an abnormal carotidography, and low plasma copper (<2 µg/dl) and ceruloplasmin levels (<2 mg/dl). After frequent seizures, he died 5 months later. The autopsy confirmed the diagnosis of Menkes' syndrome.

Infant 3. A 4.5-month-old boy was found in a coma, after having vomited the day before. Hepatomegaly and hypoglycemia (40 mg %) were noted, together with increased levels of plasma ammonium (367 mg %), BUN (40 mg %), and transaminases (GO 162 IU, GP 157 IU). There was an increased excretion of adipic acid without cetonuria. A liver biopsy revealed the presence of perilobular steatosis, and a diagnosis of "Reye's syndrome" was made. At 9 months of age the child was readmitted because of anorexia, fever, diarrhea, and muscle weakness. He had been fasting for 6 hours. He was found to be hypoglycemic (10 mg %), and died suddenly despite treatment. At the postmortem, both myocardium and liver were yellow and enlarged, with large vacuoles of perilobular steatosis. The final diagnosis was carnitine deficiency, although the carnitine blood level was not measured.

Infant 4. A 7-month-old girl was found unconscious in her crib after 5 days of fever, anorexia, and vomiting. No hepatomegaly was noted. Blood glucose was 21 mg %, and the plasma pH was 7.49. There was an increase in the levels of ammonium (746 mg %), BUN (68 mg %), and transaminases (GO 612 IU, GP 1100 IU). The Quick test was 55% of normal. Generalized amino aciduria was noted. A liver biopsy revealed microvesicular steatosis. The child survived but developed West's syndrome.

Infant 5. A 6-week-old girl developed a state of pallor and hypotonia following her first ingestion of fruit. A slight hepatomegaly was found. Blood glucose was 50 mg %. A liver biopsy showed no fructose-1-phosphate-aldolase activity. Given a sucrose- and fructose-free diet, the child developed normally and is now 10 years old.

Comments

The retrospective nature of the analysis precludes any detailed confirmation of the suspected abnormalities. Based on the available evidence, the first two infants (children 1 and 2) could be diagnosed as having suffered from a defect of the mitochondrial respiratory chain, probably affecting cytochrome c oxidase. The ensuing mitochondrial myopathy would account for the observed hypotonia, lactic acidemia, and the poor outcome.

Patients 3 and 4 could be classified as showing an impairment of fatty acid oxidation, although a primary carnitine deficiency was ruled out. The last infant showed a standard abnormality of carbohydrate metabolism that was treated with an appropriate diet.

PROSPECTIVE DETECTION OF METABOLIC ABNORMALITIES IN INFANTS WITH A HIGHER RISK OF SIDS

We have prospectively evaluated 86 infants classified as having a higher risk of SIDS. To scan for possible metabolic disorders the infants were carefully selected and subjected to a systematic series of tests, including a 15-h fasting period.

Infants Studied

Forty girls and 46 boys were admitted to the hospital to evaluate their SIDS risk factors. There were 56 siblings of sudden infant death victims (siblings), and 30 infants who had survived an apparent life-threatening event (ALTE), and for which no cause was found. The median age of the infants was 28 weeks (range 42 to 118 weeks). The criteria used for the selection of the infants included several characteristics potentially associated with metabolic abnormalities, such as the occurrence of an ALTE after an infection or a period of fasting, or when the SIDS had occurred at an unusual age—before the fourth week or after the first 12 months of life (9). Asymptomatic infants were included if they were born to families in which at least two siblings had died of SIDS or in which a sibling suffered from a metabolic abnormality. All but one of the infants were considered healthy. No medication was being given at the time of the evaluation.

Clinical Evaluation of the Infants

A detailed family and personal history was obtained for each infant, and a standard physical and neurological evaluation was made. Before initiating the fasting period, blood samples were taken to measure the levels of 3-hydroxybutyrate, transaminases, free and total carnitine, amino acids, and nonesterified fatty acids (NEFA). Urine samples were collected to determine the level of free and total carnitine, amino acids, and organic acids. The 15-h fasting test was then conducted under close medical supervision. Glycemia was monitored by hourly Dextrostix checks, and blood was taken after 9 and 11 h of fasting. Oral glucose was administered in cases of hypoglycemia. After the fifteenth hour of fasting a determination was made of 3-hydroxybutyrate, free and total carnitine, amino acids, blood glucose, lactic acid, pyruvic acid, NH_3, NEFA, and plasma pH. The presence of ketoacids, carnitine and organic acids was evaluated in the urine. Cultures of fibroblasts were performed when acyl-CoA dehydrogenasis deficiency was suspected. The findings related to enzyme activity were not yet available when this report was written.

Results

In 80 of the infants no fasting-induced hypoglycemia or abnormal metabolites were found. In the remaining six infants (one ALTE infant and five SIDS siblings) the following results emerged.

Infant 1. A 13-week-old girl was a SIDS sibling. Her brother and a cousin both died of SIDS at the age of 2.5 and 20 months, respectively. Failure to thrive, anorexia, and muscular hypotonia had been noted since the age of 9 weeks. On admission she showed global muscular hypotonia; the liver edge was felt 1 cm under the costal margin. Blood lactic acid was 29 mg/dl (normal 9–16 mg/dl), and pyruvic acid 1 mg/dl (normal 0.2–1 mg/dl). Increased levels were noted of SGOT (103 U/liter), CPK (489 IU/liter; N: 6–147 IU/liter, and LDH (1724 IU/liter; N: 162–340 IU/liter). Serum NH_3, amino acids, and free, esterified, and total carnitine levels were normal. During the fasting test blood glucose remained normal, but there was an increase in lactates (29 mg/dl) and acetone in the plasma, and two unidentified peaks of organic acids were noted in the urine. A muscle biopsy revealed such nonspecific abnormalities as fatty microvacuolar infiltrations and mitochondrial swelling. An enzymatic defect in the mitochondrial respiratory chain was suspected. Carnitine supplements were nevertheless given orally (100 mg/kg·day), accompanied by a fat-free diet. A delay in gross neuromuscular development was noted at the age of 1 year, with a persistent elevation of the level of muscular enzymes. The activity of the mitochondrial respiratory enzymes is being evaluated.

Infant 2. An 86-week-old boy, a SIDS sibling, had a sister and brother who died of SIDS at 2 and 2.5 months, respectively. A physical examination was normal. After 15 h of fasting, his blood glucose fell to 40 mg/dl, and rose slowly only after glucagon and glucose injections. There were no other abnormal findings. The fasting test had been performed less than 1 week after a viral infection. It was repeated 4 months later, at which time no abnormality was found. Two years later, the child appears to be normal.

Infant 3. A 16-week-old boy had lost two cousins to SIDS at the ages of 2.5 and

16 months. One cousin is suspected of suffering from lactic acidosis (infant 1). His physical examination was normal. The fasting test induced mild plasma lactic acidosis (27 mg/dl; normal 9–16 mg/dl), but no other abnormality was found. A muscle biopsy revealed microvascular steatosis and swollen mitochondria. Despite the lack of a precise diagnosis, oral carnitine was given for 9 months (100 mg/kg·day). At 1 year of age the child's development is normal.

Infants 4, 5, and 6. Mild dicarboxylic aciduria (adipic and 3-OH butyrate) was found in three infants: two SIDS siblings aged 9 and 23 weeks and one 33-week-old ALTE infant. The fasting test was repeated in all three infants within one month of the initial study and was found to be normal. All infants survived the first 2 years of life uneventfully, without treatment.

Comments

Infant 1 was a "floppy baby," who combined both clinically evident hypotonia and lactic acidemia. The most probable diagnosis was that of mitochondria myopathy related to the existence of a respiratory chain enzyme defect (type I or IV). As an enzymatic deficiency has not been identified, we can exclude a deficiency of MCAD or pyruvate metabolism. A defect of the fatty acid oxidation mechanisms was suspected in infant 2, because of the induced hypoglycemia. The diagnosis could not be proven, as a control fasting challenge failed to disclose any abnormality. We do not know whether the viral infection that preceded the fasting challenge contributed to the disruption of the glucose homeostasis. Deficient enzymatic activity in the mitochondrial respiratory chain was suspected in infant 3 because of a mild increase in blood lactate during fasting, abnormal findings in the muscle biopsy, and his familial relationship with infant 1, who suffered from mitochondrial myopathy. The child's clinical development could indicate that the enzymatic deficiency may be a mild one. In the last three infants (4, 5, and 6), fasting induced mild dicarboxylic aciduria but no hypoglycemia. The aciduria was not found a few weeks later during a repeat of the fasting challenges. No clinical symptom was seen, and the children's development was normal. A mild, transitory FFA oxidative defect was postulated, but we were unable to identify any metabolic abnormality in these infants.

DISCUSSION

Our retrospective study revealed that five out of 844 infants (0.6%) studied after an apparent life-threatening event suffered from a metabolic disease. Three of the children died, and one suffered from severe neurologic sequelae. Infants thought to be at higher risk of SIDS were studied prospectively to screen for unidentified metabolic abnormalities. Specific loading challenges have been advocated for the screening of acyl-CoA deficiencies, such as the administration of L-carnitine, or phenylpropionate (10). To extend the range of metabolic defects screened, we performed a fasting challenge. In infants, starvation tests lasting 15 h have been reported to require close monitoring, and to contribute efficiently to the identification of various enzymatic deficiencies (9,17,18). The finding of abnormal results in six out of 86 infants (7%) is close to the incidence of metabolic abnormalities reported in SIDS (8,16). But when the tests were controlled, no abnormality could be confirmed. Only one infant (infant 1) had a clearly abnormal response during the fasting challenge. That child was clinically abnormal, with gross delay in growth and psychomotor development, metabolic acidosis, and elevated levels of liver enzymes.

While the preliminary character of this study precludes any definite conclusions, the lack of correlation between the results of the challenge and the clinical diagnosis, together with the discrepancy between the results of the initial and control studies, raise questions as to both the nature of the abnormalities and the sensitivity of the test procedures. Within the limits of our investigation protocol, the number of SIDS or ALTE infants who suffer from a metabolic dysfunction appears to be limited.

ACKNOWLEDGMENTS

We would like to thank Professor HL Vis for his constant encouragement. The study was supported by the Fondation Nationale de la Recherche Scientifique (Grant 9.4524.87).

REFERENCES

1. Valdes-Dapena M. Sudden infant death syndrome: a review of the medical literature 1974–1979. *Pediatrics* 1980;66:597–614.
2. Sinclair-Smith CC, Dinsdale F, Emery JL. Evidence of duration and type of illness in children found unexpectedly dead. *Arch Dis Child* 1976;51:424–9.
3. Kahn A, Rebuffat E, Sottiaux M, Blum D. Management of an infant with an apparent life-threatening event. *Pediatrician* 1988;15:204–11.
4. Hoffman HJ, Damus K, Hillman L, Krongrad E. Risk factors for SIDS. Result of the National Institute of Child Health and Human Development SIDS Cooperative Epidemiological study. In: Schwartz PJ, Southall DP, Valdes-Dapena M, eds. *The sudden infant death syndrome. Ann NY Acad Sci* 1988;533:13–30.
5. Kahn A, Blum D, Muller MF, et al. Sudden infant death syndrome in a twin: a comparison of sibling histories. *Pediatrics* 1986;78:146–50.
6. Kahn A, Blum D, Rebuffat E, et al. Polysomnographic studies of infants who subsequently died of sudden infant death syndrome. *Pediatrics* 1988;82:721–7.
7. Howat AJ, Bennett MJ, Variend S, Shaw L. Deficiency of medium chain fatty acylcoenzyme A dehydrogenase presenting as the sudden infant death syndrome. *Br Med J* 1984;288:976.
8. Howat AJ, Bennett MJ, Variend S, Shaw L, Engel PC. Defects of metabolism of fatty acids in the sudden infant death syndrome. *Br Med J* 1985;290:1771–3.
9. Duran M, Hofkamp M, Rhead WJ, Saudubray JM, Wadman SK. Sudden child death and "healthy" affected family members with medium-chain acyl-coenzyme A dehydrogenase deficiency. *Pediatrics* 1986;78:1052–7.
10. Roe CR, Millington DS, Maltby DA, Kinnebrew P. Recognition of medium-chain acyl-CoA dehydrogenase deficiency in asymptomatic siblings of children dying of sudden infant death or Reye-like syndromes. *J Pediatr* 1986;108:13–18.
11. Taubman B, Hale DE, Kelly RI. Familial Reye-like syndrome: a presentation of medium-chain acyl-coenzyme A dehydrogenase deficiency. *Pediatrics* 1987;79:382–5.
12. Harpey JP, Charpentier C, Coudé M, Divry P, Paturneau-Jouas M. Sudden infant death syndrome and

multiple acyl-coenzyme A dehydrogenase deficiency, ethylmalonic-adipic aciduria, or systemic carnitine deficiency. *J Pediatr* 1987;110:881–4.

13. Johnston K, Newth CJL, Sheu KFR, et al. Central hypoventilation syndrome in pyruvate dehydrogenase complex deficiency. *Pediatrics* 1984;74:1034–40.

14. Read DTC. The etiology of the sudden infant death syndrome: current ideas on breathing and sleep and possible links to deranged thiamine neurochemistry. *Aust NZ J Med* 1978;8:322–36.

15. Burton BK, Roach ES, Wolf B, Weissbecker F. Sudden death associated with biotinidase deficiency. *Pediatrics* 1987;79:482–3.

16. Emery JL, Howat AJ, Variend S, Vawter GF. Investigation of inborn errors of metabolism in unexpected infant deaths. *Lancet* 1988;iii:29–31.

17. Pollitt RJ. Inherited disorders of straight chain fatty acid oxidation. *Arch Dis Child* 1987;62:6–7.

18. Duran M, Wadman SK. Chemical diagnosis of inherited defects of fatty acid metabolism and ketogenesis. *Enzyme* 1987;38:115–23.

DISCUSSION

Dr. Saudubray: I would like to make some comments about the difficulty in finding the right protocol for the investigation of SIDS. Of the list of the investigations you presented, I have done many over the last two years which I have found to be very questionable. For example, when you choose a 15-h fast for investigation, this is either very dangerous or absolutely useless, because if you want to investigate fatty acid oxidation during a fast, the investigation must take place at a time when fatty acid oxidation is stimulated; if the patient is still using liver glycogen stores you are not studying fatty acid oxidation. So it is a false security, because even if all measured variables are completely normal, you cannot rule out the possibility of a fatty acid oxidation defect. The same holds true for everything else. For example, amino acids in plasma are not really informative; if they are normal, what does it mean? As for carnitine, it has known incredible success; but when I reviewed my own experience after 3 or 4 years of carnitine measurement, not only for sudden infant death but for every patient with suspicion of inborn errors, I stopped measuring carnitine as a screening system; if it is low, you don't know what this means, and if it is normal, you cannot rule out the possibility of an inborn error.

Dr. Kahn: There is sufficient evidence in favor of a 15-h fast if you want to stress a child less than 1 year of age. As reported in the literature and in our own experience, a 15-h fast is not dangerous as long as you monitor the child very closely.

Dr. Holton: Can I comment on this question of the incidence of metabolic disease in SIDS patients? To answer this question we do need some systematic studies of unselected sudden infant death victims. Fortunately, three studies have been proceeding. One was reported at the Münich meeting recently, from Lyon. They had studied 109 cases of sudden infant death and had looked at available body fluids using GCMS. They also examined skin fibroblasts in these cases, using the CO_2 release assay for MCAD. In Bristol we have examined 100 cases, using almost identical methods. In Edinburgh they have looked at 200 sequential cases of sudden infant death, using the CO_2 release assay. In all these cases, over 400 now, not one metabolic disorder was detected.

Dr. Bartlett: I would like to present a dissenting view. We have done a rather limited study, looking at postmortem plasma octanoate concentrations. We studied 40 cases of sudden infant death. We found five who had raised octanoate concentrations, but of that five only one also had octanoate-carnitine present. However, we had no tissue available to confirm the diagnosis by direct enzyme assay.

Dr. Holton: I don't think it is a dissenting point of view. Metabolic disease, particularly MCAD, does cause sudden infant death, but I think only in a very small percentage.

Dr. Kahn: I agree completely with that comment. Again, let me stress that the problem of the definition of the prevalence of metabolic abnormalities in sudden infant death syndrome is a methodologically difficult one to solve. But from the clinical point of view we should not forget that, as clinicians, we also have access to information on the child's condition and on the family history that may contain a lot of information. For instance, I mentioned excessive sweating during sleep; in normal infants this is rarely seen in such studies, but in studies on 150 SIDS victims, sweating was excessive in 25%, while only 3 to 5% of the control population were reported to be sweating. The same applies to difficulty in feeding these infants. Such information could contribute to the identification of infants in whom metabolic investigations should be performed.

Dr. Roe: Part of the problem is not knowing the actual frequency of some of these disorders in the general population. It is not at all clear what the frequency of MCAD is. To make matters worse, we are further confounded by variation in the definition of sudden unexplained death in children: up to 12 months of age in my country, for example, whereas the British consider SIDS up to 24 months of age. There are a lot of variations. From the slide I showed on the situation with MCAD, one would expect to find more deaths in the second year of life than in the first. One of the things that I have found interesting while working closely with the examining medical officers is that pathologists know what SIDS is, and they will tell you precisely what the findings are or are not. When they have a sudden death and observe significant hepatic steatosis or some degree of cerebral edema at autopsy, that death is not usually considered to be SIDS. However, cases with those findings often prove to be a metabolic disorder.

Dr. Duran: I may perhaps add a comment on the age of death in children dying unexpectedly with inherited disorders of fatty acid metabolism. We know four families in which children with the medium chain acyl-CoA dehydrogenase deficiency or hydroxyacyl-CoA dehydrogenase deficiency have died. Three families had children dying in the second year of life. One family had a child who died in the first week of life. So all these children died outside the generally accepted period of sudden infant death.

Dr. Kahn: That is a comment I would like to emphasize. This is why we are also focusing mostly on those infants where a previous child died at an unusual age. We know that 85% of the infants will die of sudden infant death syndrome between 2 and 6 months of age. We also know that less than 10% occur in the first 4 weeks of life, and less than 1% of all the SIDS cases occur after 1 year of age. So whenever a child is reported to have died after the first year of age, the risk of there being a metabolic abnormality could increase, and we are therefore much more concerned with those deaths. Likewise, the prevalence of sudden death in the same families for no apparent reason is fairly small, since 97% of all siblings are normal. Whenever more than two children have died in one family with the same unexplained death we should wonder whether we are not dealing with a metabolic abnormality.

Dr. Saudubray: What is the possible influence of dietary medium chain triglyceride supplementation on the postmortem levels of decanoic, decenoic, and marginally medium chain fatty acids in plasma? Do you have any experience in this field?

Dr. Bartlett: Of the five patients in our study who had elevated octanoate concentrations, one had been on a formula containing medium chain triglycerides, but this was not the case in whom there was also octanoylcarnitine.

Dr. Duran: We don't have much experience with MCT diet in postmortem material. What we do know is that in postmortem diagnosis of MCAD deficiency, we find the unsaturated C10 fatty acid, the *cis*-4-decenoic acid, which we consider quite characteristic of this disorder.

Dr. Endres: We recently had a discussion with Dr. Ann Burchell, who published in the *Lancet* many cases of glucose-6-phosphatase deficiency in patients who had died suddenly (1). There was no agreement on the reliability of this work and I would like to ask you what you think about this publication.

Dr. Van Hoof: We have been involved in the diagnosis of more than 100 patients with type I glycogenosis. None of them developed sudden infant death syndrome.

Dr. Van den Berghe: The paper by Burchell et al. (1) claimed that glycogen storage disease type I was present in 10 of 38 cases of SIDS. Together with Dr. Van Hoof, we scrutinized this study in detail and found the following shortcomings: (1) although all children were necropsied, no information is given with respect to liver size in a disorder in which hepatomegaly is a major sign; (2) apparently neither optical nor electron microscopic examination of the liver was performed, which could have demonstrated glycogen accumulation; and (3) glucose-6-phosphatase is known to be very unstable, rendering its assay in autopsy liver highly problematic.

Dr. Hobbs: In the 1960s, Professor J. L. Emery brought me samples from 68 cot-death children which were analyzed for immunoglobulin deficiency. I regret this is one paper we did not publish, but for the record, we did not find a single abnormality.

Dr. Saudubray: Beside the true sudden infant death syndrome, we have observed sudden death several times in patients affected with respiratory chain disorders presenting with cardiomyopathy. Five patients who on admission did not appear severely ill died 5 or 6 h after admission. Of course, these were not sudden infant death syndrome cases, but when you make a diagnosis of respiratory chain disorders you must tell the parents the child is in constant danger of dying unexpectedly.

REFERENCE

1. Burchell A, et al. Hepatic microsomal glucose-6-phosphatase system and sudden infant death syndrome. *Lancet* 1989;ii:291–4.

Inborn Errors of Metabolism, edited by
J. Schaub, F. Van Hoof, and H. L. Vis.
Nestlé Nutrition Workshop Series, Vol. 24.
Nestec Ltd., Vevey/Raven Press, Ltd.,
New York © 1991.

Medium Chain Triglycerides: Advantages and Possible Drawbacks

Margit Hamosh, *Michael L. Spear, †Joel Bitman, Nitin R. Mehta,
†D. Larry Wood, and Paul Hamosh

*Department of Pediatrics and Physiology and Biophysics, Georgetown University
Medical Center, 3800 Reservoir Road, NW, Washington DC 20007; *The Medical
Center of Delaware, Newark, Delaware 19718; †Milk Secretion and Mastitis
Laboratory, USDA Beltsville, Maryland 20705, USA*

Medium chain triglycerides (MCTs) are composed of a mixture of caproic acid
(C6:0), 1–2%, caprylic acid (C8:0), 65–75%, capric acid (C10:0), 25–35%, and lauric
acid (C12:0), 1–2%. These medium chain fatty acids (MCFA) have a lower melting
point than the long chain fatty acids (16.7°C, 31.3°C, and 63.1°C for caprylic, capric,
and palmitic acids, respectively) and are therefore liquid at room temperature. These
fatty acids are much more soluble in water than are long chain fatty acids (68 mg
per 100 ml versus 0.72 mg per 100 ml at 20°C for caprylic and palmitic acids, respectively). Solubility in biological fluids is further increased because of the highly
ionized state at neutral pH of the medium chain fatty acids (1).

The metabolism of medium chain fatty acids varies greatly from that of long chain
fatty acids. The former are released from triglycerides at higher rates by digestive
enzymes: lingual (2), gastric (3), and pancreatic lipases (4). Contrary to long chain
fatty acids, the medium chain fatty acids are absorbed directly through the gastric
mucosa, a finding reported previously for suckling rats (5,6) and recently also for
the preterm infant (7). Intestinal metabolism and transport into the circulation are
also different, medium chain fatty acids being released into the portal circulation and
thus being transported chiefly to the liver, in contrast to long chain fatty acids, which
are re-esterified in the intestinal mucosa and packaged into chylomicrons prior to
their release into the lymphatics and then into the systemic circulation (4,8). Because
most of the ingested medium chain fatty acids reach the liver, they are metabolized
within hepatocytes where they are rapidly oxidized giving rise to ketone bodies, a
process facilitated by the ability of these fatty acids to cross the double mitochondrial
membrane, a process that for medium chain fatty acids, unlike for long chain fatty
acids, does not require the presence of carnitine (1). Indeed, the liver produces 10
times more CO_2 from a caprylic (C8:0) then from palmitic (C16:0) acid (1).

Thus medium chain fatty acids are mainly a rapid source of energy and contribute only little to lipogenesis (9) although it was recently reported that medium chain fatty acids can be stored in adipose tissue of orally fed infants (10).

Our understanding of MCT metabolism is based largely on animal studies, where it was reported that, in the rat, overfeeding with MCT results in diminished weight gain, fat deposition, and fat cell size (11). In the human, oxygen consumption was 12% higher after a 400-kcal meal of MCT, as compared to an increment of only 4% after an isocaloric meal of long chain triglycerides (12). The mild ketosis prevailing in the breast-fed infant (13), attributed to the medium chain fatty acid (MCFA) content of human milk, can be duplicated in infants fed formulas containing MCFA (14). The preferential incorporation of ketone bodies into brain and lung lipids (15,16) in the neonatal period suggests that MCFAs are important also as substrates for organ growth and not only as energy source.

Because of our interest in the composition of human milk fat, especially as related to length of gestation and lactation, as well as in fat digestion and absorption, we have conducted several studies relating to medium chain fatty acids and their function in the neonate. The questions we have asked were: (a) What initiates the synthesis of MCFAs in the human mammary gland? (b) To what extent are MCFAs released from triglyceride in the stomach of the newborn? (c) Are MCFAs absorbed through the gastric mucosa of the newborn? (d) Is fat absorption in the newborn improved by feeding MCT-containing formulas? and (e) What is the fate of MCT oil fed to infants as a fortifier of premature formula or human milk?

MEDIUM CHAIN FATTY ACIDS IN HUMAN MILK

Our recent studies have shown that medium chain fatty acids are present in prepartum mammary secretions (17). Furthermore, their concentration is higher in the milk secreted by mothers of preterm infants during the course of lactation than in the milk of mothers of full-term infants (18).

Medium chain fatty acids (<C16) of milk are synthesized within the mammary gland because only this tissue contains a specific enzyme, thioesterase II, that is able to terminate fatty acid synthesis at a lower carbon number, as compared to thioesterase I present in other tissues that terminates the aliphatic carbon chain at or above C16 (19,20). Because fatty acids C10:0 and 12:0 are present in much lower concentrations in prepartum mammary secretion (obtained between 70 days and 1 day before term delivery) than in colostrum of women who deliver very prematurely (at 26–30 weeks' gestation) (Table 1), we wondered what might be the trigger for MCFA synthesis in the human mammary gland. Comparison of the MCFA concentration in colostrum of women who deliver after various length of gestation shows that parturition seems to be the trigger for MCFA synthesis, since prepartum secretions obtained close to full-term delivery had much lower MCFA concentrations. Taking the milk/plasma ratio as an indicator of fatty acid origin (i.e., a ratio close to 1 indicates uptake from the circulation, and thus of dietary or fat depot origin, while a ratio >2 would indicate synthesis within the mammary gland), it is obvious

TABLE 1. *Medium chain fatty acid synthesis in the human mammary gland*

Specimen	N	Fatty acid[a] (%)			Fat (g/dl)
		C10:0	C12:0	C14:0	
Prepartum secretion (1–70 days prepartum)[b]	12	0.10	1.70	4.90	1.20
Postpartum colostrum[c]					
Very preterm infants (26–30 weeks)	18	0.26	3.09	5.52	2.00
Preterm infants (30–37 weeks)	26	0.31	3.14	5.87	1.80
Full-term infants (38–42 weeks)	6	0.27	3.10	6.81	2.20

[a] Fatty acids: C10:0, capric (decanoic); C12:0, lauric; C14:0, myristic.
[b] Prepartum secretions obtained from women who delivered at full term.
[c] Gestational age (weeks) of the infants delivered.

that MCFA synthesis is fully developed shortly after delivery, resulting in milk/plasma ratio of 16 for capric (C10:0), 17 for lauric (C12:0), and 4.3 for myristic (C14:0) acids (21) (Fig. 1).

The concentration of medium chain fatty acids in milk depends on the diet, being high in women who consume a diet rich in carbohydrates and low in fat (22–24). While this diet is natural in many parts of the world, it was recently suggested that the concentration of MCFA in the milk of American women might be augmented by increasing the carbohydrate and reducing the fat content of their diet, a process called "*in vivo* lactoengineering" (25). Recent studies suggest that high parity (10 or more children) markedly lowers the fatty acid synthesizing ability of the human mammary gland (26).

TO WHAT EXTENT ARE MCFA RELEASED FROM TRIGLYCERIDES IN THE STOMACH OF THE NEWBORN?

Lingual and gastric lipases have higher affinity for medium chain fatty acids and for long chain polyunsaturated fatty acids than for saturated long chain fatty acids (2,3). This preferential pattern of triglyceride hydrolysis is apparent already in the 1-day-old rats. In this species, milk fat content is high (>10%) and analysis of gastric contents after milk ingestion shows high levels of medium chain and long chain polyunsaturated fatty acids released through the action of lingual lipase, the only preduodenal digestive lipase in the rat (27) (Fig. 2). A similar pattern of hydrolysis of human milk fat by lingual lipase is also evident (Fig. 3). *In vitro* incubation of human milk fat with partially purified lingual lipase leads to rapid release of C10:0 and C12:0 (within 10 minutes of incubation) while long chain unsaturated fatty acids are released at lower rates (maximal hydrolysis at 30 minutes). No measurable release of C14:0 and C16:0 fatty acids was evident during this incubation time (28).

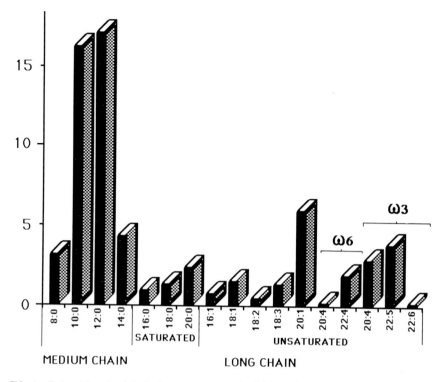

FIG. 1. Fatty acid synthesis in the human mammary gland 2 days after full-term delivery. Milk:plasma fatty acid ratios. Plasma and milk lipids were analyzed by gas-liquid chromatography. Ratios in excess of 1:0 indicate synthesis within the mammary gland. From Spear ML, et al. (21).

ARE MEDIUM CHAIN FATTY ACIDS ABSORBED THROUGH THE GASTRIC MUCOSA OF THE NEWBORN?

The very low content of C8:0 in all lipid classes, including the free fatty acids from gastric contents of milk-fed rats, indicated that this fatty acid might be directly absorbed through the gastric mucosa of suckling rats (6). Indeed, in contrast to the loss of C8:0, the free fatty acids were enriched in C10:0 and C12:0, indicating that the gastric lipolytic process released primarily medium chain fatty acids from milk triglycerides and that C10:0 and C12:0 were not absorbed completely in the stomach. These initial studies in suckling rats were followed by studies in preterm infants (7). In a recent study in which we have examined gastric digestion of formulas containing predominantly long chain fatty acids or as much as 39% medium chain fatty acids, similar results were obtained. Caprylic and capric acids (C8:0 and C10:0, respectively) were reduced in gastric triglycerides as compared with formula triglyceride, indicating preferential hydrolysis. Whereas the triglycerides of the MCT formula contained 30% C8:0 and 12% C10:0, gastric triglycerides contained only 6% of each of these fatty acids. Similarly, the triglycerides of the LCT formula

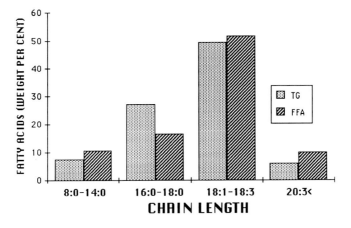

FIG. 2. Hydrolysis of rat milk in the stomach of 1-day-old pups. The pups were weaned from their mothers for 1 h and were allowed to suckle for 30 min after returning to the mothers. At the end of this period the pups were sacrificed and gastric contents removed and extracted for fatty acid analysis by gas-liquid chromatography. Adapted from Bitman J, et al. (6).

contained 3.8% C8:0 and 3.1% C10:0, whereas gastric triglycerides contained only 0.8% and 1.7% of these fatty acids, respectively. The loss of these fatty acids from the triglycerides in the stomach did not result in an increase in the percentage of these fatty acids in the free fatty acids fraction. Since these measurements were made 15 min after starting the gavage feeding, when most of the lipid was still in the stomach (94% of the MCT fed and 100% of the LCT fed), the disappearance of C8:0 and to a lesser extent of C10:0 indicates that these fatty acids had left the stomach, probably by absorption through the gastric mucosa (7). This study, which is the first to indicate that medium chain fatty acids are absorbed in the stomach of

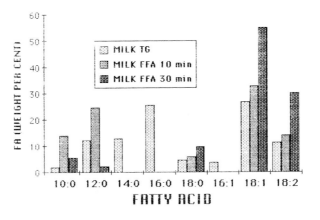

FIG. 3. Hydrolysis of human milk fat by lingual lipase. Human milk fat was incubated with partially purified lingual lipase and samples were taken for analysis of fatty acids by gas-liquid chromatography.

TABLE 2. *Fat absorption and growth rate in preterm infants fed medium chain triglyceride or long chain triglyceride formula[a]*

Formula	Dietary fat (g/kg/day)	Fat excretion (g/kg/day)	Fat absorption (%)	Weight (g/day)
Medium chain triglycerides	6.04 ± 0.54	1.04 ± 0.24	84.63 ± 3.14	23.0 ± 1.50
(n = 12)	(4.18–8.38)	(0.15–1.87)	(60.21–97.05)	(15.71–34.28)
Long chain triglycerides	5.88 ± 0.48	1.02 ± 0.26	82.81 ± 4.01	20.85 ± 1.80
(n = 12)	(3.63–7.60)	(0.18–2.29)	(49.34–97.50)	(22.42–32.85)

[a] Data are means ± SEM and ranges (in parentheses). Fat excretion and absorption were determined during a 3-day balance study. Weight gain was determined during 1 week when infants were fed either medium chain or long chain triglyceride formula. Each infant was fed each formula for 1 week. Infants were randomly assigned to start with either formula. The 12 infants studied had a gestational age of 28.7 ± 0.50 weeks (range 26–32 weeks) and postnatal age of 6.08 ± 0.81 weeks (range 2.6–12.4 weeks). From Hamosh M, et al. (7).

the newborn infant, suggests that MCTs provide a readily available energy source that can be absorbed much more rapidly than the other energy sources available to the newborn.

IS FAT ABSORPTION IN THE NEWBORN IMPROVED BY FEEDING MCT-CONTAINING FORMULA?

Medium chain fatty acids are often used in the nutritional management of premature infants (29–31). Indeed, absorption of individual medium chain fatty acids was found to be higher than that of long chain fatty acids (32). However, despite this finding, recent reports suggest similar fat absorption in infants fed MCT- or LCT-containing formulas (33–35). We have investigated this question using two formulas that were identical, except for differences in the fat blend (Mead Johnson Enfamil containing 88.3 kcal per 100 ml, 4.4% fat, 2.65% protein, and 9.71% carbohydrate; the MCT formula contained 42% of C8:0 and C10:0, and the LCT formula contained 7% of C8:0 and C10:0. Seventy-two-hour fat balance studies were conducted on days 4–7 of each formula regimen. As can be seen from Table 2, in this study, in which each infant served as his or her own control (each formula being fed for 1 week), there was no difference in fat absorption or weight gain when preterm infants were fed either MCT or LCT formula. As can be seen in Fig. 4, there was much variation among infants in the extent of fat absorption. In nine of the 12 infants studied, fat absorption ranged from 85 ot 97%. Thus, although C8:0 is rapidly absorbed from the stomach, medium chain triglycerides do not seem to improve fat absorption or weight gain in preterm infants.

WHAT IS THE FATE OF MCT OIL FED TO INFANTS AS A FORTIFIER OF PRETERM FORMULA?

Infant feeds are often supplemented with MCT oil (Mead Johnson Co.) to increase the caloric density. We wondered whether this supplement, which is not homoge-

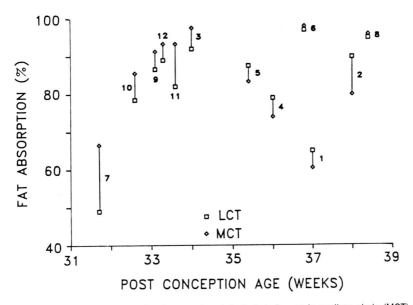

FIG. 4. Comparison of fat absorption in premature infants fed alternately medium chain (MCT) or long chain (LCT) formula. Numbers next to symbols designate individual infant numbers. From Hamosh M, et al. (7) with permission.

nized before feeding, might not be delivered in its entirety and some of the fat might be lost. As shown in Fig. 5, depending on the mode of feeding, as much as 16% of fat fed to the infant might adhere to the gavage feeding set when MCT oil is mixed with human milk prior to feeding (36). Analysis of the fatty acid composition of the residual fat showed that it was composed mainly (up to 84%) of MCFAs (C8:0 and C10:0), as compared to the fat residue in the unfortified milk feeding sets in which the fatty acid chain lengths were >C12:0 (36) (Fig. 6). Our study thus raises some concerns about the method of fortification of infant feeds, and suggests that the MCT oil be fed first followed by delivery of the feed through the feeding set. The very high loss of medium chain fatty acids indicates that the feeding sets might have special affinity for these fatty acids. Our recent studies show that the medium chain fatty acids in preterm formulas that contain high levels of this fat blend are not adhering

TABLE 3. *Characteristics of medium chain fatty acids*

High solubility in water
Rapid release from triglyceride by digestive lipases
Absorption through the gastric mucosa
Transport from the intestine to the liver as FFA in the portal circulation
Carnitine independent passage into mitochondria for oxidation
Ketogenic
Low deposition in adipose tissue
Thermogenic

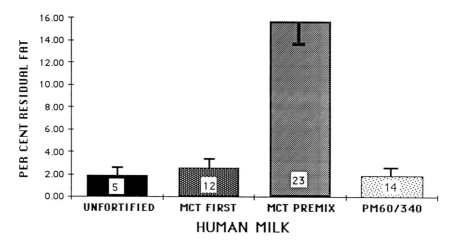

FIG. 5. Amount of fat adhering to feeding sets during intermittent feeding of fortified fresh human milk. Data are percent (mean ± SEM) of total fat adhering to feeding sets during four feeding regimens: (1) unfortified human milk; (2) MCT oil delivered first, followed by milk; (3) MCT oil premixed with milk before gavage feeding; and (4) milk fortified with PM 60/40. Numbers in each bar represent number of experiments. From Mehta NR, et al. (36) with permission.

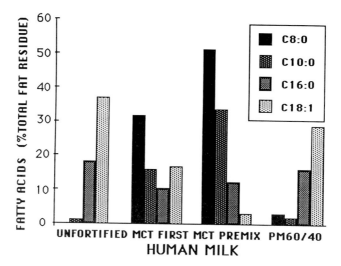

FIG. 6. Fatty acid composition of fat adhering to feeding sets during gavage feeding of fortified human milk in four feeding regimens: (1) unfortified human milk; (2) MCT oil delivered first, followed by milk; (3) MCT oil premixed with milk before gavage feeding; and (4) milk fortified with PM 60/40. C8:0 (octanoic acid) and C10:0 (decanoic acid), major components of MCT oil; C16:0 (palmitic acid) and C18:1 (oleic acid), major components of human milk fat. From Mehta NR, et al. (36) with permission.

to the gavage tubes (37), probably because of the efficient emulsification of fat during the formula preparation process.

CONCLUSION

Animal and human studies have shown that medium chain fatty acids might improve fat digestion and absorption, are a rapid energy source, and a good source of ketone bodies and are not deposited efficiently in fat depots, thus having a potential role in weight-reducing diets (Table 3, page 87). These advantages are, however, balanced by the lack of improvement in fat absorption as well as by the tendency of these fatty acids to be lost through adherence to feeding tubes. It is therefore advisable to prepare fat blends that contain 10–20% MCFA (concentrations found in human milk), and to provide MCFA as an integral part of infant formulas rather than as an oil supplement. Much additional research is needed to assess the function of these fatty acids in the nutrition of infants and children.

ACKNOWLEDGMENTS

The author's studies are supported by National Institutes of Health Grants HD-10823, 15631, and 20833 and by grants from the Mead Johnson Nutrition Division, Wyeth Laboratories, and Ross Laboratories. The expert secretarial assistance of Mrs. Barbara M. Runner is greatly appreciated.

REFERENCES

1. Bach AC, Babayan VK. Medium-chain triglycerides: an update. *Am J Clin Nutr* 1982;36:950–62.
2. Liao TH, Hamosh P, Hamosh M. Fat digestion by lingual lipase: mechanism of lipolysis in the stomach and upper small intestine. *Pediatr Res* 1984;18:402–9.
3. DeNigris SJ, Hamosh M, Kasbekar DK, Fink CS, Lee TC, Hamosh P. Human gastric lipase: secretion from dispersed gastric glands. *Biochim Biophys Acta* 1985;836:67–72.
4. Carey MC, Small DM, Blis CM. Lipid digestion and absorption. *Annu Rev Physiol* 1983;45:651–77.
5. Aw TY, Grigor MR. Digestion and absorption of milk triacylglycerols in 14-day old suckling rats. *J Nutr* 1980;110:2133–40.
6. Bitman J, Wood DL, Liao TH, Fink CS, Hamosh P, Hamosh M. Gastric lipolysis of milk lipids in suckling rats. *Biochim Biophys Acta* 1985;834:58–64.
7. Hamosh M, Bitman J, Liao TH, et al. Gastric lipolysis and fat absorption in preterm infants: effect of MCT or LCT containing formulas. *Pediatrics* 1989;83:86–92.
8. Patton JS. Gastrointestinal lipid digestion. In: Johnson LR, ed. *Physiology of the gastrointestinal tract.* New York: Raven Press, 1981;1123–46.
9. McGarry JD, Foster DW. Regulation of hepatic fatty acid oxidation and ketone body production. *Annu Rev Biochem* 1980;49:395–420.
10. Sarda P, Lepage G, Roy CC, Chessex P. Storage of medium-chain triglycerides in adipose tissue of orally fed infants. *Am J Clin Nutr* 1987;45:399–405.
11. Geliebter A, Torbay N, Brocco EF, Hashim SA, Van Itallie TB. Overfeeding with medium-chain triglyceride diet results in diminished deposition of fat. *Am J Clin Nutr* 1983;37:1–4.
12. Seaton TB, Welle SL, Warenko MK, Campbell RG. Thermic effect of medium-chain and long-chain triglycerides in man. *Am J Clin Nutr* 1986;44:630–4.
13. Lucas A, Boyes S, Bloom SR, Aynsley-Green A. Metabolic and endocrine responses to a milk feed in

that there is no difference relevant to neonatal jaundice in milk lipases or β-glucoronidase activities (1) or in the amount of milk fat (2).

Dr. Mowat: I wonder if you have any observations on the time course of development of lipase, both lingual and gastric, particularly in the more immature babies (i.e., around 24 weeks). I know that a few studies seem to start at 32 weeks. And I wonder if you have any information on what the activities of these enzymes were nearer the time of delivery.

Dr. Hamosh: We have extensive data which were published between 1981 and 1984. We measured enzyme activities starting at 25 weeks' gestation. Activity is very high from 25 weeks' gestation and there is only a slight increase after 35 weeks.

Dr. Saudubray: Do we know what are the regulatory mechanisms for the elongation of fatty acids? Is there a difference when fatty acid synthesis starts from a very short molecule, such as acetoacetyl-CoA, and when it starts from longer molecules, such as a C8, C10, or C12?

Dr. Mannaerts: Denis McGarry and Dan Foster, working in Dallas, perfused livers with [1-^{14}C]octanoate and looked where the labeled carbon atom was localized in long chain fatty acids, in order to discriminate between elongation and β-oxidation of the labeled octanoate to acetyl-CoA, and the reutilization of this acetyl-CoA for fatty acid synthesis. I think they saw very little elongation of octanoate.

Dr. Hamosh: In general, preterm infants have to be given long chain polyunsaturated fatty acids because they lack the ability to elongate and dissaturate fatty acids. We don't know at what age they acquire this ability.

Dr. Saudubray: With propionic and methylmalonic acidemias we have a good model of accumulation of propionyl-CoA, which is a very good primer for odd-numbered fatty acid synthesis.

Dr. Hobbs: We have a paradox here. In the peroxisomal diseases, where accumulation of very long chain fatty acids occurs, they must be avoided. Now we are told that the medium chain varieties may overload the peroxisomes. So we have two different ways of stressing peroxisomal patients. Do you know whether these have been studied to see if they could explain the heterogeneous expression?

Dr. Wanders: I think what Professor Van Hoof was telling us about the hypothesis that MCT and dicarboxylic acids give rise to overloading of the peroxisomal system is an attractive model. Nobody has looked at the very long chain fatty acid levels or bile acid intermediates in these patients. It is something we should do.

Dr. Van Hoof: I think that high doses of MCT need to be given to bring about a pathological accumulation of very long chain fatty acids and bile acid precursors, since MCT are widely used without clinical problems, at least according to the literature.

Dr. Hamosh: I think it would be safe when we speak about normal full-term infants, without any biochemical abnormalities, to adhere to the concentration of MCT in human milk, because after all, the human species has survived, for better or for worse, on breast milk for a long time, with a concentration of about 5–10% MCT.

REFERENCES

1. Freed LM, Moscioni D, Hamosh M, Gartner LM, Hamosh P. Breast milk jaundice revisited: no role for glucuronidase or "unstimulated lipase." *Pediatr Res* 1987;21:267A.
2. Editorial: Hamosh M, Breast milk jaundice, *J Pediatr Gastroenterol Nutr* 1990;11:145–7.

metabolite excretion. The activity of 3-methylglutaconyl-CoA hydratase was normal in all tissues tested (Dr. H. Ibel, Munich, FRG, personal communication). It can safely be concluded that in these cases 3-methylglutaconate is not derived from leucine catabolism in the liver. More investigations are inevitably needed for the elucidation of the underlying defect. An exact stereochemical characterization of urinary 3-methylglutaconate could be of help in this respect. We have recently come across several adult female 3-methylglutaconate excretors who—being healthy themselves—gave birth to neurologically handicapped children. This raises the question of a possible teratogenic effect of 3-methylglutaconate or any of its hitherto unknown precursors.

Mevalonic Aciduria

A deficiency of mevalonate kinase represents the first documented inherited disorder of cholesterol biosynthesis. As such it is a very intriguing model system for the study of regulatory mechanisms in this biosynthetic pathway. Surprisingly, none of the three patients reported so far did have a decreased plasma cholesterol level.

In vitro studies on cholesterol metabolism carried out with cultured fibroblasts also gave normal results. One of the possible explanations lies in the very high production of mevalonate—probably by an increased HMG-CoA reductase—which overcomes the decreased affinity of the enzyme and permits the mevalonate pathway to function. An argument to support this hypothesis is the level of urinary mevalonate excretion, which is exceptionally high: 167–56,200 mmol/mol creatinine. The variability of the clinical presentation—ranging from mild cerebellar ataxia with hypotonia to severe failure to thrive and early death—seems to correlate with the urinary mevalonate excretion but not with the residual enzyme activity in fibroblasts or lymphocytes (4). Organic acid analysis of these patients' urine displays a simple profile: an impressive peak of mevalonolactone is mainly observed, with a minor peak of mevalonate itself. Plasma mevalonate did not exceed values over 0.5 mmol/liter; hence metabolic acidosis due to accumulation of organic acid did not occur.

(Methyl)malònic Semialdehyde Dehydrogenase Deficiency

The catabolism of uracil, thymine, and valine proceeds via malonic and methylmalonic semialdehydes. As an example, the formation of propionyl-CoA from valine involves the action of methylmalonic semialdehyde dehydrogenase. To date a single patient with a deficiency of this enzyme has been described. A characteristic excretion profile can be observed comprising the presence of 3-hydroxypropionate, 3-hydroxyisobutyrate, 2-ethylhydracrylate, and the amino acids β-alanine and β-aminoisobutyric acid. Clinically, the patient was essentially free of symptoms (5).

Succinic Aciduria

One report has appeared in the literature. It dealt with a neonate who died at the age of 5 weeks with a complex I deficiency (6). Plasma succinate was measured on one occasion: the value was found to be 2.23 mM with a concomitant lactate of 27 mM. Urinary succinate was normal on two consecutive days, but was strongly increased on the next day. A subsequent pregnancy in this family was terminated at 22 weeks; fetal serum contained 6.3 mmol/liter succinate.

We think one should be very careful interpreting these data because (a) succinate is easily formed nonenzymatically from 2-oxoglutarate, and (b) extremely high succinate levels are usually found in serum samples that have been collected perimortally.

Fumaric Aciduria

Fumarase, an enzyme of the citric acid cycle, has been shown to be present in at least six fractions. Both cytosolic and mitochondrial forms can be distinguished. Fumaric aciduria has been described in only a few isolated cases where the enzyme defect was (a) nonexistent, (b) confined to the cytoplasm, or (c) generalized (7). It is to be expected that more variants will be found. Screening for organic acids revealed increased urinary levels of fumarate (151–772 mmol/mol creatinine) and succinate (153–194 mmol/mol creatinine). Plasma fumarate did not exceed 5.5 μmol/liter.

The clinical spectrum of fumaric aciduria ranges from speech retardation with mental regression to severe failure to thrive with cerebral atrophy and early death. In general, the clinical histories appear to be nonspecific so far.

Malonic Aciduria

Malonic aciduria is another of the "moderate" organic acidurias. Malonic acid is the main urinary metabolite (150–3,900 mmol/mol creatinine); one of the two reported patients also excreted methylmalonic acid (210 mmol/mol creatinine), probably as a result of the inhibition of methylmalonyl-CoA mutase by malonyl-CoA. A deficiency of mitochondrial malonyl-CoA decarboxylase—which plays only a minor role in the metabolism of malonyl-CoA—could be established in cultured fibroblasts. Clinically important were the following signs: (recurrent) vomiting, metabolic acidosis, and seizures (8).

Lactic Aciduria Due to Fructose-1,6-diphosphatase Deficiency

Gluconeogenesis is regulated by four key enzymes: pyruvate carboxylase, phosphoenolpyruvate carboxykinase, fructose-1,6-diphosphatase, and glucose-6-phosphatase. Defects of all enzymes are generally accompanied by severe lactic acidosis, a symptom without significance for the differential diagnosis. The deficiency of glucose-6-phosphatase, or glycogen storage disease type I, can be recognized by its clinical presentation and the secondary abnormalities of triglyceride and urate metabolism.

Fructose-1,6-diphosphatase acts in the upper half of the gluconeogenic pathway, which involves not only the metabolism of pyruvate but also that of glycerol. This opens new possibilities for the differential diagnosis, as has recently been shown. Dremsek and co-workers (9) described an increased urinary excretion of glycerol during episodes of metabolic decompensation, a finding that became more important since the description of glycerol-3-phosphate in the urine of a similar patient (10). We have studied another four patients with fructose-1,6-diphosphatase deficiency and observed glycerol-3-phosphate in all cases (for the method of detection, see Analytical Chemical Aspects).

Urinary glycerol reached values up to 90 mmol/liter, a figure comparable to those seen in glycerol kinase deficiency. A missing link in the gluconeogenic pathway from glycerol (i.e., dihydroxyacetone phosphate) could not be traced in any of the patients' urine samples. As a rule we always measure glycerol-3-phosphate in urine samples containing abnormal amounts of glycerol and lactate.

The specificity of glycerol-3-phosphate has some limitations, as exemplified by a patient with hereditary tyrosinemia type I. During episodes of hypoglycemia—probably as a result of impaired liver function—she excreted both glycerol and glycerol-3-phosphate in excess. The activity of liver fructose-1,6-diphosphatase could not be assessed, but should be subject of further studies associated with tyrosinemia.

Disorders Associated with Ketosis

Ketone bodies, which are produced by the liver, are important sources of energy to the brain, especially during starvation. Defects of ketone body utilization will thus result in a decreased energy supply to the brain, with severe clinical consequences. Two defects have been unraveled so far: (A) deficiency of succinyl-CoA:3-ketoacid CoA-transferase (11) and (B) deficiency of acetoacetyl-CoA thiolase (12).

Defect A can be suspected in children who have a permanent ketonemia in the nonfasting as well as in the fasting state. Postprandial plasma 3-hydroxybutyrate levels of 0.7–0.9 mmol/liter have been reported. Affected patients suffer from attacks of ketoacidosis without hypoglycemia. Defect B is somewhat more difficult to understand. Both acetoacetyl-CoA and 2-methylacetoacetyl-CoA are substrates for the thiolase. It has been proposed that there are two forms of the enzyme: a hepatic form and an extrahepatic form. Only the extrahepatic form is necessary for ketone body utilization. Hence a deficiency of the extrahepatic isoenzyme alone would leave the catabolism of 2-methylacetoacetyl-CoA in the liver unaffected, and consequently, no abnormal organic aciduria is observed. Clinically, a severe hypoglycemic ketoacidosis following gastroenteritis in a 10-month-old girl was observed. Intermittent ketoacidosis is not an extremely rare condition in childhood, but a sound biochemical explanation is found in only a few cases. Therefore, additional methods of investigation have to be devised for the investigation of children who suffer from recurring attacks of ketoacidosis. It will not be sufficient to relate the degree of ketosis to the glucose levels, but accurate measurements of brain ketone body consumption will be needed.

Glutaric Acidemia Type I

One of the organic acidurias accompanied by the worst clinical symptomatology is the deficiency of glutaryl-CoA dehydrogenase. The usual clinical course starts with a sudden onset of dystonia following an infection between the age of 3 months and 3 years. Patients do not recover completely and may even deteriorate further after subsequent attacks. Dystonia and choreoathetosis are among the most striking features of the disease.

Now that almost 20 cases of glutaric aciduria have been described, the large variation of the clinical presentation becomes manifest. Within one family both an acute and a chronic clinical course may occur. Even healthy affected siblings may be encountered, which stresses the need for careful family investigations (13).

Urinary glutarate in the patients reported thus far ranged from 587 to 11,800 mmol/mol creatinine with two exceptions. These were patients in whom no free glutarate could be detected on several occasions, but who permanently excreted abnormal amounts of glutarylcarnitine. Although it seems attractive to correlate these variations of metabolite excretion with those of residual enzyme activity, this did not appear to be true.

We have diagnosed three siblings with glutaryl-CoA dehydrogenase deficiency, of whom only one showed the classical clinical picture. Even this affected girl produced abnormal amounts of free glutarate exclusively during infections. During quiet periods all three siblings excreted abnormal quantities of conjugated glutarate, which was tentatively identified as glutarylcarnitine. Therefore it is advisable to analyze all patients suspected of having glutaric aciduria type I for conjugated glutarate. Another characteristic metabolite of this condition could be 3-hydroxyglutarate, a compound that is difficult to separate from the rather common 2-hydroxyglutarate, however.

Glutaric acidemia type I is theoretically accessible to dietary treatment by decreasing the intake of lysine and tryptophan. Thus far no real success has been achieved by this approach, however. Carnitine treatment is needed at least by a number of patients.

4-Hydroxybutyric Aciduria

There are data which suggest that 4-OH-butyric acid acts as a neurotransmitter. Accordingly, patients who accumulate this acid are likely to have neurological impairment. Several of the 10 or so patients diagnosed so far had a marked ataxia, hypotonia, and mental retardation. Milder variants (e.g., with speech retardation as the only clinical symptom) are now coming to light. Biochemically, all patients are diagnosed by the finding of large amounts of 4-OH-butyrate and its lactone in urine (e.g., 350 mmol/mol creatinine) and moderately increased levels of this compounds in plasma and CSF (levels in CSF always predominating over those in plasma). The activity of succinic semialdehyde dehydrogenase was deficient in lymphocyte extracts (14). Succinic semialdehyde itself was detected in trace amounts in the urine of several patients. Experimental treatment with a GABA analog has recently been proposed.

D-Glyceric Acidemia

This very rare organic acidemia has been described in only five patients. A delayed psychomotor development and neurological abnormalities were common clinical characteristics of the patients. The urinary excretion of glyceric acid was fairly high, but there was a large variation from 0.5 to 116 mmol/liter. It is important to realize that glycerate has a very bad extraction recovery with organic solvents; hence quantitative measurements have to be performed with care.

Oral loading tests with fructose (1 g/kg), dihydroxyacetone (1 g/kg), or L-serine (200 mg/kg) have been useful in provoking exaggerated glycerate excretions. D- and L-glycerate are easily separated by capillary gas-liquid chromatography of their O-acetylated (−)-methyl esters (15). It is not certain whether all patients had the same enzyme defect: only very recently a deficiency of D-glycerate kinase could be established in one of the patients (16). The human liver enzyme appeared to be very unstable and could only be assayed when the tissue had been homogenized in a special medium containing inorganic phosphate, EGTA, and glycerate. Theoretically, a deficiency of triokinase is also possible, especially in patients who do not respond to serine loading. Apparently, more studies in this area are needed.

Defect of 2-Oxobutyrate metabolism

A brother and a sister with symptoms of cyclic vomiting and ketoacidosis without hypoglycemia were found to have elevated levels of 2-OH-butyrate and 2-aminobutyrate in plasma and urine. The concentrations of both substances increased upon methionine loading, with a concomitant rise of urinary sulfur excretion. A defect of 2-oxobutyrate metabolism (dehydrogenation?) was postulated (17).

N-Acetylaspartic Aciduria

Canavan disease is a form of autosomal recessively inherited leukodystrophy with associated megalencephaly, blindness, and spasticity. The neurological findings usually appear in the first few months of life. Recently, it was shown that some cases of Canavan disease can be attributed to aspartoacylase deficiency.

This enzyme cleaves the acetyl group, yielding free aspartic acid. Affected patients excrete 800–3600 mmol/mol creatinine of N-acetylaspartate in their urine (controls <20). Cultured fibroblasts are well suited as starting material for the enzyme assay (18). N-Acetylaspartate is present only in the brain; however, its function is still unknown 30 years after its discovery. The pathogenesis of the clinical symptoms of aspartoacylase deficiency remains to be elucidated. One would expect both an increased brain N-acetylaspartate level and a decreased aspartate level. None of these phenomena have been studied up to now.

Fumarylacetoacetase Deficiency

Hereditary tyrosinemia type I due to fumarylacetoacetase deficiency is a severe disorder leading to liver disease, eventually with hepatocellular carcinoma, and renal tubular abnormalities. Both an acute and a chronic form occur. Treatment with a low-tyrosine diet does not give successful long-term results, and hence liver transplantation appears to be the ultimate form of treatment.

To make a correct diagnosis, a very careful analytical approach has to be chosen. Most patients are identified by finding an increased urinary excretion of succinylacetone, the key metabolite that is formed by reduction and decarboxylation of the primary accumulating product fumarylacetoacetate. As succinylacetone has been reported to be somewhat unstable, it is preferable to take a fresh urine sample. Furthermore, the usual ethoxime formation does not function very well for this substance: treatment with hydroxylamine will result in a stable derivative with a ring structure. Urinary excretion levels of succinylacetone may vary considerably: values from less than 1 μmol/liter to more than 500 μmol/liter for untreated patients were observed in our laboratory. In this respect it is helpful to analyze the urinary excretion of δ-aminolevulinic acid. This amino acid cannot react to form porphobilinogen due to the inhibition by succinylacetone of the corresponding enzyme. As shown in Fig. 2, the excretion of δ-aminolevulinic acid could be a more sensitive, albeit possibly less specific, parameter of tyrosinemia type I. Finally, one should be fairly liberal in assaying fumarylacetoacetase in cells of suspected patients.

One of the major problems of follow-up studies of tyrosinemia is the prediction of the moment at which hepatocellular carcinoma will develop and the timing of the liver transplantation. To date no reliable biochemical parameter has been found. Even the practical value of serial α-fetoprotein determinations has to be discussed. For the time being imaging techniques remain the sole possibility to check the condition of the patient's liver.

CONJUGATION OF ORGANIC ACIDS

Conjugation is an effective means of detoxification of potentially hazardous substances, which may be of exogenous or endogenous origin. In view of their possible

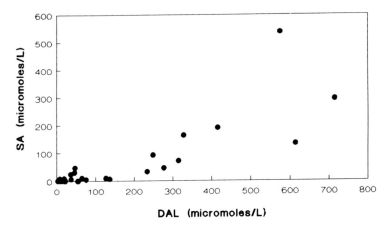

FIG. 2. Urinary excretion of succinylacetone versus that of δ-aminolevulinic acid in patients with fumarylacetoacetase deficiency. The concentration of the amino acid normalized only in those patients who were effectively treated (i.e., who had plasma tyrosine levels in the normal range).

neurotoxic action, short chain and medium chain organic acids are therefore readily conjugated. It was originally thought that only glycine conjugates were formed, as exemplified by isovalerylglycine in isovaleric acidemia, but more recent investigations have brought to light other conjugating substrates, such as carnitine and glucuronic acid. These observations have taught us many novel insights on secondary metabolic pathways (Table 2). All three conjugation reactions take place in different regions of the cell: glycine conjugation is an essentially mitochondrial process, the formation of carnitine esters is associated with the mitochondrial membrane, and glucuronidation takes place in the microsomal fraction. As virtually all catabolic

TABLE 2. *Conjugation mechanisms for short chain and medium chain organic acids in humans*

Substrate	Type of conjugate		
	Glycine ester	Glucuronide	Carnitine ester
Propionyl-CoA	+	−	+
Isovaleryl-CoA	+ +	(+)	+
3-CH₃-crotonyl-CoA	+ +	−	+
Tiglyl-CoA	+ +	−	+
Hexanoyl-CoA	+	−	+
Octanoyl-CoA	−	+	+
Valproyl-CoA	−	+ +	+
Benzoyl-CoA	+ +	+	?
Salicyloyl-CoA	+ +	+	?
7-OH-octanoyl-CoA	−	+	−
Glutaryl-CoA	−	−	+
Suberyl-CoA	+	+	−

TABLE 3. *Urinary carnitine excretion in various types of organic acidemia*[a]

Disorder	Free carnitine	Acylcarnitine	Acyl/free
Methylmalonic acidemia	32	415	13.0
Propionic acidemia	27	267	9.9
3-Ketothiolase deficiency	12	285	23.7
3-Methylcrotonylglycinuria	10	254	25.4
Isovaleric acidemia	14	240	17.1
3-Methylglutaconic aciduria I	67	219	3.3
3-OH-3-Methylglutaric aciduria	28	261	9.3
Glutaric aciduria I	19	346	18.2
Mevalonic aciduria	242	505	2.1
4-OH-butyric aciduria	251	229	0.9
Controls (20)	7–128	24–127	0.7–3.4

[a] Concentrations expressed in µmol/g creatinine.

pathways of short chain acyl-CoAs are located inside the mitochondrion, it is logical to assume that accumulating acyl-CoAs primarily react with glycine to restore the intramitochondrial CoA homeostasis. A beautiful example is given by patients with isovaleric acidemia, who start to excrete isovalerylglucuronide during attacks of metabolic decompensation only when their glycine N-acylating capacity is apparently surpassed (19).

Based on the theory of mass action, one should be able to change the pattern of conjugation by adding large amounts of a different substrate. We have achieved this by giving oral carnitine (100 mg/kg·day) to a clinically well patient with isovaleric acidemia. Subsequently, the ratio of glycine to carnitine ester in her urine changed from 96:4 to 80:20. Carnitine treatment is considered worthwhile to try only in those cases where glycine conjugation is not very effective, and secondary carnitine deficiency is thus a real threat. It can be seen from Table 3 that especially patients with propionic acidemia and glutaric acidemia type I are candidates for carnitine supplementation.

Virtually all short chain and medium chain acyl-CoAs are able to form carnitine esters by reactions catalyzed by carnitine acetyltransferase or carnitine octanoyltransferase. Apparently, there are no large differences in affinity for the various acyl-CoAs as were observed toward glycine N-acylase (20).

Formation of glucuronides has been described for a few substrates only so far. In our opinion this extramitochondrial process becomes operative only when large amounts of short chain fatty acids escape from the mitochondria. The finding of glucuronides must therefore mean that the patient is in a particularly bad condition.

REFERENCES

1. Chalmers RA, Lawson AM. *Organic acids in man.* New York: Chapman & Hall, 1982;1–523.
2. Jeneson JAL, Luyten PR, Meiners LC, Barth PG, Van Sprang FJ, Duran M. *In vivo* ¹H MRS in the

study of basal ganglia pathology associated with inborn errors of metabolism: potential for clinical use. *Proceedings of the 8th Meeting of the Society for Magnetic Resonance in Medicine*, 1989.

3. Gibson KM, Nyhan WL, Sweetman L, et al. 2-Methylgutaconic aciduria: a phenotype in which activity of 3-methylglutaconyl-coenzyme A hydratase is normal. *Eur J Pediatr* 1988;148:76–82.
4. De Klerk JBC, Duran M, Dorland L, Brouwers HAA, Bruinvis L, Ketting D. A patient with mevalonic aciduria presenting with hepatosplenomegaly, congenital anemia, thrombocytopenia, and leucocytosis. *J Inher Metab Dis* 1988;11(suppl 2):233–6.
5. Gray RGF, Pollitt RJ, Webley J. Methylmalonic semialdehyde dehydrogenase deficiency: demonstration of defective valine and β-alanine metabolism and reduced malonic semialdehyde dehydrogenase activity in cultured fibroblasts. *Biochem Med Metab Biol* 1987;38:121–4.
6. Asano K, Miyamoto I, Matsushita T, et al. Succinic acidemia: a new syndrome of organic acidemia associated with congenital lactic acidosis and decreased NADH-cytochrome c reductase activity. *Clin Chim Acta* 1988;173:305–12.
7. Zinn AB, Kerr DS, Hoppel CL. Fumarase deficiency: a new cause of mitochondrial encephalomyopathy. *N Engl J Med* 1986;315:469–75.
8. Brown GK, Scholem RD, Bankier A, Danks DM. Malonyl coenzyme A decarboxylase deficiency. *J Inher Metab Dis* 1984;7:21–6.
9. Dremsek PA, Sacher M, Stogmann W, Gitzelmann R, Bachmann C. Fructose-1,6-diphosphatase deficiency: glycerol excretion during fasting test. *Eur J Pediatr* 1985;144:203–4.
10. Krywawych S, Katz C, Lawson AM, Wyatt S, Brenton DP. Glycerol-3-phosphate excretion in fructose-1,6-diphosphatase deficiency. *J Inherited Metab Dis* 1986;9:388–92.
11. Middleton B, Day R, Lombes A, Saudubray JM. Infantile ketoacidosis associated with decreased activity of succinyl-CoA: 3-ketoacid CoA-transferase. *J Inher Metab Dis* 1987;10(suppl 2):273–5.
12. Leonard JV, Middleton B, Seakins JWT. Acetoacetyl CoA thiolase deficiency presenting as ketotic hypoglycemia. *Pediatr Res* 1987;21:211–3.
13. Amir N, Elpeleg O, Shalev RS, Christensen E. Glutaric aciduria type I: clinical heterogeneity and neuroradiological features. *Neurology* 1987;37:1654–7.
14. Gibson KM, Sweetman L, Nyhan WL, Lenoir G, Divry P. Defective succinic semialdehyde dehydrogenase activity in 4-hydroxybutyric aciduria. *Eur J Pediatr* 1984;142:257–9.
15. Duran M, Beemer FA, Bruinvis L, Ketting D, Wadman SK. D-Glyceric acidemia, an inborn error associated with fructose metabolism. *Pediatr Res* 1987;21:502–6.
16. Van Schaftingen E. D-Glycerate kinase deficiency as a cause of D-glyceric aciduria. *FEBS Lett* 1989; 243:127–31.
17. Yang W, Roth KS. Defect in alpha-ketobutyrate metabolism a new inborn error. *Clin Chim Acta* 1985; 145:173–82.
18. Matalon R, Michals K, Sebesta D, et al. Aspartoacylase deficiency and N-acetylaspartic aciduria in patients with Canavan disease. *Am J Med Genet* 1988;29:463–71.
19. Dorland L, Duran M, Wadman SK, et al. Isovalerylglucuronide, a new urinary metabolite in isovaleric acidemia. Identification problems due to rearrangement reactions. *Clin Chim Acta* 1983;134:77–83.
20. Kolvraa S, Gregersen N. Acyl-CoA:glycine N-acyltransferase: organelle localization and affinity toward straight- and branched-chained acyl-CoA esters in rat liver. *Biochem Med Metab Biol* 1986;36:98–105.
21. Chalmers RA, Roe CR, Stacey TE, Hoppel CE. Urinary excretion of l-carnitine and acylcarnitines by patients with disorders of organic acid metabolism: evidence for secondary insufficiency of l-carnitine. *Pediatr Res* 1984;18:1325–8.

DISCUSSION

Dr. Van den Berghe: I wonder if the excretion of glycerol-3-phosphate that you observed could derive from an accumulation of this compound in the liver, combined with liver lesions. Although it is biochemical dogma that phosphorylated compounds do not as a rule cross cell membranes, isolated hepatocytes have been shown to release such metabolites, including glycerol-3-phosphate (1). I should therefore like to ask you if you looked for the accumulation of glycerol-3-phosphate in the liver of your patients, and also in other conditions in which glycerol-3-phosphate may accumulate, such as hereditary fructose intolerance and following alcohol intake. Is there also an increase in the excretion of glycerol-3-phosphate during a fructose tolerance test?

Dr. Duran: We have not checked the presence of glycerol phosphate in the liver cell. I think one of the things to do would be to look at animal or human liver using *in vivo* NMR spectroscopy. We have not investigated the production of glycerol phosphate after fructose loading because we don't like to give a lot of fructose to fructose-1,6-diphosphatase-deficient patients. Finally, we have not looked at alcoholic cirrhosis.

Dr. Van den Berghe: Did you also look for excretion of glycerol-3-phosphate in children with chronic liver disease such as biliary atresia?

Dr. Duran: The only case is a patient with tyrosinemia type 1, who developed severe hypoglycemia and then started to excrete glycerol phosphate. We do not know if this was secondary to liver dysfunction or if it was due to inhibition of fructose-1,6-diphosphatase.

Dr. Krywawych: I assume that glycerol-1-phosphate does not cross the cell wall. In the patient with fructose-1,6-diphosphatase deficiency in whom we found a glycerol-1-phosphate in the urine we suspected that this compound was coming from the renal tissue as a result of renal damage. In fructose-1,6-diphosphatase deficiency there is renal involvement, and also glycerol-1-phosphate can accumulate in the kidney in this disease as it is a gluconeogenic organ. We did not perform fructose loading tests but made several measurements in this patient both during hypoglycemia and normoglycemia. The largest excretion of glycerol-1-phosphate occurred during periods of hypoglycemia.

Dr. Saudubray: I remember a very old paper from Senior, trying to explain why in glucose-6-phosphatase deficiency there is hypoketonemia. I remember he gave a hypothesis connected with glycerol phosphate accumulation in glucose-6-phosphatase deficiency. I don't agree when you state that in fructose-diphosphatase deficiency there is a ketoacidotic state. Acidosis occurs, it is true, but ketosis—not really. In many patients affected with fructose-diphosphatase deficiency there is a problem of differential diagnosis with fatty acid oxidation defects. Two patients affected with fructose-diphosphatase deficiency were referred to our unit with a possible diagnosis of fatty acid oxidation defect, because of low plasma ketone levels.

Dr. Duran: One of our patients with fructose-1,6-diphosphatase deficiency had a plasma 3-hydroxybutyrate concentration of 6 mmol/liter, together with a blood glucose of 1.5 mmol/liter. This certainly is not hypoketotic.

Dr. Saudubray: I agree, but it depends largely on the conditions of measurement. When we measured blood ketones in six patients affected with fructose-diphosphatase deficiency, using a fasting test performed when the patients were in good nutritional condition, we found that blood ketones were not very raised even when blood glucose levels were lowered. Of course, there was some accumulation but not very high compared to what we find in glycogenesis type 3, for example.

Dr. Duran: I think it is a good hypothesis to test if there is any effect of glycerol phosphate on ketogenesis.

Dr. Hobbs: You have described two serious clinical conditions that might justifiably be treated by bone marrow transplant. In glutaryl-CoA dehydrogenase deficiency you mention that the defect occurs also in the leukocytes. You could therefore devise an *in vitro* test to see if normal leukocytes would correct defective fibroblasts or another tissue grown from the patient. The other is the type 2 methylglutaconic acidemia, where the exact defect is not known. Nevertheless, it would again be possible to test *in vitro* the addition of normal leukocytes, to see if they could correct defective cells from a patient. If in either of these situations, normal leukocytes could compensate, then following a bone marrow transplantation you would have the provision of a detoxification system for that patient.

Dr. Wanders: In the first disease you treated, 3-methylglutaconic aciduria, in those patients in which the hydratase is normal, you mentioned the possibility that methylglutaconic acid comes from the other side, and you suggested some of the intermediates involved in cholesterol biosynthesis. Has cholesterol synthesis in these patients been tested? And is it normal or abnormal?

Dr. Duran: As far as I know they have normal cholesterol levels in their body fluids. Synthesis starting from precursors such as 3-hydroxy-3-methylglutaric acid has not been tested.

Dr. Saudubray: We have observed a patient with 3-methylglutaconic aciduria presenting with a very severe neurological dysfunction with myopathy. In addition to 3-methylglutaconic aciduria he had severe lactic acidosis. On muscle biopsy there was a generalized defect of the respiratory chain complex. Since you mentioned this very interesting finding of 3-methylglutaconic accumulation in mothers of microcephalic children, maybe it would be interesting to check systematically for respiratory chain disorders in these children. Have you done it?

Dr. Duran: It was checked as far as I know in only one patient, the patient from Münich. Dr. Endres could perhaps give the details.

Dr. Endres: The enzymes of the respiratory chain were normal. But this patient had a severe cardiomyopathy and died at the age of 5 months, after having already had a life-threatening event in the neonatal period. I think patients with type 2 3-methylglutaconic aciduria are so severely ill that leukocyte infusions would fail to be of any help.

Dr. Saudubray: I am not sure that your explanation of the possible teratogenic role of 3-methylglutaconic is true, because it is evident that in your two forms of the disease, one was due to hydratase deficiency and the other was not. In your first patients, the ones with hydratase deficiency, there was a very high level of 3-methylglutaconic, and these patients were not very sick. They presented with ketoacidosis but not with severe mental retardation, whereas the others were very severely retarded.

Dr. Van Hoof: Coming back to the family you report with one child excreting glutaric acid in urine while his two other sibs had low glutaryl-CoA dehydrogenase in blood cells, I presume that the activity of control enzymes has been measured in leukocytes and I suggest that the enzyme should also be assayed on cultured fibroblasts in Dr. Christensen's laboratory.

Dr. Duran: That has been done. Dr. Christensen has confirmed the diagnosis glutaryl-CoA dehydrogenase deficiency in the patient's fibroblasts.

Dr. Van Hoof: Have they performed a loading test of the fibroblasts with glutaric acid?

Dr. Duran: The dehydrogenase has been assayed using the labeled substrate, and it is deficient. This was done in fibroblast homogenates; we did not perform whole cell oxidation studies, as this is not usual in glutaric aciduria type I.

Dr. Van Hoof: It is always wise to look for substrate accumulation in living cells when an enzyme deficiency has been demonstrated *in vivo*.

Dr. Duran: Maybe I did not made myself clear enough, but all three members of this family excreted abnormal amounts of conjugated glutarate at one time or another. So the free glutarate was often very low, but the conjugated glutarate was increased in all three patients.

Dr. Van Hoof: And none of them was excreting large amounts of glutaconic acid?

Dr. Duran: We have not been able to find large amounts of glutaconic acid in other patients with glutaric acidemia type I. Also if you screen the literature on glutaric aciduria carefully, you will not find many reports dealing with increased glutaconic acid excretion.

Dr. Mowat: Could I come to fumarylacetoacetase deficiency? I understand that some Scandinavian workers found deficiency of this enzyme in normal individuals. I wonder if you could comment on that.

Dr. Duran: That is a pseudodeficiency that represents a genetic variant occurring in apparently healthy individuals. This genetic variant has important implications for the use of fumarylacetoacetase analysis in the diagnosis of tyrosinemia.

Dr. Saudubray: Do you have any idea why in some patients with tyrosinemia type 1, succinylacetone excretion is so low, contrasting with a complete absence of fumarylacetoacetase?

Dr. Duran: There has been a hypothesis for a few years that the accumulating toxic metabolites inhibit the 4-hydroxyphenyllactate dioxygenase to such an extent that no metabolite gets through to fumarylacetoacetase anymore. I don't know if this is a true hypothesis.

Dr. Jaeken: Regarding the detection of hepatoma in tyrosinemia, magnetic resonance imaging (MRI) seems to be a sensitive test. Do you have experience with this?

Dr. Duran: We have had one MR image in one of our tyrosinemia patients, but it is really difficult to follow these cases by MRI because all our patients are below the age of 3 years. You have to give them anesthesia and it is not very nice to give that every 2 or 3 months. We try to do it by ultrasound.

Dr. Sokal: As a pediatrician involved in liver transplantation, I don't see why you should delay liver transplantation in a child once you have diagnosed tyrosinemia. There is no point in waiting for transplantation and this is true for all life-threatening metabolic disorders.

Dr. Duran: No, there is no point in waiting. But, at least in our country, donor organs are so scarce that it is almost impossible to get the patients on the list for transplantation.

Dr. Hobbs: I would like to support Dr. Sokal. I think it is a mistake to wait. What we would like from you experts in genetic disease and involved with the DNA probes are tests to identify which patients are going to get the serious disease. They could then be transplanted before they suffer irreversible damage. I think that in one of the families you described there was one child of 3 years who had not yet been affected. These are the children we should be transplanting, not the ones who have progressed to end-stage disease.

Dr. Leroy: I wonder whether anyone can tell if the hepatoma in tyrosinemia patients is different from hepatoma in other conditions. Is it in any way specific? It looks as if we may be confronted by a condition here where either the liver cell is intoxicated, with the suppression of a tumor suppressor gene as a consequence, or the inborn error serves as a selecting mechanism favoring those cells in which some proto-oncogene or oncogene has become amplified. If this type of hepatoma is pathologically very similar to any other hepatoma, one can surmise that a less specific mechanism must have caused it. Maybe we missed the chance here to see some specific regulatory gene disturbances due to specific metabolic disorders of tyrosine and its derivatives.

Dr. Duran: I have no information on this.

REFERENCE

1. Van Schaftingen E, Hue L, Hers HG, et al. Extracellular metabolites in suspensions of isolated hepatocytes. *Biochem J* 1987;248:517–21.

Inborn Errors of Metabolism, edited by
J. Schaub, F. Van Hoof, and H. L. Vis.
Nestlé Nutrition Workshop Series, Vol. 24.
Nestec Ltd., Vevey/Raven Press, Ltd.,
New York © 1991.

Inborn Errors of the Urea Cycle and Other Hyperammonemias

Jean-Louis Dhondt and *Jean-Pierre Farriaux

*Laboratoire de Biochimie, Faculté Libre de Médecine, 59462, Lomme Cédex, France;
and *Service de Génétique et Maladies Héréditaires du Métabolisme, Hôpital C.
Huriez, 59037 Lille, Cédex, France*

Descriptions and studies of inborn errors of urea metabolism (Fig. 1) have greatly contributed to the knowledge of the regulation and gene expression of the enzymes involved in the urea cycle (1). Recent progress in this field has included new therapeutic approaches, a better knowledge of the mechanism of post-translational process of mitochondrial enzyme proteins, and DNA cloning of genes. For most of urea cycle enzymes, the gene for the protein has been cloned and characterized, opening up the possibility of analysis of the molecular basis for defects and new approaches to the diagnosis by DNA analysis.

However, from a medical point of view, hyperammonemia requires a rapid diagnosis workup, which is essential for instituting an adequate therapy (2). The aim of this chapter is to review recent data on the diagnosis and treatment of hyperammonemia.

CIRCUMSTANCES OF DIAGNOSIS

In urea cycle defects the signs usually appear between 2 and 4 days of age. It is likely that the rapid fatal outcome in undiagnosed patients underestimates the real incidence of urea cycle enzymopathies. Besides the classical forms with rapid onset and severe metabolic disorder, there is a wide variation in both the time of presentation and the symptoms, which may initially suggest a neurological, behavioral, or gastroenterological problem. In such cases recognition of the early symptoms of the disease is often delayed. Consequently, a family history of children dying of a metabolic disorder in the newborn period, or any history of recent alteration in diet or of unusual food avoidance, should reinforce the search for a urea cycle defect.

DIAGNOSTIC WORK-UP

Symptomatic hyperammonemia is a medical emergency demanding early recognition, specific diagnosis, and aggressive therapy. The first symptoms are feeding

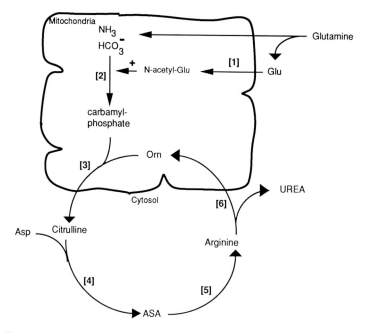

FIG. 1. The urea cycle and its defects. CPS activity deficiency can result from a lack of the carbamylphosphate synthetase I apoenzyme (EC 6.3.4.16) (*2*) or, more rarely, a deficiency in *N*-acetylglutamate synthetase (*1*). Ornithine transcarbamylase (OTC) deficiency (EC 2.1.3.3) (*3*) is the most frequent of inborn errors of urea cycle and is an X-linked disease. Citrullinemia is characterized by deficient argininosuccinate synthetase (ASS) (EC 6.3.4.5) (*4*) Argininosuccinate lyase (ASL) (EC 4.3.2.1) (*5*) deficiency is the second most common of the urea cycle disorders. Hyperargininemia is characterized by a hereditary deficiency of arginase (EC 3.5.3.1) (*6*).

difficulties, hypotonia, vomiting, lethargy, grunting respiration, and seizures; this progresses rapidly to coma and early death. The clinical presentation is associated with plasma ammoniun levels in the range of 500–2,000 μmol/liter (normal <35). A small number of routine laboratory tests can then be used to establish the diagnosis (Table 1) by excluding other metabolic situations that can be associated with hyperammonemia (Fig. 2).

Upon the discovery of symptomatic hyperammonemia, immediate therapeutic measures should be taken. Peritoneal dialysis (or hemodialysis) should be started to remove accumulated nitrogen rapidly, and sufficient energy (above 120 cal/kg·day) should be supplied to suppress endogenous proteolysis. In the meantime, the measurement of plasma amino acids and urinary orotate should differentiate the various possibilities (Fig. 2).

Once a provisional diagnosis of urea cycle enzymopathy has been made (apart from hyperargininemia), intravenous arginine supplementation (4 mmol/kg·day) and sodium benzoate (250 mg/kg·day) should be started. Final diagnosis is obtained from enzymatic investigations (Table 2).

TABLE 1. *Routine tests for the diagnostic approach to hyperammonemia*

Blood	Urine
Ammonia	pH
Glucose	Ketone bodies
Acid-base (anion gap)	DNPH test
Ketone bodies	
Lactate	(aliquot at −20°C)
Amino acids	Orotic acid

Differential Diagnosis

The prominent biochemical abnormality in urea cycle disorders is the hyperammonemia; however, many situations can be associated with hyperammonemia (Fig. 2). The identification of the underlying cause influences the prognosis for recovery and recurrence of symptoms.

1. Transient Neonatal Hyperammonemia

Batshaw *et al.* (4) reported that plasma ammonium levels are elevated in more than 50% of premature infants. Levels are approximately twice those noted in term

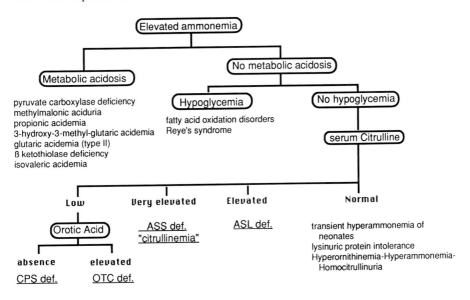

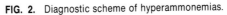

FIG. 2. Diagnostic scheme of hyperammonemias.

TABLE 2. *Tissues in which urea cycle enzymes are measurable for the diagnosis of urea cycle disorders*

	CPS	OTC	ASS	ASL	Arginase
Diagnosis	Liver	Liver, intestinal mucosa	Liver, fibroblasts	Liver, fibroblasts, erythrocytes, leucocytes	Liver, erythrocytes, leucocytes
Antenatal diagnosis	Fetal liver, chorionic villi	Fetal liver, chorionic villi (?) (RFLP[a])	Amniotic cells, chorionic villi	Amniotic cells, chorionic villi	? (Never performed)

[a] Restriction fragment length polymorphism.

infants and high levels persist for 4–8 weeks. Although they are not associated with clinical symptoms or with long-term neurologic deficits, an arginine supplementation is recommended (4,5). However, on some occasions symptomatic hyperammonemia is observed and requires aggressive therapy (6) since neurologic symptoms correlate well with levels of ammonia. There is marked central nervous system depression and most of these infants require ventilatory assistance. No specific biochemical alterations other than the hyperammonemia are noted; the plasma amino acid chromatogram is normal, and activities of urea cycle enzymes in liver are unmodified (6). The etiology of this syndrome is unknown, but it is generally attributed to a developmental delay in regulation of one of the enzymes required for urea synthesis or to a nonadaptation to nitrogen load (7). Mild hyperammonemia may also be seen during parenteral alimentation in premature infants; but differential diagnosis from "transient hyperammonemia" in sick preterm infants is not certain.

2. Hyperammonemia and Organic Aciduria

Hyperammonemia has been reported in several disorders of branched-chain amino acid metabolism, in pyruvate carboxylase deficiency (8), and in the most severe form of pyruvate dehydrogenase deficiency (9). A significant correlation between ammonia concentration and organic acid accumulation is observed (10). The secondary inhibition of ureagenesis in organic aciduria appears to be due to a functional deficiency of carbamylphosphate synthetase activity (11).

3. Reye Syndrome

Reye syndrome is probably the best situation mimicking inborn errors of the urea cycle (12); this explains the controversial reports about its pathogenesis in late 1970s. Nowadays, this syndrome should be considered a diagnosis of exclusion. Reye syndrome is generally seen in otherwise healthy children older than 2 years of age, but many cases have been reported in early infancy (13). A history of viral illness (e.g., chickenpox) and exposure to salicylates approximately 2 weeks before presentation is often found.

4. Iatrogenic Hyperammonemia

It has been stated that 20% of epileptic children treated with valproic acid can develop hyperammonemia (>60 μmol/liter) (14). In rats (15), valproic acid produces a marked reduction in hepatic CPS I activity; an inhibition of the N-acetylglutamate synthesis was also hypothesized (16). However, Morgan *et al.* (17) recommended that urea cycle defects should be sought in the diagnosis of patients with seizures and mental retardation of undetermined etiology who develop hyperammonemia after valproic acid treatment.

A syndrome of idiopathic hyperammonemia has also been described in patients who have received high-dose chemotherapy for the treatment of hematologic malignancies. It is characterized by abrupt alteration in mental status and respiratory alkalosis associated with markedly elevated ammonium levels in the absence of any identifiable cause, and frequently results in coma and death (18).

5. Dibasic Aminoaciduria

The impaired ammonia metabolism (postprandial hyperammonemia) in lysinuric protein intolerance is attributed to low plasma arginine and ornithine levels (19). Hyperornithinemia, hyperammonemia, and homocitrullinuria syndrome (HHH) is presumably due to an impairment of the transport of citrulline across the inner mitochondrial membrane.

LONG-TERM TREATMENT

It is not clear how close to normal the levels of ammonium and other metabolites must be kept to prevent mental retardation and acute episodes. The most important point is the rapidity with which infants develop symptomatic hyperammonemia at times of infection, stress, or excessive protein intake.

The morbidity remains high, presumably due to the degree of brain damage correlated with duration of neonatal hyperammonemic coma (20). Msall *et al.* (21) pointed out that even prospective treatment may not prevent cognitive impairment and suggested that asymptomatic hyperammonemia may have subtle effects on intellect. This point is illustrated by the spectrum of manifestations among female OTC heterozygotes, ranging from asymptomatic illness to recurrent episodes of coma and death, as predicted by Lyon's hypothesis (random inactivation of the X chromosomes). More frequent than initially believed are the manifestations of protein intolerance, including recurrent migraine headaches, cyclical vomiting episodes, ir-

TABLE 3. *Long-term therapy of urea cycle disorders*

	CPS/OTC	ASS	ASL	Arginase
Natural protein (g/kg·day)	0.7 (0.5–0.8)	0.7 (0.8–1.0)	1.5	Arginine-restricted diet
Essential amino acids (g/kg·day)	0.7	0.7		
Arginine (mmol/kg·day)	1.0	3–4	3–4	
Sodium benzoate (mg/kg·day)	250	250		+

ritability, ataxia, and seizures (22). Even in asymptomatic carriers, intellectual deficits have been noticed, perhaps a result of unrecognized episodic hyperammonemia (23).

The therapeutic measures include the following (Table 3 and Fig. 3):

1. *Protein restriction combined with supplements of essential amino acids (EAA) or their nitrogen-free analogues.* The need for EAA supplementation is self-evident. In addition, arginine becomes an EAA for infants with inborn errors of ureogenesis (apart from arginase deficiency). For patients with deficiencies of argininosuccinate synthetase and argininosuccinate lyase deficiency, dietary arginine supplementation promotes the synthesis of citrulline and argininosuccinate which, respectively, serve as waste nitrogen products (24). However, long-term effects of arginine therapy on chronic stimulation of growth hormone and insulin have not been evaluated. In patients with partial forms, the requirement for substrate may have a different mechanism. Wendel *et al.* (25) have recently observed a better metabolic control in a patient with a partial defect of OTC by supplying arginine in order to increase the mitochondrial ornithine to achieve critical substrate concentration for the kinetically abnormal OTC.

The keto analogs of amino acids offer at least two potential advantages. First EAA can be supplied without giving nitrogen. Second, since ketoacids are transaminated and ultimately incorporated into protein, nitrogen will be used.

2. *Stimulation of alternative pathway of waste nitrogen excretion has been extensively investigated.* This approach usually employs sodium benzoate to acylate glycine forming hippurate and sodium phenylacetate to acetylate glutamine forming phenylacetylglutamine, both of which are readily excreted in the urine (26). At a dose of 250 mg benzoate/kd·day, glycine availability seems not to be limiting for the synthesis of hippurate (27). A note of caution was raised since it has been shown in animals that benzoate potentiates ammonia toxicity. Acute benzoate toxicity can occur inadvertently, leading to irritability and vomiting mimicking hyperammonemia. At therapeutic dose, the paradoxical effect of benzoate is counterbalanced by a significant increase in waste nitrogen excretion. Nevertheless, periodical measurement of benzoate levels in plasma seems highly recommended.

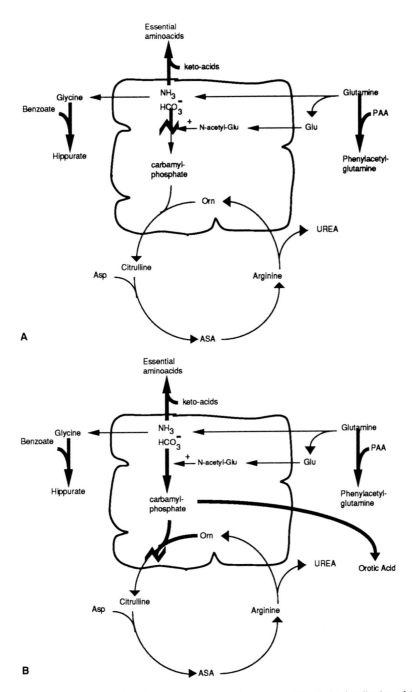

FIG. 3. Metabolic ways used to limit nitrogen accumulation according to the localization of the enzyme defect. **A:** CPS and *N*-acetylglutamate synthetase deficiency; **B:** OTC deficiency; **C:** argininosuccinate synthetase deficiency; **D:** arginosuccinate lyase deficiency. *PAA,* phenylacetic acid; *GFR,* glomerular filtration rate; *OA,* oxaloacetate; +, enzymatic activation.

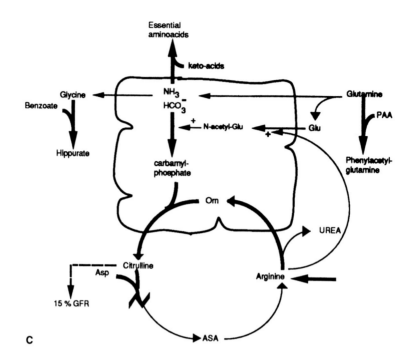

C

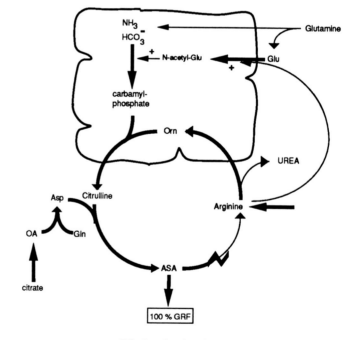

D

FIG. 3. *Continued.*

In *N*-acetylglutamate synthetase deficiency and partial CPS deficiency, administration of carbamylglutamate has been suggested (28). Because of its structural analogy with *N*-acetylglutamate, the physiologic allosteric activator of CPS, and its easy entry in mitochondria, carbamylglutamate may substitute for the decreased or nonexistent *N*-acetylglutamate in the first case, while in the second, stimulation of the remaining CPS may increase the rate of urea synthesis.

In argininosuccinate lyase deficiency, argininosuccinic acid, the substrate of the defective enzyme, is ideally suited as a waste nitrogen product. It contains the two nitrogen atoms destined for excretion as urea and has a renal clearance equal to glomerular filtration rate. Argininosuccinic acid is not toxic (29) and is dependent on the provision of adequate arginine and citrulline carbon skeletons. An arginine supplement of 3–4 mmol/kg·day is sufficient to meet these needs. With arginine supplementation, a high protein intake is expected to be well tolerated (30) and avoids the deleterious effects of severe protein restriction (29). Citrate supplementation has also been used successfully to improve waste nitrogen excretion. Indeed, citrate is cleaved in the cytosol to oxaloacetate, which is transaminated to aspartate at the expense of glutamine. Aspartate is required as substrate with citrulline to form argininosuccinic acid. Aspartate becomes an "essential" substance in this disease.

Hyperargininemia represents a different situation since elevated levels of arginine or its metabolites [guanidino compounds (31)] are thought to lead to a progressive neurologic disorder characterized by epilepsy, pyramidal spasticity, and mental retardation, which gives the disease a particular clinical picture. Hyperammonemia may be absent, but intercurrent hyperammonemia can result in episodes of vomiting and lethargy. Therapy has been directed at reducing hyperammonemia and hyperargininemia by protein restriction or by an arginine-free diet. However, the addition of benzoate has also been suggested (32) to permit a more varied diet than is possible with an amino acid mixture alone.

3. *Protective effect of L-carnitine* has been evoked by several authors (33,34). Ohtani *et al.* (34) reported data suggesting that OTC-deficient patients had a secondary carnitine deficiency and O'Connor *et al.* reported that L-carnitine prevents the paradoxical effect of benzoate on ammonia toxicity (35). Oral administration of L-carnitine (50–100 mg/kg·day) was proposed.

Other Therapeutic Problems

A side effect of the dietary treatment is anorexia and food refusal, often observed in such patients, which may necessitate nasogastric or gastrostomy tube feeding. Generalized food aversion is often observed. Hyman *et al.* (36) have suggested that an increased serotonin turnover secondary to either hyperammonemia or high-carbohydrate low-protein diets can explain a serotonin-dependent appetite suppression.

The Future

Liver transplantation is the only available form of enzyme replacement therapy for patients with severe defects in the urea cycle. However, new problems may appear which may clarify some physiologic aspects of the urea cycle. For example, Tuchman (37) reported a case of CPS deficiency who underwent a successful liver transplantation. Interestingly, citrulline levels failed to increase, confirming that citrulline probably originates from the gut, the only organ other than the liver that has CPS and OTC activities. Consequently, citrulline supplementation was continued in this case.

In the future, gene therapy may become possible. Cloned genes can be transferred into cells. Transgenic mouse is a model for the study of tissue specificity of gene expression; OTC deficiency in mouse (*sfp-ash*) has been corrected by gene transfer (38).

CONCLUSION

Although screening methods have been developed using blood or urine specimens, the cost-benefit ratio of mass screening for urea cycle disorders is particularly unfavorable. "The patients with neonatal onset will become ill before routine screening is performed. On the other hand, the patients with late onset forms of urea cycle disorders may escape screening in the neonatal period" (39). Clinical information and simple routine laboratory tests, *including ammonia determination*, allow rapid orientation of the diagnosis to enable the patient to be managed correctly initially. Final diagnosis is a matter of more sophisticated investigation not immediately necessary for the institution of the treatment. In summary, the crucial point remains that the possibility of hyperammonemia should be considered at all.

Whatever the defect, variability in residual enzyme activity and clinical presentation (lethal neonatal or delayed onset form) points toward a variety of mutations in the enzyme molecule. Recent developments in molecular genetics will provide new tools for the diagnosis of these diseases. However, correct identification of the index case and the preservation of tissue for DNA extraction are prerequisites for optimal utilization of these new techniques.

REFERENCES

1. Farriaux JP. *Le cycle de l'urée et ses anomalies*. Pains: Doin Ed, 1978.
2. Dhondt JL, Farriaux JP. Diagnosis and management of the urea cycle enzymopathies. In: Benson PF, ed. *Screening and management of potentially treatable genetic metabolic disorders*. Lancaster UK: MTP Press, 1984;143–59.
3. Batshaw ML, Brusilow SW. Treatment of hyperammonemic coma caused by inborn errors of urea synthesis. *J Pediatr* 1980;97:893–900.
4. Batshaw ML, Wachtel RC, Cohen L, et al. Neurologic outcome in premature infants with transient asymptomatic hyperammonemia. *J Pediatr* 1986;108:271–5.
5. Nakamura S, Kondo Y, Ogata T, et al. Blood ammonium level in low birth weight infants in relation to arginine intake. *Acta Paediatr Jpn* 1988;30:692–5.
6. Ballard RA, Vinocur B, Reynolds JW, et al. Transient hyperammonemia of the preterm infant. *N Engl J Med* 1978;299:920–5.
7. Beddis IR, Hughes EA, Rosser E, Fenton JCB. Plasma ammonia levels in newborn infants admitted to an intensive care baby unit. *Arch Dis Child* 1980;55:516–20.

8. Coude FX, Ogier H, Marsac C, Munnich A, Charpentier C, Saudubray JM. Secondary citrullinemia with hyperammonemia in four neonatal cases of pyruvate carboxylase deficiency. *Pediatrics* 1981;68:914.
9. Brown GK, Scholem RD, Hunt SM, Harrison JR, Pollard AC. Hyperammonemia and lactic acidosis in a patient with pyruvate dehydrogenase deficiency. *J Inher Metab Dis* 1987;10:359–66.
10. Coude FX, Ogier H, Grimber G, et al. Correlation between blood ammonia concentration and organic acid accumulation in isovaleric and propionic acidemia. *Pediatrics* 1982;69:115–7.
11. Walser M, Stewart PM. Organic acidaemia and hyperammonemia: a review. *J Inher Metab Dis* 1981; 4:177–82.
12. Yokoi T, Honke K, Funabashi R, et al. Partial ornithine transcarbamylase deficiency simulating Reye syndrome. *J Pediatr* 1981;99:929–31.
13. Bellman MH, Ross EM, Miller DL. Reye's syndrome in children under three years old. *Arch Dis Child.* 1982;57:259–63.
14. Iinuma K, Hayasaka K, Narisawa K, Tada K, Hori K. Hyperamino-acidaemia and hyperammonemia in epileptic children treated with valproic acid. *Eur J Pediatr* 1988;148:267–9.
15. Marini AM, Zaret BS, Beckner RR. Hepatic and renal contributions to valproic-induced hyperammonemia. *Neurology* 1988;38:365–71.
16. Coude FX, Rabier D, Cathelineau L, Grimber G, Parvy P, Kamoun PP. A mechanism for valproate-induced hyperammonemia. *Pediatr Res* 1981;15:974–5.
17. Morgan HB, Swaiman KF, Johnson BD. Diagnosis of argininosuccinic aciduria after valproic acid-induced hyperammonemia. *Neurology* 1987;37:886–7.
18. Mitchell RB, Wagner JE, Karp JE, et al. Syndrome of idiopathic hyperammonemia after high-dose chemotherapy: review of nine cases. *Am J Med* 1988;85:662–9.
19. Coude FX, Ogier H, Charpentier C, et al. L'intolérance aux protéines avec lysinurie: une hyperammoniémie sévère par carence en L-arginine. *Arch Fr Pediatr* 1981;38:829–35.
20. Batshaw ML. The diagnosis of ornithine transcarbamylase deficiency. *J Pediatr Gastroenterol Nutr* 1985;4:4–6.
21. Msall M, Monahan PS, Chapanis N, Batshaw ML. Cognitive development in children with inborn errors of urea synthesis. *Acta Paediatr Jpn* 1988;30:435–41.
22. Batshaw ML, Msall M, Beaudet AL, Trojak J. Risk of serious illness in heterozygotes for ornithine transcarbamylase deficiency. *J Pediatr* 1986;108:236–41.
23. Batshaw ML, Roan Y, Jung AL, Rosenberg LA, Brusilow SW. Cerebral dysfunction in asymptomatic carriers of ornithine transcarbamylase deficiency. *N Engl J Med* 1980;302:482–5.
24. Brusilow SW. Arginine, an indispensable amino acid for patients with inborn errors of urea synthesis. *J Clin Invest* 1984;74:2144–8.
25. Wendel U, Wieland J, Bremer HJ, Bachmann C. Ornithine transcarbamylase deficiency in a male: strict correlation between metabolic control and plasma arginine concentration. *Eur J Pediatr* 1989;148:349–52.
26. Batshaw ML, Thomas GH, Brusilow SW. New approaches to the diagnosis and treatment of inborn errors of urea synthesis. *Pediatrics* 1981;68:290–7.
27. Barshop BA, Breuer J, Holm J, Leslie J, Nyhan WL. Excretion of hippuric acid during sodium benzoate therapy in patients with hyperglycinaemia or hyperammonemia. *J Inher Metab Dis* 1989;12:72–9.
28. O'Connor JE, Jorda A, Grisolia S. Acute and chronic effects of carbamyl glutamate on blood urea and ammonia. *Eur J Pediatr* 1985;143:196–7.
29. Farriaux JP, Dhondt JL, Formstecher P, et al. Etude anatomo-pathologique d'un cas néo-natal d'argininosuccinylurie. *Acta Neurol Belg* 1976;76:26–34.
30. Donn SM, Thoene JG. Prospective prevention of neonatal hyperammonemia in argininosuccinic aciduria by arginine therapy. *J Inher Metab Dis* 1985;8:18–20.
31. Marescau B, Qureshi IA, De Deyn P, et al. Guanidino compounds in plasma, urine and cerebrospinal fluid of hyperargininemic patients during therapy. *Clin Chim Acta* 1985;146:21–7.
32. Qureshi IA, Letarte J, Ouellet R, Batshaw ML, Brusilow Q. Treatment of hyperargininemia with sodium benzoate and arginine-restricted diet. *J Pediatr* 1984;104:473–6.
33. Costell M, Miguez MP, O'Connor JE, Grisolia S. Effect of hyperammonemia on the levels of carnitine in mice. *Neurology* 1987;37:804–8.
34. Ohtani Y, Ohyanagi K, Yamamoto S, Matsuda I. Secondary cartinine deficiency in hyperammonemic attacks of ornithine transcarbamylase deficiency. *J Pediatr* 1988;112:409–14.
35. O'Connor JE, Costell M, Grisolfa S. The potentiation of ammonia toxicity by sodium benzoate is prevented by L-carnitine. *Biochim Biophys Acta* 1987;145:817–24.
36. Hyman SL, Porter CA, Page TJ, et al. Behavior management of feeding disturbances in urea cycle and organic acid disorders. *J Pediatr* 1987;111:558–62.

37. Tuchman M. Persistent acitrullinemia after liver transplantation for carbamylphosphate synthetase deficiency. *N Engl J Med* 1989;320:1498–9.
38. Briand P, Cavard C, Grimber G, Kamoun P. Mouse enzyme deficiency corrected by gene transfer. *4th International Congress of Inborn Errors of Metabolism*, Sendai (Japan), 1987.
39. Saudubray JM, Ogier H, Charpentier C, et al. A programmed screening for hyperammonemias: strategy and results. In: Naruse H, Irie M. eds. *Neonatal screening*. Amsterdam: Excerpta Medica, 1983; 382–7.

DISCUSSION

Dr. Wang: We are concerned about detection of carriers and about prenatal diagnosis of urea cycle abnormalities, but we have some difficulties just using enzyme determination. What is your comment about this kind of determination? Can detection of carriers with enzyme determinations be useful for heterozygote detection or even for prenatal diagnosis?

Dr. Dhondt: Phenomenal advances in molecular biology have changed the way in which we obtain the diagnosis and, of course, the detection of carriers has also improved. About the detection of carriers for OTC deficiency, the main problem is to have the index case very well documented, because the DNA analysis looks for the polymorphism. Since all the mutations are probably different, it is not possible to search directly for the abnormal gene. Without documentation of the index case, DNA analysis is informative in only 10% of the carriers, except where other biochemical investigations are taken in account (i.e., protein loading test). Consequently, tissue samples have to be taken from any patients who die with a suspected metabolic disease, for eventual DNA analysis.

Dr. Endres: I would like to take the opportunity to advertise some enzymatic methods of my co-worker Dr. Shin. With these more sensitive methods it is possible to use blood cells and chorionic villi for the postnatal and prenatal diagnosis of urea cycle disorders (UCD) (1). Concerning postnatal diagnosis activities of the two mitochondrial enzymes, carbamylphosphate synthetase and ornithine transcarbamylase, are measurable in leukocytes. In contrast, the argininosuccinate synthetase activity is not detectable in blood cells but can be detected in cultured fibroblasts. The determination of the argininosuccinate lyase and arginase activity in red blood cells is an excellent method for diagnosing the respective homozygotes as well as the heterozygotes. Concerning prenatal diagnosis, application of these methods to chorionic villi demonstrated that they might be suitable for the antenatal detection of all five urea cycle disorders.

Dr. Hobbs: I have a question concerning the white cell and red cell content of the other two enzymes. Do you think there is sufficient content of enzyme to detoxify patients if we exchange transfuse their blood with normal white and red cells, which is very easy.

Dr. Endres: I am afraid that the enzyme content is not high enough for sufficient ammonia detoxication.

Dr. Hobbs: The red cell mass is enormous, and might detoxify the blood sufficiently to save the brain. The other question is: your colleagues in Paris have described cellular immune deficiency with orotic aciduria because of an associated defect in nucleic acid synthesis. Have you encountered this, and do you know the frequency with which it occurs among all orotic aciduria?

Dr. Endres: I have no idea at all.

Dr. Saudubray: I can give a short comment because it was my friend Claude Griscelli who published this case. This is a completely different inborn error due to a specific defect in orotic acid catabolism: hereditary orotic aciduria. In orotic aciduria secondary to urea cycle defects, as in OTC deficiency, there is no immune deficiency.

Dr. Jaeken: Let me tell you something about our experience with the transient neonatal hyperammonemia syndrome. We have seen 13 patients during the last 10 years, all preterm neonates, from 31 to 36 weeks of gestational age. All had a respiratory distress syndrome and went into deep coma with complete apnea and required ventilatory support; only some spinal reflexes remained. Eight died due to cerebral hemorrhage and the others survived, four of them with completely normal development and one with cerebral palsy. We have evidence that in this disorder there is hepatic hypoperfusion. There is no enzymatic deficiency or developmental delay in enzymatic activity of the urea cycle. In our experience this disease is even more frequent than congenital urea cycle defects.

Dr. Dhondt: I am glad to have this information because the explanation of a delayed maturation of enzymes was not very good. What is really important to remember is that in transient neonatal hyperammonemia, if the child survives, there is no severe long-term effect from the hyperammonemia itself. The reverse situation occurs in heterozygotes for OTC, where the chronic hyperammonemia has subtle effects on brain development. I think this is one of the reasons why we need to use very aggressive therapy like liver transplantation as early as possible in urea cycle disorders to prevent such developmental problems.

Dr. Van den Berghe: Maybe I missed the point, but you said that you did not find data concerning the amount of amino nitrogen that was accounted for by the excretion of orotate. This surprises me since one molecule of carbamyl phosphate, synthesized from ammonia in the mitochondria but flowing over in the cytoplasm in urea cycle disorders, and one molecule of aspartate yield one molecule of orotic acid.

Dr. Dhondt: Perhaps I did not explain myself enough. I never found any evaluation of orotate as a waste nitrogen compound.

Dr. Saudubray: Sodium benzoate therapy has been advocated as a good method of detoxication in the acute phase of hyperammonemia, but I am not sure that it really works. Consider from a quantitative point of view the catabolism of 6 g protein and 1 g nitrogen: 1 g of nitrogen is 71 mmol; when you give sodium benzoate at a dose of 250 mg/kg, it means that in a 3- to 4-kg neonate you give a total amount of approximately 12 to 14 mmol. So when you compare 70 mmol from the catabolism of 30 g of muscle to 14 mmol of sodium benzoate I can't understand how this therapy can work. It is the same kind of question you stressed. Do you have some comments?

Dr. Dhondt: I agree with you and for this reason I was very interested in the recent report from Batshaw about the use of phenylacetate or phenylbutyrate because it looks from these data better than the benzoate therapy.

Dr. Vis: You claim that high blood levels of ammonia, either permanent or transient, are toxic for the brain. What level do you think may be tolerated by premature newborns over a period of several weeks without deleterious effects? The question is of importance because premature babies receiving parenteral amino acid mixtures sometimes present very high levels of ammonia in blood. I don't think this problem has been given enough attention in the literature.

Dr. Dhondt: We don't know exactly what ammonia level is toxic in the long term. Even in asymptomatic transient hyperammonemia it has been proposed that arginine should be added to prevent such an effect.

Dr. Jaeken: I think that below 150 μmol/liter there is no clinical problem at all, but there is probably no clear cutoff value.

Dr. Schaub: You recommend peritoneal dialysis. In many hospitals this technique is not available in newborns. Is there another form of treatment like exchange transfusion for newborns in hyperammonemic crisis?

Dr. Dhondt: The Johns Hopkins hospital group has shown that peritoneal dialysis is the most effective system for clearing ammonium, more effective than exchange transfusion.

Dr. Endres: Sometimes you can even increase the level of ammonium by exchange transfusions because the blood you give contains a lot of ammonium.

Dr. Saudubray: I have observed more than 70 patients with urea cycle defects in the neonatal period. My policy now is not to treat such patients. I disagree completely with Batshaw's treatment policy in neonates because more than 80% of their patients are very severely mentally retarded. Therefore, it is not reasonable to treat a neonate who will spontaneously die within 3 days of life. This is my policy. It does not seem reasonable to me to treat patients with urea cycle defects presenting with the very severe neonatal form.

Dr. Sokal: The liver enzymes are heterogeneously distributed across the liver acinus. The urea cycle enzymes are located in the periportal zone, whereas other ammonium detoxification systems, such as glutamine synthetase, are located in the perivenular zone. Ammonium ions "escaping" the urea cycle are detoxified by glutamine synthetase in the perivenular zone. It is likely that in urea cycle enzyme defects, the latter system has an enhanced activity. Is there any evidence that this could lead to a secondary lack of glutamate which is the substrate for this reaction, and would it help the patient to give additional glutamate or α-ketoglutarate?

Dr. Wanders: Carbamyl glutamate could be used in the urea cycle defects, because in these conditions limited amounts of protein are given and hence intramitochondrial glutamate levels will be low; consequently, the N-acetylglutamate levels will also be low, because N-acetylglutamate arises from glutamate and acetyl-CoA. So by giving carbamyl glutamate you might speed up CPS to the greatest degree and so effectively remove ammonia. I would therefore suggest that in the other enzyme deficiencies it would also be good to use carbamyl glutamate.

Dr. Dhondt: This should be a possibility, similar to arginine supplementation since arginine stimulates carbamyl phosphate synthesis.

Dr. Wanders: With regard to the stimulation by arginine, it is very doubtful whether this also happens *in vivo* because the K_i of arginine is in the micromolar range and the normal concentration in mitochondria is far above this K_i.

Dr. Dhondt: However, carbamyl glutamate is an analog and we are always a little anxious about using nonnatural products.

Dr. Roe: I just want to elaborate on a point and also ask a question. My comment is related to our experience with ASL deficiency and citrate administration. We know that in that ASL deficiency, plasma citrulline levels are extremely high, aspartate levels low, and ASA is high. With the administration of citrate the citrulline level drops and ASA levels go up. But more important one can see the resolution of hepatomegaly in that disease and appetite returns. This all suggest a very fundamental problem with intermediary metabolism and the TCA cycle that may apply to several disorders. We agree with the importance of the use of arginine. I am not so convinced about benzoate, phenylacetate, and phenylbutyrate. One of my concerns is there seems to be no documentation in the literature regarding the dose of arginine used for supplementation.

Dr. Widhalm: Dr. Thalammer introduced the modified Murphy test for arginine-succinate deficiency into the Austrian screening program. By means of this test about 14 patients have been detected with arginine-succinate lyase deficiency but without or with only mild hyperammonemia. These patients had been treated for several years with arginine and within the last year with citric acid. I would like to ask if anybody has experience with mild hyperammonemia and a definite-succinate lyase deficiency.

Dr. Baerlocher: We have observed two children with argininosuccinic aciduria and only slight hyperammonemia. They have grown up with no special problems. May I ask Dr. Saudubray if he includes argininosuccinic aciduria among the disorders of the urea cycle in which he would not begin any treatment. My experience is not so bad with this disorder. We recently observed a child with a severe neonatal form of argininosuccinic aciduria and severe hyperammonemia. We started peritoneal dialysis on the third day without any effect on the hyperammonemia. Only when arginine was given 12 h later did the hyperammonemia rapidly diminish and finally normalize. The child is at the moment quite well. On the third day, ultrasonography revealed dense kidney parenchyma reflecting nephrocalcinosis. Orotic acid was very high in the urine at this time but diminished under treatment with arginine. We therefore suggest that orotic acid crystals may have been responsible for the ultrasonographic findings.

Dr. Saudubray: I agree. Maybe argininosuccinic aciduria is a little bit different from the other urea cycle defects because you have a very effective way of nitrogen clearance through argininosuccinic acid excretion itself. But until now if you consider the Johns Hopkins group's long-term results there is no 10-year-old patient with normal psychomotor development having presented with a urea cycle defect in the neonatal period. The true problem in the neonatal period confronted with hyperammonemia is to separate the following three conditions rapidly: transient hyperammonemia, urea cycle defect, and organic aciduria. In the first condition (transient hyperammonemia) you have to treat, of course, because the patient can die but he can also improve and develop normally afterward. In this condition the clinical context is evident; it is a clinical diagnosis, not a biological one. As stated by Dr. Jaeken, all the patients affected with transient hyperammonemia are premature babies. This is not a clinical condition encountered in full-term neonates. Patients with organic acidurias also have to be treated, whereas those with urea cycle defects do not have to be.

Dr. Dhondt: I cannot totally agree on an ethical point of view because it is difficult to refuse treatment in such patients. I remember our first OTC-deficient patient, who was in poor condition at the start but now is totally normal. Of course, that will represent only 5–10% of patients, but how can one refuse the possibility of treatment even if only a few patients will have normal development?

Dr. Krywawych: My comment is an addition to the points raised on argininosuccinic aciduria. In our patient with argininosuccinic acid lyase deficiency a diagnosis was made at 48 h after birth and treatment was started within 3 days after birth. During the neonatal period this child was treated with arginine supplements and citrate to replenish the oxaloacetate which was being excreted and lost as part of the argininosuccinic acid. In later life benzoate supplements were also included in the treatment regime. Since that time, this patient has experienced only three crisis periods but was promptly treated and the plasma ammonia was rapidly brought under control. His plasma ammonia levels have generally been maintained below 100 μmol/liter. He is now 6 years old and is neurologically delayed. We do not know whether this has been caused by some toxic properties of argininosuccinic acid, by the chronically mildly raised plasma ammonia levels, or whether this patient may have suffered some degree of neurological damage during the three brief crisis periods. I would like to ask whether anyone here has any experience of children with argininosuccinic aciduria presenting with an acidosis. In the three cases we have seen profound acidosis was present with only a mildly raised lactate and some indication of a raised plasma chloride. I would also wish to ask whether the administration of benzoate to these patients could lead the formation of benzoyl carnitine, carnitine loss, and interference with fatty acid metabolism.

Dr. Roe: In response to the question about whether benzoyl carnitine is formed, this is apparently not a substrate for carnitine acyltransferase, as we are completely unable to identify any benzoylcarnitine in patients on benzoate therapy.

REFERENCE

1. Shin YS, Kruis B, Heininger U, Endres W. Radioisotopic methods for assay of the enzymes in the urea cycle: first trimester diagnostic possibilities for urea cycle disorders using chorionic villi sampling. *J Inher Metab Dis* 1987;10(suppl 2):314–6.

Inborn Errors of Metabolism, edited by
J. Schaub, F. Van Hoof, and H. L. Vis.
Nestlé Nutrition Workshop Series, Vol. 24.
Nestec Ltd., Vevey/Raven Press, Ltd.,
New York © 1991.

Theoretical and Practical Aspects of Preventing Fetal Damage in Women with Phenylketonuria

Stephen Krywawych, M. Haseler, and D. P. Brenton

University College and Middlesex School of Medicine, Department of Medicine, The Rayne Institute, 5 University Street, London WC1E 6JJ, United Kingdom

The problem of mental retardation in children born to mothers with phenylketonuria (PKU) was first raised in 1956 at the 23rd Ross Pediatric Conference in Columbus, Ohio, by the late Charles E. Dent, and subsequently reported in the proceedings in 1957 (1). Six years later a high incidence of mental retardation was described among 14 children born to three mothers with PKU (2). These findings of mental retardation, microcephaly, congenital heart disease, and other organ defects were confirmed in other studies (3–5). Perry *et al.* (6) drew attention to the unrecognized PKU patients presenting at antenatal clinics. They described two sisters with plasma phenylalanine levels at around 1 mmol/liter who between them had nine non-PKU children with an impaired IQ. In 1980, Lenke and Levy (7) reviewed a survey of 155 mothers with PKU who had 423 offspring and 101 spontaneous abortions (including many of those reported earlier in the literature). Spontaneous abortion, mental retardation, microcephaly, congenital heart disease, and low birth weight became recognized as the major clinical problems associated with maternal PKU. With the introduction of screening of newborns for phenylketonuria in the 1970s, resulting in a population of young successfully treated adults with PKU by the late 1980s, a widespread problem of maternal phenylketonuria has emerged. Any attempts at treating this condition to prevent damage to the developing fetus requires an understanding of the placental transport of amino acids, embryonic development, and the mechanisms of fetal damage.

PLACENTAL TRANSPORT OF AMINO ACIDS

Transport of amino acids from the maternal circulation to the fetal side serves to provide for fetal metabolic (anabolic) requirements and to a much smaller extent to satisfy the metabolic requirements of the trophoblast (8). With the exception of cystine, taurine, glutamic, and aspartic acid, all other amino acids are actively transported from the maternal to the fetal side. Unlike the fetal surface, the maternal surface of the trophoblast has microvilli which structurally resemble the brush border of intestinal and renal epithelium and is in direct contact with maternal blood. Investigations on human placental brush border membrane vesicles have demonstrated three transport mechanisms: the A system, the L system, and the ASC system (9). The first system, the A system, transports proline, glycine, and α-amino isobutyric acid and is inhibited by methylalanine. The second system, the L system, demonstrates preference for the aromatic and the large neutral amino acids (e.g., leucine, phenylalanine, tyrosine, and methionine) and is inhibited by 2-aminonorborane-2-carboxylic acid, but not significantly by methylalanine. Finally, the third system acts upon the basic and short chain neutral amino acids (e.g., alanine, serine, threonine, and glutamine) and is inhibited by both 2-aminonorborane-2-carboxylic acid and methylalanine. In guinea pig placenta, membrane transporters have been shown to exist on both the maternal and fetal sides of the trophoblast but only unidirectional transport at the maternal interface is sodium dependent (10,11). The K_m value for phenylalanine at the fetal side was threefold higher than on the maternal side. Transport studies in membrane vesicles from term human placenta indicate that saturation of placental phenylalanine transport is unlikely at phenylalanine concentrations seen in affected PKU mothers, but competitive inhibition of tyrosine and tryptophan may occur.

With the exception of threonine, all maternal plasma amino acid concentrations fall in pregnancy (12). On the other hand, transport of amino acids across the placenta produces higher fetal than maternal values, the ratio between the two differing for different amino acids. In our patients, for maternal plasma phenylalanine concentrations ranging from 112 to 657 μmol/liter the fetal/maternal phenylalanine ratio averaged 1.6:1. This gradient is still maintained at much higher maternal values than 657 μmol/liter. The higher fetal/maternal plasma phenylalanine ratio has been shown to occur from early pregnancy (13,14). To maintain fetal values below 500 μmol/liter, maternal phenylalanine values require to be kept below 300 μmol/liter. It is of course still debatable how low the fetal values need to be to ensure a normal child.

EMBRYONIC DEVELOPMENT

Rapid development of the fetus occurs during organogenesis, 3–8 weeks after fertilization. At 5 weeks postfertilization the 10-somite embryo develops a contracting heart, still a simple tube within a pericardium, and by 8 weeks the development to an adult heart form is virtually complete. Neural crest cells may also contribute to the cardiac development. The heart is therefore most vulnerable during the initial 8 weeks, and congenital heart disease has been shown to occur at an increased incidence in those babies born to mothers in whom the plasma phenylalanine concentration has remained above 900 μmol/liter. In our experience two of three infants resulting from pregnancies conceived before diet when mother's plasma phenylal-

anine concentration was high in the first trimester had severe congenital heart malformations and died. The third may also have more minor heart defects.

The neural folds meet anteriorly at 3 weeks, and complete posterior closure occurs
at 4 weeks. However, neural tube defects appear to be uncommon in untreated
maternal phenylketonuria (15,16). The very high incidence of microcephaly and mental retardation, however, probably has its origins during the first trimester since poor
control then may still result in microcephaly even if later control is satisfactory (16,
17).

The formation of the trachea begins at 3 weeks and major malrotation of the midgut
occurs later, between 6 and 12 weeks. Esophageal atresia, diaphragmatic hernia,
and malrotation have been described in maternal PKU and certainly originate during
the first trimester (7).

MECHANISMS OF FETAL DAMAGE

From the data on 53 offspring in untreated pregnancies (18), some authors argued
that there is a graded effect of maternal plasma phenylalanine concentrations on the
brain development of the offspring (19,20). However, for other defects it is possible
that there is a threshold value of around 600 μmol/liter for maternal plasma phenylalanine concentration, below which congenital malformations may not occur more
commonly than in the normal population.

From the postnatal treatment of homozygous patients with phenylketonuria it is
evident that the neurological system is vulnerable to phenylalanine in the young child
but less so in the older child and young adult. It is likely that similar mechanisms
of damage to nervous tissue operate in the fetal state as in the postnatal period. The
precise mechanism for the postnatal damage has not been elucidated, but an inadequate supply of some amino acids to the brain, deranging protein synthesis or neurotransmitter synthesis, is likely to be a factor contributing to brain damage (21).
High plasma phenylalanine concentrations in rats have been shown to decrease the
entry of related long chain neutral amino acids into brain (22–24). Similarly, the
transport of methionine, leucine, tyrosine, valine, and glutamine but not arginine
and lysine was inhibited at the ovine blood-brain barrier by increased concentrations
of phenylalanine (25). This interference occurs as a result of competition by different
amino acids for a common carrier across the blood-brain barrier. Three carrier systems for the transport of amino acids have been identified; one for the short chain
neutral amino acids, the second for the long chain neutral amino acids, and the third
for the basic amino acids (26).

Phenylalanine undergoes facilitated transport by a carrier that is also active on
the branched-chain amino acids tryptophan, tyrosine, histidine, methionine, and glutamine. The carrier at the blood-brain barrier is similar to that of the L-system of
Christensen (27) but with much lower K_m values. At the normal plasma amino acid
concentrations this carrier is almost saturated, and therefore not only is the flux of
an amino acid across the blood-brain barrier sensitive to any changes in its concen-

tration, but is also influenced by changes in the concentration of other competing amino acids.

There is limited experimental information in animals concerning the kinetic parameters of amino transport at blood-brain barrier in the developing fetus. The blood-brain barrier depends on the development of tight junctions between capillary endothelial cells forming an impermeable barrier to water-soluble substrates. As the development of such a barrier occurs in early gestation, it is reasonable to assume that the transport of amino acids may be important in the pathology of brain damage in the developing fetus in maternal phenylketonuria. During fetal development these amino acid imbalances are likely to be further exacerbated by the generation of the placental gradient for phenylalanine from maternal to fetal side. The exact mode of damage by the brain amino acid imbalance is unknown, but its effect may be directed on neuron replication, protein synthesis, axonal and dendritic development and growth, myelation, or neurotransmitter metabolism.

Low concentrations of dopamine and serotinin have been found in the cerebrospinal fluid (CSF) and in the brain tissue of homozygous subjects with PKU when plasma phenylalanine concentrations were elevated (28). Furthermore, a reciprocal relationship has been observed between the concentration of plasma phenylalanine and that of plasma and CSF serotonin and dopamine and their metabolites (29–32). Phenylalanine may inhibit dopamine and serotonin synthesis by restricting the entry of their precursors tyrosine and tryptophan into brain or even possibly by inhibiting the enzymes involved in the synthesis of these monoamines (33–37). Disturbed monoamine synthesis is more likely to be responsible for the reversible behavioral and psychological problems observed in treated patients with phenylketonuria on occasions when the plasma phenylalanine concentration is elevated, but may also be related to the permanent irreversible neurological damage seen in untreated patients with PKU.

Specific interventions through the administration of selected amino acids to correct the deficiency of such amino acids in the brain of patients with phenylketonuria has been proposed as a therapeutic approach (38). The supplementation with branched-chain amino acids of normal diets fed to young rats with induced hyperphenylalaninemia has markedly improved their maze-learning techniques (39). Similar branched-chain supplements fed to maternal rats with induced phenylketonuria have restored normal birth weights in the offspring (40). These branched-chain amino acid supplements may act by restricting phenylalanine entry into brain, thereby preventing it from exerting its toxic effects, or simply by correcting a deficiency of branched-chain amino acids caused by the inhibition of their transport across the placenta or into the CNS. Recently, the exodus of small neutral amino acids from brain tissues has been shown to be inhibited in rats with induced hyperphenylalaninemia (41). This is thought to occur because the normal exchange of large neutral amino acids in the L-system for proline, alanine, and glycine accumulated intracellularly by the sodium-dependent A system is inhibited by the elevated concentrations of phenylalanine; this also explains the lower concentrations of these three amino acids in the plasma from patients with phenylketonuria (42). In view of the uncertainty as to whether low blood concentrations of glycine affect the supply of glycine as a neurotransmitter in brain it has been proposed that these nonessential amino acids should also receive attention (41).

Clearly, more work is required on designing the composition of diet for treatment of phenylketonuria and maternal phenylketonuria. Consideration must also be given to spreading the intake of the amino acid supplement over a longer duration so as to minimize wide fluctuations in plasma amino acid concentrations caused by swallowing of large quantitites of rapidly absorbed amino acid mixtures.

TREATMENT AND MANAGEMENT

A phenylalanine-restricted diet is introduced preconceptionally as the means of treatment to prevent *in utero* fetal damage in maternal PKU. It is essential that all pregnancies are planned. This can be effective only if patients understand the harmful effects that a mother's high phenylalanine may have on the brain and heart of the developing fetus and how this can be averted by dietary manipulation. Management therefore really starts with counseling given to teenage girls with PKU. To avoid unwanted pregnancies the importance of contraception should be discussed. Patients are encouraged to explain their condition to their future husbands and to bring them for similar counseling.

If the patient has been off dietary restriction for several years, the reintroduction of the diet is likely to require hospital admission to reacquaint the patient with using the diet and collecting Guthrie samples twice weekly for phenylalanine estimations. Full amino acid analyses are carried out monthly. It is not possible to define an absolute threshold value for maternal plasma phenylalanine concentration below which there is no risk to the fetus. Earlier attempts to keep the maternal values below 500 µmol/liter were not always successful in the first trimester and would have allowed fetal phenylalanine concentrations to rise above 800 µmol/liter, a value higher than acceptable in the treatment of young growing children with PKU. Maternal values <250 µmol/liter are needed to keep the fetal values <400 µmol/liter. The first trimester is a period of extensive organ development and lowest maternal tolerance to phenylalanine. Pregnancy nausea and vomiting may be a problem in dietary control. Tolerance gradually increases into the second and third trimesters, coinciding with the increased phenylalanine requirement for growth in the rapidly growing fetus and the development of the phenylalanine hydroxylase enzyme in fetal liver between 16 and 20 weeks. A very rapid rise in tolerance has been observed in our patient with a twin pregnancy. From about 18 weeks the diet administered to all our patients is further supplemented with 2–3 g of tyrosine daily to produce a total intake of 8 g daily.

OUTCOME OF TREATMENT

At University College Hospital we have now looked after 11 pregnancies in seven mothers with 12 children born (one twin pregnancy). None has inherited phenylketonuria. Of the three conceptions where diet began at 7, 12, and 7 weeks, two infants died of congenital heart disease and the third child was considered to have suffered possible supraventricular tachycardias in infancy. The crucial nature of dietary control in the first trimester as far as congenital malformations is concerned is self-evident from what has been said about embryonic development. The marked decline in congenital heart disease with preconception diet is clear from Lenke and Levy (7), Levy and Waisbren (18), and Drogari et al. (16). None of the nine children born at University College Hospital after preconception diet has a cardiac abnormality or other congenital defect (but see below). These results are consistent with the view that damage to the fetus occurs as a result of high maternal phenylalanine concentrations and not as a result of damage to the sperm or ovum preconceptionally or from unforseen complications that may occur during dietary restriction during pregnancy.

The data of Drogari et al. (16), collected from many centers including our own, indicated that both birth weight and head circumference at birth are related to phenylalanine concentration at conception, which in turn is related to two factors. First, preconception diet obviously lowers the phenylalanine at conception, and this group presumably remains much better controlled in the first 8 weeks than those not on diet where pregnancy is not diagnosed and dietary control not established until 8 weeks or later. Second, the phenylalanine at conception also reflects the severity of the mother's PKU, whether treated or untreated, since lower phenylalanine concentrations are likely to be more easily achieved by diet in mothers with milder forms of the disease. Phenylalanine concentrations at conception therefore are likely to correlate closely with first-trimester control. Indeed, from our own data we can show correlations between birth weight and head circumference with maternal plasma phenylalanine concentration in the first trimester. It is surprising perhaps that first-trimester control is so important to the overall growth and head size of the baby. To look independently at the effects of second- or third-trimester control is difficult. The practical difficulties of first-trimester control relate to the fact that it is the period of lowest phenylalanine tolerance and it produces the highest mean values for phenylalanine of any trimester.

The postnatal development of the children born to the PKU mothers is being closely followed at University College Hospital by Dr. Anne Stewart. Of the nine infants born after preconception diet, eight are progressing normally. Minor neurological signs have frequently been noticed in these on very careful neonatal examination, but all have disappeared with time. Intellectual assessment is also being carefully assessed and so far the children are in the normal range for tests appropriate to their age group. There remains one exception—one child out of the nine is grossly abnormal, with seizures and profound developmental delay. At the age of 18 months this child has minimal head control. Investigations at University College Hospital and at the Hospital for Sick Children, Great Ormond Street, have failed to find a cause. The child appears much more profoundly abnormal than usual for the offspring of mothers with untreated PKU. The mother's first pregnancy was ectopic and terminated with emergency surgery. For that pregnancy and the second she started diet preconception. Analysis of her amino acids in pregnancy has shown no differences from the findings in PKU mothers on diet where the pregnancy outcome has been normal. Although this baby's grossly abnormal development does not seem to be due to the mother's PKU or its management, it is a cautionary reminder to us that we may not have all the answers yet to maternal phenylketonuria, and follow-up of the offspring of PKU mothers for years to come is essential.

REFERENCES

1. Dent CE. Relation of biochemical abnormality in development of mental defect in phenylketonuria. Etiological factors in mental retardation. *23rd Ross Pediatric Research Conference,* November 1956. Columbus, Ohio, 1957;32.
2. Mabry CC, Denniston JC, Nelson TL, Son CD. Maternal phenylketonuria: a cause of mental retardation in children without the metabolic defect. *N Engl J Med* 1963;269:1404–8.
3. Mabry CC, Denniston JC, Goldwell TG. Mental retardation in children of phenylketonuric mothers. *N Engl J Med* 1966;275:1331–6.
4. Fisch RO, Walker WA, Anderson JA. Prenatal and postnatal consequences of maternal phenylketonuria. *Pediatrics* 1966;37:979–86.
5. Fisch RO, Doeden D, Lansky LL, Anderson JA. Maternal phenylketonuria. *Am J Dis Child* 1969; 118:847–58.
6. Perry TL, Hansen S, Tischler B, Richards FM, Sokol M. Unrecognised adult phenylketonuria. *N Engl J Med* 1973;289:395–8.
7. Lenke RL, Levy HL. Maternal phenylketonuria and hyperphenylalaninaemia. *N Engl J Med* 1980; 303:1202–8.
8. Yudilevich DL, Swiery JH. Transport of amino acids in the placenta. *Biochim Biophys Acta* 1985;822; 169–201.
9. Yudilevich DL, Boyd CAR. Amino acid transport in animal cells. Manchester: Manchester University Press, 1987;138–45.
10. Yudilevich DL, Eaton BM. Amino acid carriers at maternal and fetal surfaces of the placenta by single circulation paired tracer dilution. Kinetics of phenylalanine transport. *Biochim Biophys Acta* 1980; 595:315–9.
11. Eaton BM, Mann GE, Yudilevich DL. Transport specificity for neutral and basic amino acids at maternal and fetal interfaces of the guinea pig placenta. *J Physiol (Lond)* 1982;328:245–58.
12. Young M, Prenton MA. Maternal and fetal plasma amino acid concentration during gestation and in retarded fetal growth. *J Obstet Gynaecol* 1969;76:333–44.
13. Soltesz G, Harris D, Mackenzie IZ, Anysley-Green A. The metabolic and endocrine milieu of the human fetus and mother at 18–21 weeks of gestation. I. Plasma amino acid concentrations. *Paediatr Res* 1985; 19:91–3.
14. Fowler B, Horner R, Wraith JE, Sardharwalla IB. Maternal PKU fetal blood and tissue amino acid concentrations in mid-trimester. *Abstracts of 26th SSIEM Symposium,* Glasgow, 1988.
15. Fisch RO, Burke B, Bass J, Ferrara TB, Mastri A. Maternal phenylketonuria: chronology of the detrimental effects on embryogenesis and fetal development. *Pediatr Pathol* 1986;5:449–61.
16. Drogari E, Smith I, Beasley M, Lloyd JK. Timing of strict diet in relation to fetal damage in maternal phenylketonuria. *Lancet* 1987;ii:927–30.
17. Smith I, Macartney FJ, Erdohazi M, et al. Fetal damage despite low phenylalanine diet after conception in a phenylketonuric woman. *Lancet* 1979;i:17–19.
18. Levy HL, Waisbren SE. Effects of untreated maternal phenylketonuria and hyperphenylalaninaemia on the fetus. *N Engl J Med* 1983;309:1269–74.
19. Buist NRM, Tuerck J, Lis E, Penn R. Effects of untreated maternal phenylketonuria and hyperphenylalaninaemia on the fetus. *N Engl J Med* 1984;311:52–3.
20. Kirkman HN, Hicks RE. More on untreated hyperphenylalaninaemia. *N Engl J Med* 1984;311:1125.
21. Tourian A, Sidbury JB. Phenylketonuria and hyperphenylalaninaemia. In: Stanbury JB, Wyngaarden JB, Frederickson DS, Goldstein JL, Brown MS, eds. *The metabolic basis of inherited disease,* 5th ed. New York: McGraw-Hill, 1983;270–86.

22. Pratt OE. Transport inhibition in the pathology of phenylketonuria and other inherited metabolic diseases. *J Inher Metab Dis* 1982;5(Suppl 2):75–81.
23. Partridge WO, Oldendorf WH. Transport of metabolic substrates through the blood barrier. *J Neurochem* 1977;28:5–12.
24. McKean C, Boggs D, Peterson N. The influence of high phenylalanine and tyrosine on the concentrations of the essential amino acids in brain. *J Neurochem* 1968;15:235–41.
25. Brenton DP, Gardiner RM. Transport of L-phenylalanine and related amino acids at the ovine blood brain barrier. *J Physiol (Lond)* 1988;402:497–514.
26. Collarini EJ, Oxender DL. Mechanisms of transport of amino acids across membranes. *Annu Rev Nutr* 1987;7:75–90.
27. Christensen HN. On the development of amino acid transport systems. *Fed Proc* 1973;32:19–28.
28. McKean CM. The effects of high phenylalanine concentrations on serotonin and catechalamine metabolism in the human brain. *Brain Res* 1972;47:469–76.
29. Curtius HC, Vollmin JA, Baerlocher K. The use of deuterated phenylalanine for the eludication of the phenylalanine-tyrosine metabolism. *Clin Chim Acta* 1972;37:277–85.
30. Curtius HC, Wiederwieser A, Viscontini M, et al. Serotonin and dopamine synthesis in phenylketonuria. *Adv Exp Med Biol* 1981;133:277–91.
31. Krause W, Halminski M, McDonald L, et al. Biochemical and neuropsychological effects of elevated plasma phenylalanine in patients with treated phenylketonuria. *J Clin Invest* 1985;75:40–8.
32. Butler LJ, O'Flynn ME, Seifert WE, Howell RR. Neurotransmitter defects and treatment of disorders of hyperphenylalaninemia. *J Pediatr* 1981;98:729–33.
33. Udenfriend S. The primary enzymatic defect in phenylketonuria and how it may influence the central nervous system. In: Anderson JA, Swaiman KF, eds. *Phenylketonuria and allied metabolic diseases.* Washington DC: Dept. of Health, Education and Welfare, 1967;1–8.
34. Lovenberg W, Jéquier E, Sjoerdsma A. Tryptophan hydroxylation in mammalian systems. *Adv Pharmacol* 1968;6A:21–35.
35. Tong JH, Kaufman S. Tryptophan hydroxylase: purification and some properties of the enzyme from rabbit hindbrain. *J Biol Chem* 1975;250:4152–8.
36. Bowden JA, McArthur CL. Possible biochemical model for phenylketonuria. *Nature* 1972;235:230.
37. Paere CM, Sandler M, Stacey RS. Decreased 5-hydroxytryptophan decarboxylase activity in phenylketonuria. *Lancet* 1958;ii:1099–101.
38. Pratt OE. A new approach to the treatment of phenylketonuria. *J Ment Defic Res* 1980;24:203–17.
39. McSwigan JD, Vorhees CB, Brunner RL, Butcher RE, Berry HK. Amelioration of maze deficits from induced hyperphenylalaninemia in adult rats using valine, isoleucine and leucine. *Behav Neural Biol* 1981;33:378–84.
40. Brunner RL, Vorhees CV, McLean MS, Burchewr RE, Berry HK. Beneficial effect of isoleucine on fetal brain development in induced phenylketonuria. *Brain Res* 1978;154:191–5.
41. De Cespedes C, Thoene JG, Lowler K, Christensen HN. Evidence for inhibition of exodus of small neutral amino acids from non brain tissues in hyperphenylalaninemic rats. *J Inher Metab Dis* 1989; 12:166–80.
42. Efron ML, Song Kong E, Visakorpi J, Feller FX. Effects of elevated plasma phenylalanine levels on other amino acids in phenylketonuria and normal subjects. *J Pediatr* 1969;74:399–405.

DISCUSSION

Dr. Wang: Is there any difference between the fetal outcome of maternal typical PKU and maternal atypical PKU?

Dr. Krywawych: The data presented here and other published work indicates that congenital abnormalities in the developing fetus are associated with raised maternal phenylalanine levels at conception and during pregnancy. Congenital heart damage occurs predominantly at maternal plasma phenylalanine concentration above 600 μmol/liter at conception and in pregnancy. For the intellectual development there appears to be a graded effect, whereby the abnormality occurs at lower maternal plasma phenylalanine concentrations but its frequency increases with increasing phenylalanine concentration. Plasma phenylalanine concentrations in this unsafe lower range would be expected not only in treated typical classical phenylketonuric subjects but also in the milder atypical ones untreated.

Dr. Endres: I think there is a confusion of the nomenclature. Atypical PKU, as you, Dr. Krywawych, define it, is mild PKU or hyperphenylalaninemia called non-PKU HPA, and what you, Dr. Wang, mean is tetrahydrobiopterin (BH_4)-deficient hyperphenylalaninemia or "atypical PKU." Nobody can answer your question because up to now we don't have a patient with such a disease old enough to become pregnant. I think the prognosis for such a pregnancy would be rather uncertain. There is no experience in treating a woman during pregnancy with neurotransmitter precursors and BH_4.

Dr. Schaub: For the clinician it is important to hear what you recommend: What blood level of phenylalanine do you recommend in maternal PKU?

Dr. Krywawych: Previously, we aimed at controlling the maternal blood phenylalanine level at a concentration of 500 μmol/liter. Currently, we have reduced this figure still further to a value of between 120 and 300 μmol/liter.

Dr. Casaer: Dr. Krywawych, you mentioned that you were surprised to see that these infants have microcephaly at birth. I am not surprised, since if there is a negative effect of phenylalanine early in gestation, this might interfere with the neural crest cells. From this layer of cells other neurons divide and from here they will migrate. Thus a toxic effect that interferes with this division and migration can result in microcephaly.

Dr. Casaer: Dr. Krywawych, you explained to us in your paper that phenylalanine had a negative effect on some of the neurotransmitters. It is important to realize that neurotransmitters early in gestation function more as trophic factors than as real neurotransmitters, and thus they can interfere with growth and development of the brain. In this respect did you see any differences in the effect of phenylalanine, according to the period of gestation in which you had difficulty in controlling the maternal blood level of phenylalanine?

Dr. Krywawych: We have not actually studied these differences related to control and gestational age. In all the cases where we have experienced poor control of the maternal blood phenylalanine concentration, this period of poor control was confined to conception and the first trimester.

Dr. Saudubray: Everybody shares the opinion that it is very important to keep phenylalanine blood levels under 400–600 μmol/liter at the time of conception. But the problem from a practical point of view is that the time of conception does not depend only on the physician (!). So the real difficulty in day-to-day practice is maintaining the phenylalanine level under 500 μmol/liter sometimes for many months. I remember a paper on the use of oral phenylalanine ammonialyase in PKU which resulted in a lowering of the phenylalanine levels by a few milligrams per 100 ml. Do you have an opinion on this therapy in addition to the diet?

Dr. Krywawych: No, I do not have an answer to this. We have not tried this on our patients. We have attempted at conception and during pregnancy to maintain the plasma phenylalanine level at 300 μmol/liter by diet alone. This is extremely difficult but becomes easier into the second and third trimesters. As better control of maternal plasma phenylalanine results in a more favorable outcome for the pregnancy, maybe your proposal should be given more serious consideration.

Dr. Hobbs: Having worked on isoamylases I think there are some lessons to be learned. We chose by chance to use pig pancreatin. This is immunologically identical to the human enzyme, so most patients do not make antibodies to it. For almost any other animal you make antibodies to the enzyme, and if you choose bovine pancreatin it could be useless. It would generate antibodies that could prevent the enzyme from working. My conviction would be that if you try these enzymes they might work for 6 weeks and then fail. There was an attempt to treat hyperammonemia in liver disease with a urease, and it does not work after a few weeks. The human being makes antibodies and stops the enzyme working.

Dr. Van den Berghe: I would not be as negative as Dr. Hobbs with respect to enzyme replacement therapy with purified enzyme preparations. In two inborn errors of purine metabolism, adenosine deaminase deficiency (1) and purine nucleoside phosphorylase deficiency, good clinical results have been obtained with polyethylene glycol (PEG)–modified enzymes, given intramuscularly. PEG attachment to the enzymes markedly decreases their clearance from the circulation, their attack by degradative enzymes, and their antigenicity. PEG-modified enzymes are thus valuable in lowering the concentration of toxic metabolites in plasma.

Dr. Endres: I would like to underline what Professor Saudubray said. I think young women or girls with PKU never know when they will become pregnant. And you remember the figures Dr. Krywawych showed us: among the offsprings of those mothers who had phenylalanine levels between 3 and 10 mg/dl (170–570 μmol/liter), 21% had IQs below 75 and 24% had microcephaly. This 3–10 mg range is very great. The question arises as to whether these babies, the 21% or 24%, are to be found mainly in the upper part of this range or whether they are spread throughout the range. So what we don't know at the moment is where the safe limit is. Is it sufficient enough to say that the diet has to be restricted in phenylalanine in order to keep the plasma level of phenylalanine below 10 (570 μmol/liter) or, as in our prospective study in Germany, below 5 mg/dl (285 μmol/liter). But I am not sure whether 5 mg is low enough.

Dr. Krywawych: I agree that we are not certain exactly what the safe limit is. We have decreased our earlier recommended limit still further from 500 μmol/liter. The phenylalanine concentration on the fetal side of the placenta, which is always higher than that on the maternal side, is probably the most important factor to consider.

Dr. Holton: I am not sure what significance one can attach to animal experiments on the competitive inhibition of amino acid transport into brain. For a number of years we look at the question of the effect of histidine on the transport of amino acids into brain, and found that it has exactly the same effect as phenylalanine on the transport of other amino acids. You said that the blood-brain barrier is established very early in the fetus. I wonder whether you could put a time to that? We have been looking at fetal cerebrospinal fluid amino acids and we have found high levels, a completely different pattern to those of infants.

Dr. Krywawych: I cannot put a precise time on the development of the blood-brain barrier. It is dependent on the formation of tight junctions that have been identified histologically early in gestation. I agree that it is very difficult to extrapolate from animal experiments to the human condition. However, from the V_{max} and pK values for these amino acid carriers in humans it can be calculated that in histidinemia, tyrosine and tryptophan influx is decreased to only 50 to 60% of normal, whereas in phenylketonuria it is decreased to about 20%. To attain the same degree of inhibition for tyrosine and tryptophan in phenylketonuria as occurs in histidinemia, the plasma phenylalanine concentration would have to be maintained at approximately 450 μmol/ liter.

Dr. Vis: Available information from the literature, as well as the data shown by Dr. Krywawych, point to the fact that one of the conditions for a mother with PKU to enable her to give birth to a normal newborn is very strict dietetic management. When a PKU patient informs me that she wants to become pregnant, I always prescribe a very strict dietetic treatment for a test period of 2 months, before conception, to evaluate the compliance of the mother-to-be. The dietetic prescription for a pregnant woman with PKU is not easy to establish, because besides phenylalanine restriction, a very precise balance needs to be maintained between the intakes of various other nutrients. We don't know that much about the nutritional requirements of the fetus. For instance, diets low in phenylalanine are usually also low in taurine, which is not synthesized by the fetus, although that nutrient is essential for the development of the fetal brain. Trace element intakes also need to be monitored. Most PKU diets, for example, are low in selenium. I would like to ask at what time of the day plasma phenylalanine levels need to be measured. The authors suggest that levels below 400 μmol/liter (6.5 mg/dl) or even 600 μmol/liter (10 mg/dl) are safe. However, phenylalanine levels in blood are sometimes extremely variable during the day (postprandial levels for instance). Further to this, I would like to emphasize Dr. Eggermont's comment about the risk in case of fetal heterozygosity. Even in the normal fetus the enzymatic machinery responsible for the conversion of phenylalanine to tyrosine comes into action very slowly. We all know of transient hyperphenylalaninemia in premature newborns. This phenomenon is quite certainly even more important in the heterozygous fetus.

Dr. Krywawych: At the moment I do not think that we really know what the complete composition of the diet should be. Regarding the taurine requirement of the fetus, from investigations on placental transport there is some evidence suggesting that taurine does not cross the placenta. The timing of blood sampling complicates data, for it is not always possible to time the collection of samples at precisely the same point in relation to the ingestion of food. Fluctuations of plasma amino acid levels do occur in relation to feeds. Future diets may need to look toward a slower and more even release of amino acids into the blood. Consideration also needs to be given to a more balanced dietary amino acid composition so as to restore in the plasma concentration more normal ratios of the individual amino acids relative to phenylalanine.

REFERENCE

1. Hershfield MS, Buckley RH, Greenberg ML, et al. Treatment of adenosine deaminase deficiency with polyethylene glycol-modified adenosine deaminase. *New Engl J Med* 1987;316:589–96.

Inborn Errors of Metabolism, edited by
J. Schaub, F. Van Hoof, and H. L. Vis.
Nestlé Nutrition Workshop Series, Vol. 24.
Nestec Ltd., Vevey/Raven Press, Ltd.,
New York © 1991.

Inborn Errors of the Metabolism of Branched-Chain Amino Acids

Jean Marie Saudubray, *H. Ogier, T. Billette de Vilmeur,
J. P. Bonnefont, S. Lyonnet, F. Herve, A. Munnich, [†]D. Rabier,
[†]M. Coude, and [†]C. Charpentier

*Département de Pédiatrie, Clinique de Génétique et INSERM U-12; *Hôpital Robert
Debré, 48 Boulevard Serrurier, 75019 Paris; [†]Département de Biochimie et INSERM
U-75, Hôpital Necker—Enfants-Malades, 149 Rue de Sèvres, 75743 Paris, France*

METABOLIC PATHWAYS OF BRANCHED-CHAIN AMINO ACIDS

The three essential neutral branched-chain amino acids, L-leucine, L-valine, and
L-isoleucine, are unique among the amino acids in that they undergo oxidation to a
greater extent in the peripheral tissues than in the liver. Transamination is the initial
metabolic step, resulting in branched-chain 2-oxo acids. Hypervalinemia and hy-
perleucine-isoleucinemia have been identified as disorders of branched-chain amino
acid transamination in extremely rare cases. The next step is an irreversible oxidative
decarboxylation to the corresponding acyl-CoA derivatives. All three branched-
chain 2-oxo acids are decarboxylated by a single mitochondrial multienzyme complex, called branched-chain 2-oxo-acid dehydrogenase.

This multienzyme complex resembles pyruvate and 2-oxoglutarate dehydrogenase
complexes in composition (three catalytic components: E_1 = branched-chain 2-oxo
acid decarboxylase, E_2 = branched-chain acyltransferase, and E_3 = dihydrolipoyl
dehydrogenase), cofactor requirement, and regulation. The branched-chain 2-oxo
acid dehydrogenase complex activity is deficient in patients with maple syrup urine
disease (branched-chain ketoaciduria, leucinosis). Immunologic and recombinant
DNA techniques have shown that the E_1 and eventually the E_2 component of the
complex are affected (1,2). A deficiency of E_3, which is a common catalytic subunit
for all three 2-oxo-acid dehydrogenase complexes, produces a syndrome with features of congenital lactic acidosis, branched-chain ketoaciduria, and 2-oxoglutaric
aciduria (3).

Leucine Metabolism

Leucine is further metabolized to acetoacetate and acetyl-CoA and hence into the
Krebs cycle. Specific enzymes deficiencies at every stage of this metabolic pathway

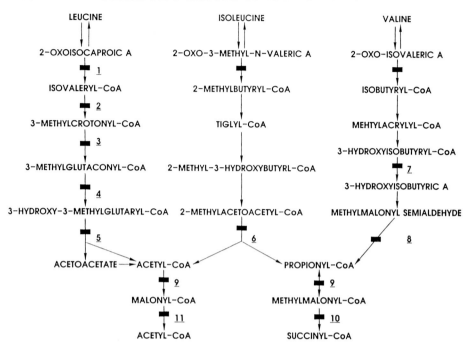

FIG. 1. Metabolism of branched-chain amino acids showing the position of the known inherited metabolic disorders. *1*, BCAA decarboxylase; *2*, isovaleryl-CoA dehydrogenase (FAD-ETF) (isovaleric aciduria); *3*, 3-methylcrotonyl-CoA carboxylase; *4*, 3-methylglutaconyl-CoA hydratase; *5*, 3-hydroxy-3-methylglutaryl-CoA lyase; *6*, 2-methylacetoacetyl-CoA thiolase; *7*, 3-hydroxyisobutyryl-CoA deacylase; *8*, methylmalonyl-semialdehyde dehydrogenase; *9*, propionyl-CoA carboxylase (biotin) (propionic aciduria); *10*, methylmalonyl-CoA racemase and mutase (B_{12}) (methylmalonic aciduria); *11*, malonyl-CoA decarboxylase. From Ogier H, et al. (13).

are known. Isovaleryl-CoA produced by the oxidative decarboxylation step of leucine is metabolized by a specific mitochondrial FAD-ETF-dependent dehydrogenase to 3-methylcrotonyl-CoA (Fig. 1, step 2). A defect in this dehydrogenase activity may occur secondary to apoenzyme mutation (isovaleric acidemia) or to FAD-ETF system dysfunction (glutaric aciduria type II).

3-Methylcrotonyl-CoA is carboxylated by a specific biotin-dependent acyl-CoA carboxylase (BMCC) to form 3-methylglutaconyl-CoA (step 3). Deficient activity of this enzyme leads to 3-methylcrotonylglycinuria. Variants are known, including defects in biotin metabolism that are responsible for multiple carboxylase deficiency (MCD). Isolated and biotin-resistant BMCC deficiency is much less common than that of MCD.

3-Hydroxy 3-methylglutaconyl-CoA is metabolized to 3-hydroxy-3-methylglutaryl-CoA by 3-methylglutaconyl-CoA hydratase (step 4). Defective activity leads to 3-methylglutaconic aciduria. However, there are at least two distinct disorders among patients affected with 3-CH_3-glutaconic aciduria, as most of them display a normal hydratase activity in fibroblasts. These diseases responsible for major developmental delay are not amenable to treatment (see Duran et al., *this volume*).

3-Methylglutaryl-CoA is converted to acetoacetate and acetyl-CoA by a specific lyase (HMG-CoA lyase) (step 5). In addition to its role in leucine degradation, HMG CoA lyase is involved in the cycle of ketogenesis, which explains most of the clinical manifestations of this enzyme deficiency (see Bartlett et al., *this volume*).

Isoleucine/Valine Metabolism: The Propionyl-CoA Pathway

The metabolism of valine and isoleucine is of particular interest since both are major precursors of propionyl-CoA and methylmalonyl-CoA. A deficiency of L-valine catabolism at the step of 3-hydroxyisobutyryl-CoA deacylase (Fig. 1, step 7) and methylmalonic semialdehyde dehydrogenase (Fig. 1, step 8), respectively, have been observed in only one and two patients (see Duran et al., *this volume*). In addition, two patients with malonyl-CoA decarboxylase deficiency (step 11) have been described. The latter enzyme serves an important function in the mitochondria by preventing accumulation of malonyl-CoA from acetyl-CoA through propionyl-CoA carboxylase (4).

The final unique step in the metabolism of L-isoleucine involves the ketolysis process at the cleavage of 2-methylacetoacetyl-CoA to acetyl-CoA and propionyl-CoA (step 6). L-Valine is also metabolized ultimately to propionyl-CoA and thus these two BCAA form the major precursors of propionyl-CoA. Other amino acid precursors, including threonine and methionine, are also metabolized to this intermediate via 2-oxybutyryl-CoA (Fig. 2). The β-oxidation of fatty acids containing odd numbers of carbon, which are minor components of dietary fats and body lipids, yield propionyl-CoA, too. Through the peroxisomal β-oxidation, the side chain of cholesterol is also a minor precursor of propionate. Finally, the potential importance of propionate synthesis by gut bacteria is of interest in disorders of propionate metabolism (5).

Propionyl-CoA is carboxylated to D-methylmalonyl-CoA by a mitochondrial biotin-dependent carboxylase enzyme (step 9). This carboxylation is readily reversible. It is also of interest that either *n*-butyryl-CoA or acetyl-CoA can substitute for propionyl-CoA to yield ethylmalonyl-CoA or malonyl-CoA, respectively. A defect in propionyl-CoA carboxylase activity results in propionyl-CoA accumulation and hence propionic acidemia. Propionyl-CoA accumulation also occurs in MCD due to defective activities of all three biotin-dependent carboxylases.

D-Methylmalonyl-CoA is converted by methylmalonyl-CoA racemase into the L-isomer, which in turn is converted into succinyl-CoA by the vitamin B_{12}-dependent methylmalonyl-CoA mutase (step 10). The succinyl-CoA subsequently enters the Krebs cycle. Deficient activity of the apomutase enzyme leads to methylmalonic aciduria, and because of the requirement by the apomutase for adenosylcobalamin, abnormal B_{12} metabolism leads to variant forms of methylmalonic aciduria.

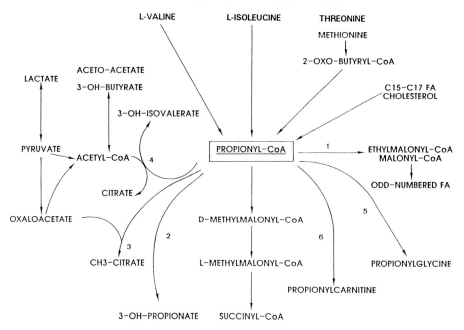

FIG. 2. Metabolism of propionyl-CoA: major alternative pathways in case of propionyl-CoA accumulation. *1*, acetyl-CoA carboxylase; *2*, β- or ω-oxidation; *3*, citrate synthase; *4*, acetyl-CoA and propionyl-CoA condensation and reduction; *5–6*, glycine-*N* acylase and carnitine-*N* acylase. (From Ogier H, et al. (13).

In this chapter we consider only the four main inborn errors of BCAA: MSUD, IVA, PA, and MMA.

METABOLIC CONSEQUENCES OF INBORN ERRORS OF BRANCHED-CHAIN AMINO ACIDS

Maple Syrup Urine Disease

Maple syrup urine disease (MSUD) is due to an inherited deficiency of the branched-chain 2-oxo acid dehydrogenase activity, affecting the metabolism of all three branched-chain 2-oxo amino acids. This defect produces marked increases in plasma, urinary, and CSF branched-chain amino acids (3). Smaller amounts of the respective 2-hydroxy acids, especially of 2-hydroxyisovaleric acid, are formed by reduction of the oxo acids. L-Alloisoleucine is constantly found in blood from MSUD patients. This compound is endogenously formed from (3*S*)2-oxo-3-methyl-*n*-valeric acid through nonenzymic racemization to (3*R*)2-oxo-3-methyl-*n*-valeric acid and further transamination to L-alloisoleucine (3).

The leucine/2-oxoisocaproic acid pair is the most toxic of the branched-chain metabolites. Probably 2-oxoisocaproic acid is the main neurotoxic substance. In maple syrup urine disease, leucine and 2-oxoisocaproate are always present in plasma in about equimolar concentrations (6,7). Valine and isoleucine are of less clinical significance.

Isovaleric Aciduria

Isovaleric aciduria is the first organic aciduria described using GC-MS. It is caused by a defect in isovaleryl-CoA dehydrogenase (IVCoA-DH), leading to an accumulation of isovaleryl-CoA (IVCoA) and its by-products. Biochemically, the disease is characterized by a greatly increased excretion in the urine of *N*-isovalerylglycine (IVG) and 3-hydroxyisovaleric acid (3OHIVA), which are diagnostic. The concentration of free isovaleric acid (IVA) is usually increased in both blood and urine, but normal levels have been reported. In this disorder, the majority of the accumulating IVCoA is conjugated with glycine to IVG by the action of glycine *N*-acylase, which shows a high affinity for the IVCoA as a substrate (8). IVG thus formed is rapidly excreted in the urine (9). IVCoA accumulation also favors isovalerylcarnitine (IVC) synthesis by carnitine *N*-acylase, which leads to high IVC urinary excretion (10). Considering the treatment of this condition, these two alternative pathways are of interest as they allow the transformation of the highly neurotoxic IVA into nontoxic by-products with a high renal clearance.

Propionic Acidemia

Isolated propionic acidemia (PA) is secondary to a defect in the synthesis or structure of the apoenzyme propionyl-CoA carboxylase (PCC). The enzyme has the structure $\alpha_4\beta_4$, with the alpha chain containing a biotin prosthetic group. Irrespective of the clinical phenotype, severe reduction but not complete absence of PCC activity (1–5%) has been found in cultured skin fibroblasts of all patients. Two complementation groups have been demonstrated, pcc A and pcc BC, the latter further divided into two subgroups pccB and pccC, which showed intragenic complementation. At the molecular level, pcc A and pcc BC correspond to the genes named PCCA and PCCB coding for the alpha and beta subunits of PCC, respectively. The β chain is unstable in the absence of the alpha chain (11,12). These data account for the heterozygote expression in PCC deficiency. Mean PCC activity in fibroblast extracts or peripheral blood leukocytes from pcc A heterozygotes is 50% of that in controls. This contrasts with PCC activity in pcc C heterozygotes, which is indistinguishable from that of controls, the latter data being consistent with compensatory balancing rates of synthesis and degradation for the two subunits in pcc C heterozygotes. Theoretically, beside the common biotin-nonresponsive PA, and independently of combined carboxylase deficiency, a biotin-responsive form of PA may exist. However, the first reports are confusing and its existence remains uncertain.

Biochemically, PA is characterized by greatly increased concentrations of free propionate in blood and urine. However, this major sign may fail and the diagnosis is based on multiple organic acid by-products present in the urine. Methylcitrate and 3-hydroxypropionate are major diagnosis metabolites. The latter product is formed either by β- or ω-oxidation of propionyl-CoA. Methylcitrate arises via condensation of propionyl-CoA with oxaloacetate by the action of citrate synthase. Otherwise, organic aciduria could include low levels of tiglylglycine, tiglic acid, and propionylglycine. During ketotic episodes, 3-hydroxyvaleric acid is formed via propionyl-CoA and acetyl-CoA condensation and reduction. Some lactate, 3-hydroxybutyrate, methylmalonate, 2-methyl-3-hydroxybutyrate, and several other organic acids may be present (13).

Methylmalonic Acidemia

Deficient activity of methylmalonyl-CoA apomutase and, because of the requirement by the apomutase for adenosyl cobalamin (AdoCbl), defects at any step of AdoCbl metabolism, can lead to methylmalonic acidemia (MMA). Nine classes of MMA are defined on the basis of complementation studies. Approximately one half of patients have a mutase apoenzyme defect further divided into mut^o and mut$^-$ groups. Mut^o group is B_{12} nonresponsive both *in vivo* and *in vitro* and CRM −. Mut$^-$ group is usually B_{12} nonresponsive *in vivo*, partially responsive *in vitro* and CRM +. It corresponds to a defective coenzyme-apoenzyme affinity. Recently, the human mutase gene has been cloned and assigned to chromosome 6 and the first molecular characterization of normal and mutant mutase are henceforth available (14). The remaining patients are cobalamin variants. Among them, Cbl A and Cbl B types implicate AdoCbl synthesis. CblA is due to a defect in mitochondrial cobalamin reductase and CblB to defective AdoCbl transferase. All Cbl A patients and 40% of Cbl B are B_{12} responsive. Cbl C, D, and F are characterized by reduced function of both methylmalonyl-CoA mutase and methionine synthase, resulting in combined methylmalonic aciduria and homocystinemia. Cbl C and D are due to a defect in cytoplasmic reduction of Cob(III)alamin. Most but not all patients are B_{12} responsive *in vivo*. The Cbl F is due to abnormal lysosomal release of cobalamin (15). Only one patient has been described with this defect.

Biochemically, impairment of mutase activity leads to accumulation of methylmalonyl-CoA and secondary propionyl-CoA, which is reflected by the presence in blood and urine of greatly increased amounts of MMA and PA. Propionyl-CoA metabolites such as methylcitrate, 3-hydroxypropionate, and 3-hydroxyisovalerate are usually found in the urine. Vitamin B_{12} deficiency must be excluded when excessive amounts of urinary MMA are found, even more so in infants who are breast-fed by a mother who is either a strict vegetarian (16) or is suffering from subclinical pernicious anemia. Some patients without B_{12} deficiency have also been found (especially in the neonatal period) with methylmalonic aciduria 10–50 times the normal level. However, they are "well babies," and no confusion with the true congenital MMA should occur if the proper analytical procedures of organic aciduria are employed.

Secondary Metabolic Disorders Common to PA and MMA

Propionyl-CoA and its metabolites are known to produce a variety of metabolic disturbances which have major effects on intermediary metabolism (inhibition of citrate synthase, pyruvate dehydrogenase complex, *N*-acetylglutamate synthetase, the glycine cleavage system, and pyruvate carboxylase). These inhibitions may explain some clinical features common to both disorders, such as hypoglycemia, mild hyperlactacidemia, hyperammonemia, and hyperglycinemia (13).

Patients affected with PA or MMA have increased acylcarnitines in blood and urine in which propionylcarnitine is the major metabolite. Thus a relative insufficiency of L-carnitine may occur in a state of continual propionyl-CoA accumulation.

Odd-carbon number fatty acids are precursors of propionyl-CoA, but propionyl-CoA can replace acetyl-CoA or *n*-butyryl-CoA as "primer" for *de novo* long chain fatty acid synthesis leading to the formation of odd-numbered fatty acids via malonyl-CoA and ethylmalonyl-CoA. By competition with malonyl-CoA, methylmalonyl-CoA is responsible for the accumulation of methyl-branched long chain fatty acids. This secondary effect has recently been studied in erythrocytes and reported as a potentially useful means for long-term assessment of these disorders (17).

CLINICAL PRESENTATION

Children with MSUD, IVA, PA, and MMA have in common many clinical and biochemical symptoms, which can be divided into three schematic presentations: a severe neonatal onset form, with metabolic distress; an intermittent late onset form; and a chronic progressive form presenting as hypotonia, failure to thrive, and developmental delay. In addition to these three presentations, the prospective data gathered by the Massachusetts metabolic disorders newborn screening program and the systematic screening of siblings have demonstrated the relative frequency of asymptomatic forms mainly for MMA (18). Most of the severe neonatal MMA forms belong to mut° class and are B_{12} unresponsive *in vivo*. Many late onset forms belong to CbLA or CbLB classes. There is an extremely rare thiamin-responsive MSUD which is always present with a late onset form (19).

Severe Neonatal Onset Form

The general presentation of this form can be summarized as a neurological distress "intoxication type" with ketoacidosis and belongs to type II of the classification of the neonatal inborn errors of metabolism (20) (Tables 1 and 2). An extremely evocative clinical setting is that of a full-term baby born after a normal pregnancy and delivery who, after an initial symptom-free period, undergoes a relentless deterioration that has no apparent cause and is unresponsive to symptomatic therapy. The interval between birth and clinical symptoms may range from hours to weeks, depending on the nature of metabolic block, and is not necessarily correlated to the

TABLE 1. *Five neonatal types of inherited metabolic distress*

Type	Clinical symptoms	Acidosis	Ketosis	Hyperlact-acidemia	Hyperam-monemia	Most frequent diagnoses
I	Neurological distress	0	+	0	0	Maple syrup urine disease
II	Neurological distress	+	+	0	+	Organic acidurias
III	Neurological distress	+	+	+	0	Congenital lactic acidemias
IVA	Neurological distress	0	0	0	+	Urea cycle defects
IVB	Neurological distress	0	0	0	0	Nonketotic hyperglycinemia, sulfite oxidase deficiency, peroxisomal disorders, respiratory chain defects
V	Hepatomegaly, liver dysfunction, seizures	+	+	+	0	Gluconeogenesis defects, galactosemia, tyrosinemia type I, α_1-antitrypsin deficiency

protein content of the feeding. Typically, the first reported sign is poor sucking and diminished feeding, after which the child sinks into an unexplained coma despite supportive measures. At a more advanced stage, neurovegetative problems with respiratory distress, hiccup, apneas, bradycardia, and hypothermia may appear. In the comatose state, most patients have characteristic changes in muscle tone and involuntary movements. Generalized hypertonic episodes with opisthotonus are frequent, and boxing or pedaling movements as well as slow limb elevations, spontaneously or upon stimulation, are observed. Another suggestive neurological pattern

TABLE 2. *Clinical presentation before treatment in 69 neonates[a]*

	MSUD ($n = 26$)	MMA ($n = 18$)	PA ($n = 15$)	IVA ($n = 10$)
Symptom-free period (days)	5	2.9	2.1	3.7
Feeding refusal	100	61	100	100
Coma	100	100	100	100
Hypertonia and abnormal movements	100	100	93	90
Ketosis	100	83	87	100
Dehydration	15	100	100	20
Acidosis	0	94	87	90
Hyperammonemia	19	100	100	100
Hypocalcemia	0	72	73	70

[a] Data are expressed as the percentage of *n*, the total number of patients.

is axial hypotonia and limb hypertonia with large amplitude tremors and myoclonic jerks which are often mistaken for convulsions. In contrast, true convulsions occur late and inconsistently. The EEG often shows a periodic pattern in which bursts of intense activity alternate with nearly flat segments.

Dehydration is a frequent finding in propionic and methylmalonic acidemia. A moderate hepatomegaly may be observed in IVA, PA, and MMA. Sometimes, the importance of vomiting associated with abdominal distension and constipation may suggest gastrointestinal abnormalities such as pyloric stenosis or intestinal obstruction. In isovaleric acidemia, a strong "sweaty feet" odor of urine and skin is constantly present in sick neonates as well as in late onset acute episodes. In MSUD concomitantly with the onset of neurologic symptoms the infants start emitting an intensive (sweet, caramel-like) maple syrup–like odor.

In IVA, PA, and MMA, laboratory abnormalities include metabolic acidosis (pH < 7.30) with increased anion gap, associated with ketonuria (Acetest 2 to 3 + when it is checked before, or early at the beginning of intravenous glucose infusion). However, ketoacidosis can be moderate and transient and is often responsive to symptomatic therapy. Hyperammonemia is a constant finding. When it is very high (>800 μmol/liter) it can induce a respiratory alkalosis and lead to the erroneous diagnosis of a urea cycle defect. Moderate hypocalcemia (<1.7 mmol/liter) and hyperlactacidemia (3–6 mmol/liter) are frequent symptoms. The physician should be wary of attributing marked neurological dysfunction merely to these findings. Blood glucose can be reduced or elevated. In some patients it may reach 20 mmol/liter or more before glucose administration. If associated with glycosuria, ketoacidosis, and dehydration, it may mimic insulin-dependent diabetes. Neutropenia, thrombocytopenia, nonregenerative macrocytic anemia, and pancytopenia are other frequent findings and often responsible for confusion with sepsis.

The final diagnosis is made by identifying specific abnormal metabolites by GLC-MS of blood and urine. Free carnitine plasma levels are constantly low, with abnormal excretion of specific acylcarnitine. By contrast, plasma and urine amino acid chromatography are often normal or may show a non specific profile such as a slight increase in glycine.

In MSUD, the dinitrophenylhydrazine test is strongly positive, whereas urine tests for acetone may be negative. None of our patients with maple syrup urine disease had an initial blood pH less than 7.30 (20). The diagnosis is confirmed by serum amino acid chromatography, which displays an elevation of the branched chain amino acids leucine (usually higher than 2 mmol/liter), valine, isoleucine, and the presence of alloisoleucine (3).

Intermittent Late Onset Form

In approximately one third of the patients, the disease presents with a late onset after a symptom-free period commonly longer than 1 year, or even in adolescence or adulthood. Recurrent attacks are frequent and in between the child may seem entirely normal. This makes the diagnosis difficult if adequate investigations have not been performed during the acute attack itself. Onset of acute disease may be precipitated by an infection or even severe constipation. Excessive protein intake, and all conditions that enhance protein catabolism, may exacerbate such decompensations. However, sometimes no overt cause is found. Recurrent attacks of coma and lethargy with ataxia are the main presentations of these late onset acute forms. The most frequent variety of coma is that presenting with ketoacidosis accompanied by low, normal, or high blood glucose levels, the latter condition mimicking insulin-dependent diabetes. Exceptionally, ketosis may be absent. Hyperammonemia is rarely encountered in attacks of ketoacidosis that occur later in infancy or childhood. Unlike patients with PA and MMA, patients with IVA are mostly normoglycinemic. Although most recurrent comas are not accompanied by neurological signs, we have observed PA, MMA, and MSUD patients who presented with acute hemiplegia and hemianopsia mimicking a cerebrovascular accident or cerebral tumor. A few patients with MMA developed acute extrapyramidal disease and corticospinal tract involvement after metabolic decompensation. The neurologic findings resulted from bilateral destruction of the globus pallidus with variable involvement of the internal capsule. This complication is not related to a specific gene defect, as it was observed irrespective of mutant class type and *in vivo* cobalamin responsivity (21). Cerebellar hemorrhage has also been observed in IVA, PA and MMA patients. These disorders must therefore be considered in the diagnostic list of metabolic strokes after respiratory chain disorders and urea cycle defects.

These apparent initial manifestations have frequently been preceded by other premonitory symptoms which had been missed or misdiagnosed. These symptoms include acute ataxia, unexplained episodes of dehydration, persistent anorexia, chronic vomiting associated with failure to thrive, hypotonia, and progressive developmental delay. Severe hematological manifestations are frequent in IVA, PA, and MMA, mostly concomitant with ketoacidosis and coma, sometimes as the presenting problem. Neutropenia is regularly observed in both neonatal and late onset forms of IVA, PA, and MMA. Thrombocytopenia occurs only in infancy and anemia only in the neonatal period. Recurrent infections are common and there appears to be a special relationship with *Candida*. Chronic mucocutaneous candidiasis is frequent and reflects the clinical status of the patient. Toxic metabolites might suppress the cellular immune system (22). Some children with frequent infections sustain a concurrent mild generalized hypogammaglobulinemia which improves when metabolic control is achieved (23).

Chronic Progressive Forms

Persistent anorexia, chronic vomiting, failure to thrive, and osteoporosis are frequent revealing signs. This "digestive" presentation is easily mistaken for cow's milk protein intolerance, celiac disease, late onset chronic pyloric stenosis, or fructose intolerance, particularly as these symptoms start after weaning and diversification of food. The anorexia is a prominent feature of these disorders. Some patients present with severe hypotonia, muscular weakness, and poor muscle mass and can simulate congenital or metabolic myopathies. Cardiomyopathy has been observed in PA and MMA. As plasma carnitine levels are severely lowered, as in IVA (24), the diagnosis of idiopathic systemic or muscular carnitine deficiency must be questioned in such patients. Nonspecific developmental delay and progressive psychomotor retardation as well as seizures can also be observed during the course of the disease. However, these rather unspecific symptoms are rarely observed as the only presenting symptom.

Complications

Skin Disorders

We have observed patients (with PA and with MMA) who presented a generalized staphyloccal cutaneous epidermolysis concomitant with an ultimate metabolic decompensation leading to death despite supportive measures. Rajnhere described severe skin lesions with vesicobullous and eczematous eruption in a PA patient. Complete healing of the skin was accomplished within a week by daily infusions of fresh frozen plasma (25).

Renal Complications

With early diagnosis and appropriate treatment, an increasing number of patients with the most severe forms of MMA are surviving longer. As a result, long-term complications are becoming apparent. Chronic renal impairment in MMA is becoming increasingly recognized, although only a few cases have been documented (26). However, in some patients affected with the subacute form, renal complications can be the presenting symptom. A transient tubular dysfunction presenting as a pseudocystinurialysinuria is also frequently observed in the severe neonatal form of PA, whereas it is not present in IVA and MMA (27). Acute pancreatitis have been recently described in MMA, PA, IVA, and MSUD (34).

TREATMENT AND PROGNOSIS

Over the past three decades, several hundred patients have been observed. Evidence is accumulating that the central nervous system dysfunction often associated with such organic acidurias can be prevented by early diagnosis, emergency treatment, and then by compliance to the restricted diet. This aspect is important in view of a more radical therapeutic development such as liver transplantation, which represents a real hope for the most severe cases of PA and MMA, who have to deal with recurrent life-threatening episodes of metabolic acidosis.

As discussed earlier in this chapter, patients affected with BCAA disorders are divided into neonatal onset forms and late onset forms. This heterogeneity of manifestation is reflected in the variety of therapeutic management strategies. Neonatal onset forms require early toxin removal. Thereafter, the restricted food pattern, essential to limit formation of organic acid by-products, is applied to survivors of the newborn period as well as to the patients affected with the late onset form. In both, the prevention and early treatment of recurrent episodes of metabolic imbalance is crucial. Each of these recurrent episodes is life-threatening and parents must be taught to recognize early warning signs and have an immediate plan for intervention.

The emergency management of BCAA disorders in the neonate has two main goals: toxin removal and promotion of anabolism. Toxin removal is achieved with blood exchange transfusions and peritoneal dialysis in IVA, PA, and MSUD; and with hydration and exchange transfusions in MMA (28). Additionally, thiamine 50 mg/day in MSUD, glycine 500 mg/kg·day in IVA, biotin in PA, and vitamin B_{12} in MMA should be tried in all cases, although the neonatal forms of these defects are rarely vitamin responsive. L-Carnitine (200 mg/kg) is systematically given in IVA, PA, and MMA. Additional treatment such as insulin or growth hormone may be considered. Anabolism is met by early effective continuous enteral nutrition with a protein-free diet. A special amino acid mixture free of precursors is added to the formula immediately in MSUD and as soon as ammonia levels are below 80 μmol/liter in IVA, PA, and MMA (3,13,20,28).

Long-term dietary treatment is aimed at reduction of toxic metabolites accumulated, in parallel with maintenance of normal development, nutrition status, and prevention of catabolism. In IVA, leucine intake can be increased up to 800 mg/day during the first year and then most of children can tolerate 20–30 g/day of vegetable protein if associated with oral L-glycine and L-carnitine therapy. In most PA and MMA early onset forms, the intake of valine must be severely restricted to 250–500 mg/day for the first 3 years of life, subsequently slowly increased to 600–800 mg/day by the age of 6–8 years. Supplementation with a synthetic amino acid mixture containing none of the amino acid precursors is generally recommended, although still controversial. In general, these infants are severely anorexic and the diet must be totally delivered through a nocturnal gastric drip feeding using a peristaltic pump. Long-term carnitine treatment may be considered. Metronidazole has recently been found to be effective in reducing excretion of propionate metabolites because of its activity against gut anaerobic bacteria (29). In MSUD, the BCAA intake has to be adjusted according to their plasma levels, which have to be monitored several times a week during the first weeks of life; later in life the intervals can be prolonged to 2–4 weeks. Leucine blood levels ranging from 0.1 to 0.5 mmol/liter are sufficient for normal growth and appear to prevent neurologic damage. In our experience, these levels can be achieved in most of the severe neonatal forms with a daily leucine intake ranging 400–600 mg/day during the first 5 years of life. There is, however, a considerable interindividual variation of the BCAA requirements during the first 3 months of life.

The long-term outcome of classic maple syrup urine disease under dietary therapy is still uncertain as both mental retardation and cerebral palsy are common. The outcome depends on early diagnosis and management. However, the most recent reviews (1,12,22,30–32) suggest that normal somatic growth and normal psychomotor development can be achieved if early diagnosis and treatment, subsequent long-term management, and meticulous attention to catabolic states accompanying even minor illnesses are guaranteed. A reasonable number of children with classic maple syrup urine disease are now developing normally and are performing well in the early elementary school grades (30).

Most of the late onset forms are easier to manage, patients tolerate up to 1.5–2 g/kg·day of protein, and amino acid mixtures are no longer necessary. In all CblA and 40% of CblB patients, hydroxocobalamin at a dose of 1 mg IM/day is very efficient. Some patients have gradually interrupted chronic B_{12} therapy without apparent discomfort. In MSUD, since some variants may respond to thiamin (19), a prolonged trial with supraphysiologic amounts of thiamin (20–200 mg/day) may be given, although additional treatment, such as a reduction of dietary branched-chain amino acids, must not be omitted (3). These late onset forms, as well as the vitamin-responsive forms, have an excellent long-term prognosis, although they may decompensate at any age and in unpredictable situations (33).

GENETIC COUNSELLING

All forms of MSUD, IVA, PA, and MMA are autosomal recessive disorders. The true incidences are estimated about 1/50,000 for MMA, 1/100,000 for PA and MSUD, and 1/200,000 for IVA. All forms of MSUD, IVA, PA, and MMA can be diagnosed early in pregnancy through the measurement of the defective enzyme activity in uncultured chorionic villi, and for IVA, PA, and MMA, through the direct measurement of abnormal metabolites accumulated in amniotic fluid as early as week 12 of gestation (3,13).

REFERENCES

1. Danner DJ, Armstrong N, Heffelfinger SC, Sewell ET, Priest JH, Elsas LJ. Absence of branched chain acyl-transferase as a cause of maple syrup urine disease. *J Clin Invest* 1985;75:858–60.
2. Hu C-WC, Chitayat D, Berns L, Braver D, Muhlbauer B. Peculiar odours in newborns and maternal prenatal ingestion of spicy food. *Eur J Pediatr* 1985;144:403.
3. Wendel U. Disorders of branched chain amino acid metabolism. In: Fernandes J, Saudubray JM, Tada K, eds. *Inborn metabolic diseases: diagnosis and treatment.* Berlin: Springer-Verlag, 1990;263–70.
4. Haan EA, Scholem RD, Croll HB, Brown GK. Malonyl coenzyme A decarboxylase deficiency. Clinical biochemical findings in a second child with a more severe enzyme defect. *Eur J Pediatr* 1986;144:567–70.
5. Bain MD, Jones M, Borrielo SP, et al. Contribution of gut bacterial metabolism to human metabolic disease. *Lancet* 1988;1:1078–9.
6. Langenbeck U, Wendel U, Mench-Hoinowski A, et al. Correlations between branched-chain amino acids and branched-chain alpha-keto acids in blood in maple syrup urine disease. *Clin Chim Acta* 1984;88:283–91.
7. Snyderman SE, Glodstein F, Sansaricq C, Norton PM. The relationship between the branched chain amino acids and their alpha-ketoacids in maple syrup urine disease. *J Pediatr* 1984;18:851–3.
8. Bartlett K, Gompertz D. The specificity of glycine-*N* acylase and acylglycine excretion in the organic acidemia. *Biochem Med* 1974;10:15–23.

9. Krieger I, Tanaka K. Therapeutic effects of glycine in isovaleric acidemia. *Pediatr Res* 1976;10:25–9.
10. Chalmers RA, Roe CR, Stacey TE, Hoppel CR. Urinary excretion of L-carnitine and acyl-carnitine by patients with disorders of organic acids metabolism: evidence for secondary insufficiency of L-carnitine. *Pediatr Res* 1984;18:1325–8.
11. Lamhonwah AM, Gravel RA. Propionic acidemia: absence of alpha-chain mRNA in fibroblasts from patients of the pccA complementation group. *Am J Hum Genet* 1987;41:1124–31.
12. Lam Hon Wah AM, Lam KF, Tsui F, Robinson B, Saunders ME, Gravel RA. Assignment of the alpha and beta chains of human propionyl-CoA carboxylase to genetic complementation groups. *Am J Hum Genet* 1983;35:889–99.
13. Ogier H, Charpentier C, Saudubray JM. Organic acidemias. In: Fernandes J, Saudubray JM, Tada K, eds. *Inborn metabolic diseases: diagnosis and treatment*. Berlin: Springer-Verlag, 1990;271–99.
14. Ledley FD, Lumetta M, N-Guyen PN, Kolhouse JF, Allen RH. Molecular cloning of L-methylmalonyl-CoA mutase: gene transfer and analysis of mut-cell lines. *Proc Natl Acad Sci USA* 1988;85:3518–21.
15. Surtees RAH, Leonard JV. Inborn errors of cobalamin metabolism. In: Fernandes J, Saudubray JM, Tada K, eds. *Inborn metabolic diseases: diagnosis and treatment*. Berlin: Springer-Verlag, 1990;607–21.
16. Higginbottom MC, Sweetman L, Nyhan WL. A syndrome of methylmalonic aciduria, homocystinuria, megaloblastic anemia and neurological abnormalities in a vitamin B12-deficient breast-fed infant of a strict vegetarian. *N Engl J Med* 1978;299:317–23.
17. Wendel U. Abnormality of odd-numbered long-chain fatty acids in erythrocytes membrane lipids from patients with disorders of propionate metabolism. *Pediatr Res* 1989;25:147–50.
18. Ledley FD, Levy HL, Shih VE, Benjamin R, Mahoney MJ. Benign methylmalonic aciduria. *N Engl J Med* 1984;16:1015–8.
19. Duran M, Wadman SK. Thiamine-responsive inborn errors of metabolism. *J Inher Metab Dis* 1985;8(suppl 1):70–5.
20. Saudubray JM, Ogier H, Bonnefont JP, et al. Clinical approach to inherited metabolic diseases in the neonatal period: a 20-year survey. *J Inher Metab Dis* 1989;12(suppl 1):1–17.
21. Heidenreich R, Natowicz M, Hainline BE, et al. Acute extrapyramidal syndrome in methylmalonic acidemia: "metabolic stroke" involving the globus pallidus. *J Pediatr* 1988;113:1022–7.
22. Müller S, Falkenberg N, Mönch E, Jakobs C. Propionacidaemia and immunodeficiency. *Lancet* 1980;2:551–2.
23. Wolf B, Hsia YE, Sweetman L, Gravel R, Harris DJ, Nyhan WL. Propionic acidemia: a clinical update. *J Pediatr* 1981;99:835–46.
24. Berry GT, Yudkoff M, Segal S. Isovaleric acidemia: medical and neurodevelopmental effects of long term therapy. *J Pediatr* 1988;113:58–64.
25. Rajnhere JR, Van Gennip AH, De Nef JJEM, Jakobs AJM. *Unusual skin disorder during treatment of a baby with propionic acidemia*. Leeds, UK: Society for Study of Inborn Errors of Metabolism. Sept. 1982. Abstract.
26. Walter JH, Michalski A, Wilson WM, Leonard JV, Barratt TM, Dillon MJ. Chronic renal failure in methylmalonic acidemia. *Eur J Pediatr* 1989;148:344–8.
27. Parvy P, Bardet J, Rabier D, Kamoun P. Pseudo-cystinuria-lysinuria in neonatal propionic acidemia. *Clin Chem* 1988;34:2158.
28. Saudubray JM, Ogier H, Charpentier C, et al. Neonatal management of organic aciduras: clinical update. *J Inher Metab Dis* 1984;7:2–9.
29. Thompson GN, Chalmers RA, Walter JH, et al. The use of metronidazole in management of methyl-malonic and propionic acidemias. *Eur J Pediatr* 1990;169:408–11.
30. Clow CL, Reade TM, Scriver CR. Outcome of early and long-term management of classical maple syrup urine disease. *Pediatrics* 1981;68:856–62.
31. Naughten ER, Saul IP, Roche G, Mullins C. Early diagnosis and dietetic management in newborn with maple syrup urine disease—birth to six weeks. *J Inher Metab Dis* 1985;8(suppl 2):131–2.
32. Wendel U. Acute and long-term treatment of children with maple syrup urine disease. In: Adibi SA, Fekl W, Langenbeck U, Schauder P, eds. *Branched-chain amino and ketoacids in health and disease*. Basel: Karger, 1984;335–47.
33. Rousson R, Guibaud P. Long term outcome of organic acidurias: survey of 105 French cases (1967–1983). *J Inher Metab Dis* 1984;7(suppl 1):10–12.
34. Kahler S, Woolf D, Leonard J, Lawless S, Zaritsky A, Sherwood WJ. Pancreatitis and organic acidurias. *28th Congress of the Society for the Study of Inborn Errors of Metabolism*. Birmingham, UK. Sept, 1990:abstr.

DISCUSSION

Dr. Wendel: You told us that there is no hyperlactacidemia in neurological distress "intoxication type II" (organic acidurias). In some cases there is lactic acidosis.

Dr. Saudubray: Yes, you are right. I tried in this presentation to emphasize the leading symptoms. The problem is to find the leading symptom and to choose from among the constellation of signs the best hallmark of the disorder. Lactic acidosis is not a leading symptom when you have this clinical presentation with ketosis, metabolic acidosis, and hyperammonemia.

Dr. Casaer: I should like to ask whether focal clinical signs, secondary to brain edema during metabolic deterioration, are seen more frequently in younger infants than in older infants and children. The reason I ask this is that there is some clinical evidence that brain edema can remain more focalized in young infants, while in older infants and children it has the tendency very quickly to become a diffuse edema of the whole brain.

Dr. Saudubray: I have never observed localizing neurological signs in neonates. I guess this is because the patient is deteriorating very rapidly, so he is hospitalized immediately in the intensive care unit and has no time to develop neurological symptoms. I don't know the exact pathogenesis of this very strange case of hemianopsia and hemiplegia. In some patients the diagnosis of cerebral tumor was very strongly considered until a CT scan and even ventriculography and encephalography were performed.

Dr. Wendel: You told us that there are no congenital malformations in patients with branched-chain organic acidurias. That is true. But I would like to stress that fetuses affected with propionic acidemia accumulate large amounts of odd-numbered fatty acids in body lipids, including brain. At 22 weeks of gestation various tissue lipids contain 6–7% of C15 and C17 fatty acids compared to about 1% in normal controls. We do not know the relevance of the odd-chain fatty acids accumulated in the fetal brain for the later psychomotor development. Most probably, during severe tissue catabolism such as after birth, the breakdown of adipose tissue during lipolysis might contribute to excessive accumulation of propionyl-CoA leading to symptoms of severe intoxication.

Dr. Saudubray: Odd-numbered fatty acids represent a very important source of propionyl CoA. Through stable isotope studies performed by Thompson and us in methylmalonic and propionic acidemia we were able to show that approximately one third of the propionyl CoA turnover comes from protein catabolism, one third comes from gut bacteria (anaerobic flora), and the final third probably comes from lipolysis. We are now doing experiments with the C13 propionate turnover to demonstrate this important source of propionate production.

Dr. Wang: I am interested by your methylmalonic acidemia group. During the past 3 years we have had four cases of MMA, and only one of them was responsive to vitamin B_{12}; the other three belong to the *mut* group. One of these persisted with minimal enzyme activity, while the other two had total deficiency of mutase activity. The outcome is that two of them died eventually, and one has psychomotor retardation. What is the outcome of your 31 MMA patients?

Dr. Saudubray: Our 31 MMA patients were collected over 20 years, so you cannot compare the patients we found in 1967 and the patients we found last year or yesterday. So collectively about two thirds of our patients (19 or 20) are mutase deficient, B_{12} unresponsive, with a complete absence of methylmalonyl-CoA mutase activity. Among this first group we need to divide the patients we observed in the first 10 years of our survey (i.e., in the late 1960s and the 1970s) from the patients we have observed in the 1980s. We have now changed our management completely, and we systematically insert a nasogastric tube immediately after the diagnosis, whatever the infant's appetite. We teach the parents to feed the child for a minimum of 20 h out of 24. Since we started with this method the patients are doing very well. Of course, it is a major constraint for the parents, but they don't have the terrible problem of feeding their child. These children are not anorectic at all, because they are not fed orally. They grow well because they are permanently in an insulin-secreting state. So since the 1980s these patients have been doing well. In the second group, composed of patients with the variant forms of methylmalonic aciduria (I mean either some B_{12} variants, CBLA, CBLB, or two patients with a minus mutation) the prognosis is good. It is very easy to manage these patients because they need only a slightly protein restricted diet and B_{12} therapy.

Dr. Brodehl: I also was interested in the long-term outcome of these patients. How are the patients with MSUD on long-term treatment?

Dr. Saudubray: I have had very good experience with the long-term outcome of MSUD patients. I feel it is really easy to manage these patients. It is as easy as PKU. You have to make a distinction between the 1960s and 1970s and the 1980s, of course, because our management has greatly improved. My general impression of the outcome in patients who have been treated since the beginning of the 1980s is good. I have five patients now attending regular school, in the regular level, and two of them are very bright, first in the class. So I am pretty sure that the results are even better than in PKU, because we are managing MSUD patients more carefully than the PKU ones. In PKU it is not acutely dangerous in the day-to-day management if plasma levels over 12 mg/dl occur, because there are no immediate symptoms. In MSUD, on the other hand, you get immediate consequences of daily variations in control.

Dr. Wendel: Clinicians need tools for monitoring patients on long-term treatment, not only methods for making diagnoses. In four out of six of our patients with propionic acidemia and methylmalonic acidemia there was a relative abundance of odd-chain fatty acids in erythrocyte lipids, while two extremely well treated patients had normal odd-chain fatty acid levels, which are about 0.7% of the total fatty acids. In one patient with methylmalonic aciduria and a very high odd-chain fatty acid level of over 5%, efforts were made to improve metabolic control. When oral treatment with metronidazole was started in order to reduce the propionate production by the gut bacteria, the level of odd-chain fatty acids came down very much to below 2%. To me the odd-chain fatty acid content in various lipids seems to be a valuable long-term measure of control in patients with disorders of propionate metabolism, and could be a useful indicator of disease severity in individual patients and hence a possible indicator of prognosis, like glycosylated hemoglobin (HbA_1) in diabetes.

Dr. Saudubray: I guess this must be one of the most convenient ways of monitoring long-term therapy of methylmalonic and propionic acidemia. In our prospective protocol in which we are starting to study the value of metronidazole therapy for the long-term management of methylmalonic and propionic acidemia we shall check the concentration of odd-numbered fatty acids in erythrocytes as an indicator of metabolic equilibrium.

Dr. Roe: I would like to ask about the late onset of propionic aciduria. I recently encountered a family in which a previously asymptomatic child presented for the first time at 2 years of age with ketoacidosis. His elder sibling of 4 years had propionic acidemia and this 2-year-old turned out to have the condition as well. His mother was pregnant and the fetus was also affected. I found it very unusual that the child was growing reasonably well. It is clearly a very mild form. I wonder if you have experience with similar types of families and if there is any explanation for the difference.

Dr. Saudubray: I have no explanation for this. I don't know of any similar situations. In my experience patients with late onset forms of propionic acidemia are in very bad health because paradoxically they presented with very severe hypotonia and may have destroyed their brain at the first attack. But I have no fortuitous association, within the same family, of one severe case and one mild case. Maybe you have to look at the possibility of composite heterozygocity with a combination of two different mutations. We observed in an MSUD family the coexistence of a mild form and severe neonatal form. The father was a compound heterozygote, both for the classical mutation and for another mild variant form as well. The mother was a classical heterozygote for the classical form. So they produced two kinds of children: one with the classical neonatal form due to true homozygocity with the classical mutation, and the other a heterozygote compound like the father.

Dr. Otten: Do you use tube feeding only for neonates? How long do you do it for, and do you expect that these children will ever eat by themselves?

Dr. Saudubray: When I teach the family what is in effect a management contract, I explain that it will last for a minimum of 5 years. After 1 year I reevaluate the tolerance of the nasogastric tube. If it is badly tolerated, we perform a gastrostomy for 5 years. Why 5 years? Because it is the most important period for the rapid growth. During this period you have very important variations in anabolism, depending on intercurrent infectious diseases. Feeding by gastric tube minimizes these variations.

Dr. Dufour: What is the cause of dehydration in MMA and PA?

Dr. Saudubray: The cause of dehydration is methylmalonic acidemia is very clear. Methylmalonic acid, secondary to accumulation of methylmalonic CoA, is a "cul-de-sac" of metabolism. The organism is unable to use this methylmalonic acid. The only way for detoxication is excretion through the urinary flow. The renal clearance of methylmalonic acid is very high. Dehydration is due to this very high renal clearance inducing enhanced diuresis. When you look carefully at these patients, both neonates and older children during an acute attack in the late onset forms, very frequently dehydration contrasts with enhanced diuresis. This association suggests that it is an osmotic mechanism. In propionic acidemia the situation is not so clear. Maybe the same explanation can be given for methyl citrate.

Inborn Errors of Metabolism, edited by
J. Schaub, F. Van Hoof, and H. L. Vis.
Nestlé Nutrition Workshop Series, Vol. 24.
Nestec Ltd., Vevey/Raven Press, Ltd.,
New York © 1991.

Genetic Diseases of Neurotransmitter Metabolism

Jaak Jaeken and Paul Casaer

Department of Pediatrics, Divisions of Nutrition and Metabolism, and of Neurology, University of Leuven, University Hospital Gasthuisberg, Herestraat 49, B-3000 Leuven, Belgium

Although there are many (established and putative) neurotransmitters, known diseases due to hereditary defects in the metabolism of these substances are rather few. The established neurotransmitter systems can be divided into *amino acidergic* [mainly the inhibitory γ-aminobutyrate (GABA) and glycine, and the excitatory aspartate and glutamate], *cholinergic* (acetylcholine), *monoaminergic* (mainly adrenaline, dopamine, noradrenaline, and serotonin), and *purinergic* (adenosine, ADP, AMP, and ATP), while increasing numbers of peptides are considered putative neurotransmitters. Possibly involved in neurotransmission and/or neuromodulation are the *N*-acetylamino acids and *N*-acetyl peptides. This chapter deals with hereditary diseases in the metabolism of glycine, GABA, dopamine, and *N*-acetylaspartate.

NONKETOTIC HYPERGLYCINEMIA

Nonketotic hyperglycinemia, probably the most frequent of the known genetic diseases of neurotransmitters, was first reported in 1963 (1). It has to be differentiated from the ketotic hyperglycinemia syndrome occurring in disorders of organic acid metabolism such as methylmalonic and propionic acidemia (2).

Clinical Picture

The majority of patients present with a generalized hypokinesia, hypotonia, and hyporeflexia within a few hours or days after birth. As a rule there is rapid progression to coma and apnea requiring artificial ventilation. Seizures are a prominent feature of this disease, presenting mostly as myoclonic jerks. The electroencephalogram shows early diffuse disturbances with a typical periodicity or burst suppression pattern. However, this pattern is not pathognomonic since it can also occur in newborns with herpes encephalitis or anoxia. After a few weeks hypsarrhythmia may follow. About half of these patients die rapidly (in a few days or weeks), while in the others death ensues after several years of evolution toward severe spasticity accompanied by extreme psychomotor retardation and intractable convulsions. Different degrees of involvement may be seen in the same family.

Apart from this classical neonatal form, atypical presentations have been reported with a later onset and a more benign clinical picture (3) or with a rapid "degenerative" course (2). Recently, Schiffman et al. (4) discovered a transient hyperglycinemia in two neonates with convulsions; the outcome was favorable. Inheritance is autosomal recessive.

Biochemical Defect

The metabolic marker of this disease is increased glycine in the cerebrospinal fluid (5). There are also increases of glycine in plasma (inconstant) and urine. Hyperglycinemia and hyperglycinuria secondary to organic acid disorders or to treatment with the antiepileptic drug dipropylacetate (6) are not associated with hyperglycinorachia.

The basic defect is in the glycine cleavage system of brain and liver. This system, located in the mitochondria, is the major catabolic pathway of glycine. It is composed of four protein components: P-protein (a pyridoxal phosphate-dependent glycine decarboxylase), H-protein (a lipoic acid–containing protein), T-protein (a tetrahydrofolate-requiring enzyme), and L-protein (a lipoamide dehydrogenase). These components interact to degrade glycine to CO_2 and NH_3. In nonketotic hyperglycinemia, defects have been identified in each of these proteins except the L-protein. Most patients with the classical neonatal form have an abnormality of the P-protein. The extent of the glycine cleavage defect may differ in brain and hepatic mitochondria (3). As the glycine cleavage system exists in placenta, prenatal diagnosis seems feasible on chorionic villi. It is not detectable in fibroblasts and amniocytes.

Treatment

No effective treatment is known. Strychnine blocks glycinergic inhibition and it has been used with moderate success in a few patients with the milder form of the disease; those with the classical phenotype do not respond (7).

Glycine may have excitatory effects on cortical neurons via facilitation of *N*-methyl-D-aspartate excitation. *N*-Methyl-D-aspartate receptor inhibition has therefore been proposed as a possible treatment for nonketotic hyperglycinemia (4).

INBORN ERRORS OF GABA METABOLISM

Three genetic diseases due to a defect in the brain GABA metabolism have been reported: pyridoxine-responsive convulsions, considered to be the consequence of

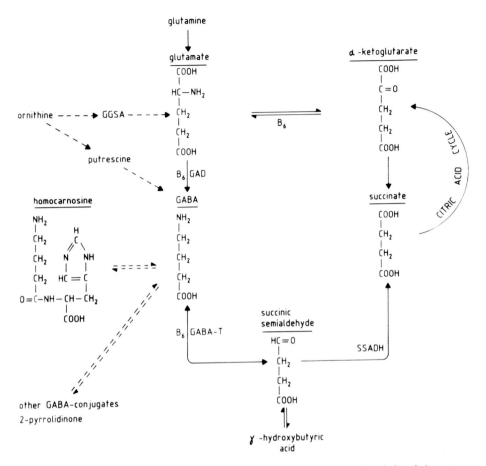

FIG. 1. Schematic representation of the brain metabolism of GABA. *B6*, pyridoxal phosphate coenzyme; *GGSA*, glutamic acid-γ-semialdehyde; *GAD*, glutamic acid decarboxylase; *GABA T*, GABA transaminase; *SSADH*, succinic semialdehyde dehydrogenase. *Dashed arrows* indicate reactions postulated.

a GABA synthesis defect (glutamate decarboxylase deficie.   nd two defects in the GABA catabolism: GABA transaminase deficiency and   nic semialdehyde dehydrogenase deficiency (Fig. 1).

Pyridoxine-Responsive Convulsions

This disorder was first reported in 1954 (8). It is a rare cause of convulsions in early childhood (9).

Clinical Picture

Typical pyridoxine-responsive convulsions have to be differentiated from the more recently identified atypical presentation. The typical form satisfies the following criteria:

Onset of convulsions before or shortly after birth (10)
Rapid response to pyridoxine
Refractoriness to other anticonvulsants
Dependence on a maintenance dose
Absence of pyridoxine deficiency (11)

The disease may start as intrauterine convulsions as early as the fifth month of pregnancy. Some patients have suffered from peripartal asphyxia probably as a consequence of this disorder. The seizures are intermittent at onset but may proceed to status epilepticus. There is a pronounced hyperirritability that can alternate with flaccidity. Abnormal eye movements are often reported (nystagmus, "rolling" eyes, miosis, and/or poor reaction of the pupils to light).

The atypical presentation (12,13) differs from the typical one by:

Later onset of the attacks (up to the age of 14 months)
Prolonged seizure-free intervals without pyridoxine (as long as 5 months)
The need for larger pyridoxine doses in some of these patients
Higher incidence

All types of seizures can be observed; long-lasting seizures and repeated status epilepticus are most common, but brief convulsions (generalized or partial), atonic attacks, and infantile spasms also occur.

Biochemical Defect

Pyridoxine-responsive convulsions are considered to be due to brain GABA deficiency resulting from a genetic defect at the pyridoxal phosphate coenzyme binding site of glutamate decarboxylase, the rate-limiting enzyme in GABA synthesis (15). Yoshida et al. (16) presented evidence but no definitive proof of glutamate decarboxylase deficiency in their patient. Brain GABA has been measured (postmortem) in only one patient (17) and cerebrospinal fluid GABA in another (18); values were low in both patients. No data are available on cerebrospinal fluid homocarnosine concentrations.

Treatment

The disease responds promptly to pyridoxine but is refractory to other antiepileptic medications. The minimum effective daily dose is at least 10 times the minimum daily amount recommended for healthy infants and usually varies between 10 and

100 mg orally. Treatment with isoniazid increases the minimum effective dose. The convulsions cease within a few minutes when pyridoxine is administered parenterally, and within a few hours when it is given orally. In the same patient the effect of a single dose lasts for a consistent period (usually 2–5 days) and is independent of the amount or method of administration. When treatment is interrupted, the seizures return, although there might be exceptions to this rule (delayed "maturation" of enzyme activity?) (18).

In case of (suspected) intrauterine convulsions, treatment of the mother with pyridoxine is effective (around 100 mg/day). In later onset presentation, doses of 100–200 mg may be necessary to control the seizures. Here also the minimum effective maintenance dose has to be determined individually. In the absence of early appropriate treatment, severe psychomotor retardation is the rule and if untreated the disease runs a fatal course, at least in the neonatal form.

In conclusion, a trial of pyridoxine should be performed in all unclear seizure disorders with onset before the age of 15 months.

Gamma-Aminobutyric Acid Transaminase Deficiency

Gamma-aminobutyric acid transaminase deficiency was first reported in 1984 in a brother and sister from a Flemish family (19). No other patients seem to have been described since then.

Clinical Picture

Both patients showed feeding difficulties from birth, often necessitating gavage feeding. They had a pronounced axial hypotonia and generalized convulsions. A high-pitched cry and hyperreflexia were present during the first 6–8 months. Further evolution was characterized by lethargy and psychomotor retardation (neither patient attained the level of a 4-week-old infant). Corneal reflexes and reaction of the pupils to light remained normal. A remarkable, continued acceleration of length growth was noted from birth to death (Fig. 2). This was explained by increased fasting plasma growth hormone levels (8–39 ng/ml; normal < 5); these could be suppressed by oral glucose. In one of the patients, head circumference showed a rapid increase during the last 6 weeks (from the 50th to the 97th percentile).

Biochemical Defect

Using ion-exchange chromatography with fluorescence detection (20), we found very high free GABA concentrations in the cerebrospinal fluid of the index patient (up to 60 times the median control value). Total GABA, homocarnosine (a GABA-histidine dipeptide), and "unidentified" GABA compounds (total GABA minus

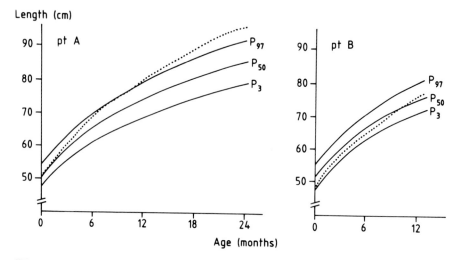

FIG. 2. Longitudinal growth of siblings with GABA transaminase deficiency. From Jaeken J, et al. (19).

homocarnosine and free GABA), as well as β-alanine, were only slightly increased in the plasma and urine. Liver GABA and β-alanine concentrations were normal.

This metabolic pattern could be explained by a decrease of GABA transaminase activity. In liver this activity was 18% of the median control value: 0.07 μmol/mg protein·h (median 0.38, range 0.31–0.69 in 10 controls); and in lymphocytes 2.2%— 48 pmol/mg protein·h (median control value 2,154, range 936–4,176, n = 6). In the patient's healthy sibling it was 24%, in her father 17%, and in her mother 40%. It can be assumed that the same enzymatic defect exists in the brain since GABA transaminases of human brain and of peripheral tissues have the same kinetic and molecular properties (21). β-Alanine seems to be an alternative substrate for GABA transaminase, hence its increase in this disease (22).

GABA transaminase activity is not expressed in fibroblasts (23) and thus prenatal diagnosis based on enzyme analysis of amniotic fluid cells is not feasible; however, activity is present in chorionic villous tissue (24). The pattern of occurrence in this family as well as the enzyme data strongly suggest autosomal recessive inheritance of GABA transaminase deficiency.

Treatment

We found no clear-cut biochemical or clinical response after administration of pharmacological doses of pyridoxine, the precursor of the coenzyme of GABA transaminase, not with picrotoxin, a potent noncompetitive GABA antagonist (25). To be efficient, any treatment should probably be started before birth. Outcome was fatal in both children at ages 1 year and 2 years, 7 months.

Succinic Semialdehyde Dehydrogenase Deficiency

Succinic semialdehyde dehydrogenase deficiency was first reported as γ-hydroxy-butyric aciduria in 1981 (26). It has been documented in at least 15 patients (27–29).

Clinical Picture

The clinical picture comprises nonprogressive ataxia, hypotonia, mild to marked psychomotor retardation, and less frequently, hyperactivity, choreoathetosis, autistic features, convulsions, hyporeflexia, nystagmus, and oculomotor apraxia. Clinical symptomatology as well as metabolite accumulation tend to decrease with age, at least in some patients (30).

Biochemical Defect

The hallmark feature is the increase in urine, plasma, and cerebrospinal fluid of γ-hydroxybutyrate formed by the reduction of accumulating succinic semialdehyde (Fig. 1). γ-Hydroxybutyrate can be higher in cerebrospinal fluid than in plasma and is extremely increased in some patients (31). It is a neuropharmacologically active compound. With currently used methods it is not detectable in the plasma of controls, but small amounts are present in urine (32). Cerebrospinal fluid GABA may (30) or may not be increased (27). Cerebrospinal fluid homocarnosine levels are increased. In about half of the patients, an increase in plasma glycine is mentioned. The enzyme defect, succinic semialdehyde dehydrogenase deficiency, has been demonstrated in lymphocytes and lymphoblasts; enzyme activity in intact cells has ranged from 3.7 to 11% of the mean control value (29). Enzyme activity is absent in control human fibroblasts but present in chorionic villous tissue (24).

Treatment

In an attempt to reduce the accumulation of γ-hydroxybutyrate in a 2-year-old Italian girl with this disease, we used the antiepileptic drug γ-vinyl GABA. This substance is known to cause an irreversible inhibition of GABA transaminase, the enzyme preceding succinic semialdehyde dehydrogenase. This treatment (75 mg/kg·day) has now been given for 2.5 years and has been accompanied by a significant and sustained clinical and biochemical improvement; ataxia and hyperactivity have decreased, electroencephalograms have improved, and the levels of cerebrospinal fluid γ-hydroxybutyrate have dropped to about 25% of the pretreatment value (27). This disease runs a much more benign course than GABA transaminase deficiency and no fatal outcome has been mentioned (at the time of writing the oldest reported patient is 11 years). Inheritance is autosomal recessive.

DOPA-RESPONSIVE HEREDITARY PROGRESSIVE DYSTONIA

Segawa et al. (33) first reported a variant of dystonia called "hereditary progressive dystonia with marked diurnal fluctuation." A remarkable feature of this disease is a complete or pronounced alleviation of the symptoms with small doses of L-dopa (34,35). At least 80 patients are presently known.

Clinical Picture

Age at onset of the dystonia is mostly between 1 and 10 years. It starts in the lower extremities mostly with gait difficulties and often remains limited to the extremities with no or minimal axial dystonia. In most patients (not in all!) there is a marked diurnal fluctuation of symptoms characterized by worsening of symptoms and increasing fatigue throughout the day, and marked benefit after sleep. Symptoms noted in a minority of patients are scoliosis, opisthotonus, dysarthria, dysphagia, postural tremor, and/or intermittent eye deviation. There is a great variability in the severity of the disorder. Some patients have been misdiagnosed for as long as 12 years as having cerebral palsy (36). It seems that the age of onset is earlier in girls and that they are generally more severely involved than boys. Available data strongly suggest dominant inheritance with low penetrance in most families.

Biochemical Defect

The precise biochemical defect underlying this disease is still unknown. The dramatic response to L-dopa suggests a dysfunction of dopaminergic systems in the basal ganglia of the brain. No consistent abnormalities of the catecholamines and their metabolites have been found in the cerebrospinal fluid of these patients. De Jong (37) found a biological half-life of dopamine reduced to about 50% of that of the control in three children with this disease after oral loading with deuterated L-tyrosine. This could point to an impaired dopamine storage in the basal ganglia. Recently, cerebrospinal fluid concentrations of homovanillic acid, 5-hydroxyindoleacetic acid, and biopterin were found to be decreased in five patients (38).

Treatment

Low doses of L-dopa (5–30 mg/kg·day) cause a marked improvement with complete or almost complete remission of symptoms, usually within days or weeks. Progressive improvement continues to occur for months in some cases without increase in dosage. On withdrawal of L-dopa there is immediate recurrence of symptoms. Although no long-term adverse effects of L-dopa therapy have been seen in this disease, it should be given at the minimum effective dose.

CANAVAN'S SPONGIFORM LEUKODYSTROPHY: ASPARTOACYLASE DEFICIENCY

Canavan reported on an early onset cerebral spongy degeneration in 1931 (39). This disorder was further delineated in 1949 by Van Bogaert and Bertrand (40). The basic defect was identified as aspartoacylase deficiency by Matalon et al. (41).

Clinical Picture

Onset is usually in the first 6 months of life. The main features are psychomotor retardation, hypotonia followed by hypertonia, excessive crying, seizures, and blindness. Macrocephaly is common. Progressive deterioration leads to a decorticate condition and death within a few years. Histologic changes involve astrocytic swelling and vacuolation of the myelin. Genetic transmission is autosomal recessive.

Biochemical Defect

The key feature is accumulation of N-acetylaspartic acid in the body fluids, levels in the cerebrospinal fluid being much higher than in the serum (42). The normal function of N-acetylaspartic acid is not well understood. It is abundant in brain, where its concentration is second only to glutamic acid in the free amino acid pool and is higher than that of GABA.

The enzymatic defect was discovered by Hagenfeldt et al. (43), who found aspartoacylase deficiency in fibroblasts from a boy with leukodystrophy. It was the achievement of Matalon et al. (41) to link this defect with Canavan's disease. Since aspartoacylase activity is present in cultured amniotic cells and chorionic villi, it is likely that the assay for this enzyme can be used for prenatal diagnosis (41).

Treatment

It has been proposed that N-acetylaspartic acid serves as a transporter of acetyl groups from mitochondria to the cytosol for lipogenesis. Therefore, in an attempt to supply alternative substrate for lipogenesis in the brain, a ketogenic diet was given to one patient for 5 months. No improvement was seen (43). No other treatment is available.

ACKNOWLEDGMENT

This work was supported by the Nationaal Fonds voor Wetenschappelijk Onderzoek Grant 3.0026.75.

REFERENCES

1. Mabry CC, Karam A. Idiopathic hyperglycinemia and hyperglycinuria. *South Med J* 1963;56:1444–5.
2. Nyhan WL. Nonketotic hyperglycinemia. In: Stanbury JB, Wyngaarden JB, Fredrickson DS, Goldstein JL, Brown MS, eds. *The metabolic basis of inherited disease.* New York: McGraw Hill, 1983;561–9.
3. Singer HS, Valle D, Hayasaka K, Tada K. Nonketotic hyperglycinemia: studies in an atypical variant. *Neurology* 1989;39:286–8.
4. Schiffmann R, Kaye EM, Willis III JK, Africk D, Ampola M. Transient neonatal hyperglycinemia. *Ann Neurol* 1989;25:201–3.
5. Perry TL, Urquhart N, MacLean J, et al. Nonketotic hyperglycinemia: glycine accumulation due to absence of glycine cleavage in brain. *N Engl J Med* 1975;292:1269–73.
6. Jaeken J, Corbeel L, Casaer P, Carchon H, Eggermont E, Eeckels R. Dipropylacetate (valproate) and glycine metabolism. *Lancet* 1977;ii:617.
7. Gitzelmann R, Steinmann B, Otten A, et al. Nonketotic hyperglycinemia treated with strychnine, a glycine receptor antagonist. *Helv Paediatr Acta* 1977;32:517–25.
8. Hunt AD, Stokes J, McCrory WW, Stroud HH. Pyridoxine dependency: report of a case of intractable convulsions in an infant controlled by pyridoxine. *Pediatrics* 1954;13:140–5.
9. Minns R. Vitamin B6 deficiency and dependency. *Dev Med Child Neurol* 1980;22:795–9.
10. Bejsovec M, Kulenda Z, Ponca E. Familial intrauterine convulsions in pyridoxine dependency. *Arch Dis Child* 1967;42:201–7.
11. Coursin DB. Vitamin B6 deficiency in infants: a follow-up study. *Am J Dis Child* 1955;90:344–8.
12. Stephenson JBP, Byrne KE. Pyridoxine responsive epilepsy: expanded pyridoxine dependency? *Arch Dis Child* 1983;58:1034–6.
13. Goutieres F, Aicardi J. Atypical presentations of pyridoxine-dependent seizures: a treatable cause of intractable epilepsy in infants. *Ann Neurol* 1985;17:117–20.
14. Scriver CR, Cullen AM. Urinary vitamin B6 and 4-pyridoxic acid in health and in vitamin B6 dependency. *Pediatrics* 1965;36:14–20.
15. Scriver CR. Vitamin B6 dependency and infantile convulsions. *Pediatrics* 1960;26:62–74.
16. Yoshida T, Tada K, Arakawa T. Vitamin B6-dependency of glutamic acid decarboxylase in the kidney from a patient with vitamin B6-dependent convulsions. *Tohoku J Exp Med* 1971;104:195–8.
17. Lott IT, Coulombe T, Di Paolo RV, Richardson Jr EP, Levy HL. Vitamin B6-dependent seizures: pathology and chemical findings in brain. *Neurology* 1978;28:47–54.
18. Kurlemann G, Löscher W, Dominick HC, Palm GD. Disappearance of neonatal seizures and low CSF GABA levels after treatment with vitamin B6. *Epilepsy Res* 1987;1:152–4.
19. Jaeken J, Casaer P, De Cock P, et al. Gamma-aminobutyric acid-transaminase deficiency: a newly recognized inborn error of neurotransmitter metabolism. *Neuropediatrics* 1984;15:165–9.
20. Böhlen P, Schechter PJ, Van Damme W, Coquillat G, Dosch JC, Koch-Weser J. Automated assay of γ-aminobutyric acid in human cerebrospinal fluid. *Clin Chem* 1978;24:256–60.
21. White HL, Sato TL. GABA-transaminases of human brain and peripheral tissues: kinetic and molecular properties. *J Neurochem* 1978;31:47–7.
22. Grove J, Schechter PJ, Tell G, et al. Increased gamma-aminobutyric acid (GABA), homocarnosine and β-alanine in cerebrospinal fluid of patients treated with γ-vinyl GABA (4-amino-hex-5-enoic acid). *Life Sci* 1981;28:2431–9.
23. Gibson KM, Sweetman L, Nyhan WL, et al. Succinic semialdehyde dehydrogenase deficiency: an inborn error of gamma-amino-butyric acid metabolism. *Clin Chim Acta* 1983;133:33–42.
24. Sweetman FR, Gibson KM, Sweetman L, et al. Activity of biotin-dependent and GABA metabolizing enzymes in chorionic villus samples: potential for 1st trimester prenatal diagnosis. *Prenat Diagn* 1986;6:187–94.
25. Olsen RW. GABA-benzodiazepine barbiturate receptor interactions. *J Neurochem* 1981;37:1–13.
26. Jakobs C, Bojasch M, Monch E, Rating D, Siemes H, Hanefeld F. Urinary excretion of gamma-hydroxybutyric acid in a patient with neurological abnormalities. The probability of a new inborn error of metabolism. *Clin Chim Acta* 1981;111:169–78.
27. Jaeken J, Casaer P, De Cock P, François B. Vigabatrin in GABA metabolism disorders. *Lancet* 1989;i:1074.
28. Jaeken J, Casaer P, Haegele K, Schechter PJ. Normal and abnormal central nervous system GABA metabolism in childhood. *J Inher Metab Dis* 1990;(in press).
29. Pattarelli PP, Nyhan WL, Gibson KM. Oxidation of (U-^{14}C) succinic semialdehyde in cultured human

lymphoblasts: measurement of residual succinic semialdehyde dehydrogenase activity in 11 patients with 4-hydroxybutyric aciduria. *Pediatr Res* 1988;24:455–60.
30. Rating D, Hanefeld F, Siemes H, et al. 4-Hydroxybutyric aciduria: a new inborn error of metabolism. I. Clinical review. *J Inher Metab Dis* 1984;7(Suppl I):90–2.
31. De Vivo DC, Gibson M, Resor LD, Steinschneider M, Aramaki S, Cote L. 4-Hydroxybutyric acidemia: clinical features, pathogenetic mechanisms, and treatment strategies. *Ann Neurol* 1988;24:304.
32. Gibson KM, Nyhan WL, Jaeken J. Inborn errors of GABA metabolism. *BioEssays* 1986;4:24–7.
33. Segawa M, Hosaka A, Miyagawa F, Nomura Y, Imai H. Hereditary progressive dystonia with marked diurnal fluctuation. *Adv Neurol* 1976;14:215–33.
34. Deonna T. DOPA-sensitive progressive dystonia of childhood with fluctuations of symptoms: Segawa's syndrome and possible variants. *Neuropediatrics* 1986;17:81–5.
35. Casaer P, Casteels-Van Daele M, Jaeken J, et al. Segawa syndroom. Dopa Gevoelige "Progressieve dystonie van het kind met sterke diurne fluctuatie": drie nieuwe observaties. *Belg Verenig Kindergeneeskd* 1988;20:97–9.
36. Boyd K, Patterson V. Dopa responsive dystonia: a treatable condition misdiagnosed as cerebral palsy. *Br Med J* 1989;298:1019–20.
37. De Jong APJM. Development of new mass spectrometric methods for the study of catecholamines. Investigation of patients with Segawa's disease. Thesis, Utrecht University, The Netherlands, 1988.
38. Fink JM, Barton N, Cohen W, Lovenberg W, Burns RS, Hallett M. Dystonia with marked diurnal variation associated with biopterin deficiency. *Neurology* 1988;38:707–11.
39. Canavan M. Schilder's encephalitis periaxialis diffusa. Report of a child of sixteen and one half months. *Arch Neurol Psychiatry* 1931;25:229.
40. Van Bogaert L, Bertrand I. Sur une idiotie familiale avec dégénérescence spongieuse du neuraxe. *Acta Neurol Belg* 1949;49:572.
41. Matalon R, Michals K, Sebesta D, Deanching M, Gashkoff P, Casanova J. Aspartoacylase deficiency and *N*-acetylaspartic aciduria in patients with Canavan disease. *Am J Med Genet* 1988;29:463–71.
42. Kvittingen EA, Guldal G, Borsting S, Skalpe IO, Stokke O, Jellum E. *N*-Acetylaspartic aciduria in a child with a progressive cerebral atrophy. *Clin Chim Acta* 1986;158:217–27.
43. Hagenfeldt L, Bollgren I, Venizelos N. *N*-Acetylaspartic aciduria due to aspartoacylase deficiency: a new aetiology of childhood leukodystrophy. *J Inher Metab Dis* 1987;10:135–41.

DISCUSSION

Dr. Mannaerts: L-Dopa is not only a precursor of dopamine but also of noradrenaline and adrenaline. So the defect in dopa-responsive hereditary progressive dystonia is not necessarily a dysfunction of dopaminergic transmission.

Dr. Jaeken: We have not analyzed this in this disease, but several groups have measured other catecholamine compounds and found normal levels.

Dr. Casaer: In a recent discussion, Dr. Segawa from Tokyo stressed that a more systematic study of catecholamines before, during, and after treatment could perhaps be helpful in understanding some of the underlying mechanisms. From analysis in our observations no clear-cut picture has emerged.

Dr. Dhondt: I think you definitely have to add biopterin deficiency to that list, because it is a real inborn error of the metabolism of neurotransmitters and probably is one of the best models for the dopamine and serotonin defect.

Dr. Endres: Concerning the treatment of undiagnosed seizures with pyridoxine I would like to propose that pyridoxal phosphate levels should be determined in cerebrospinal fluid (CSF) as well as in serum before giving pyridoxine. We have developed a very sensitive method and we sometimes find a very low CSF level in the presence of a normal serum level of pyridoxal phosphate.

Dr. Saudubray: I have a general comment and a question. I guess we can make a distinction between the disorders affecting the synthesis of neurotransmitters and the disorders affecting the catabolism of the neurotransmitters. Of course, as already suggested by Dr. Dhont, it is important to include in the list the disorders affecting the synthesis of biopterin, dihydropteridine reductase deficiency, and even PKU. It is important because in the clinical presentation of PKU offspring, one hypothesis for explaining mechanisms of congenital malformations is the abnormal synthesis of neurotransmitters. Along this line neurotransmitters could be considered as substances necessary for brain development, and we could expect to find congenital malformations as frequent findings in this first category. By contrast, in the second category, including the disorders of catabolism, I feel a little disappointed when faced with the very large variety and the nonspecificity of the clinical symptoms due to these disorders. But there are absolutely no congenital malformations suggesting that consequences of these disorders start after birth.

My question is about the physiological significance of acetyl amino acids. You presented Canavan's disease with acetylaspartaturia, which is a model of accumulation of acetyl amino acids. More generally, do you feel that this is a new field of investigation for inborn errors?

Dr. Jaeken: The significance of these acetyl amino acids and acetyl peptides is not understood. I think we can detect defects in the metabolism of these compounds by doing strong acid hydrolysis of the CSF. For example, we recently found a child with a large increase of alanine in the CSF after hydrolysis; in this child an accumulation of acetyl alanine has to be excluded.

Dr. Van Hoof: Dr. Jaeken makes an excellent point by insisting on cerebrospinal fluid analysis for the detection of abnormal metabolites. Did you note the accumulation of GABA in patients on valproate therapy? As you know, this drug inhibits ω-hydroxyacyl-CoA oxidation (1). 4-Hydroxybutyrate is thus expected to accumulate and this would reduce GABA transamination.

Dr. Jaeken: No, we have never observed this. But it could perhaps be below the detection level.

Dr. Saudubray: I have a comment on γ-hydroxybutyrate aciduria. This compound has been used and may still be used as an anesthetic drug. I remember some babies born from mothers who had been anesthetized with this compound. These babies were completely floppy. My other comment is on the "transience" of nonketotic hyperglycinemia. I totally disagree with Goodman's last paper (2). It is very unwise to treat nonketotic hyperglycinemia. I have personally observed three patients with the so-called "transient" nonketotic hyperglycinemia, and these patients are now mentally retarded after 4 years of life.

Dr. Jaeken: I agree with you. It remains uncertain whether the convulsions are the consequence of the increased CSF glycine in "transient" neonatal hyperglycinemia.

Dr. Schaub: This definition of "transient" is based on what? On the clinical picture? Or is it a biochemical definition?

Dr. Saudubray: The early clinical presentation is identical to the classical type of nonketotic hyperglycinemia with severe hypotonia, myoclonic jerks, and "bursts suppression" on the EEG. In CSF and sometimes in the blood you find high levels of glycine. In contrast to the usual course of the severe form of nonketotic hyperglycinemia, these patients get an unexpected improvement and all the symptoms can resolve. Glycine in CSF decreases slightly and can reach normal levels. But the long-term outcome is poor and all three patients I have observed have developmental delay.

Dr. Schaub: I think there may be a slight improvement with strychnine therapy as in the case of Gitzelmann and Baerlocher. Can Dr. Baerlocher comment on this case. What is the long-term outcome?

Dr. Baerlocher: The child you mention has a severe form of nonketotic hyperglycinemia. It survived spontaneously for the first 6 months and has since been treated successfully over 10 years with strychnine by Professor Gitzelmann. He has treated two more children (twins) with strychnine; both also showed some improvement but deteriorated rapidly after discontinuation of strychnine and died thereafter (3,4).

Dr. Jaeken: Regarding the transient type, the CSF glycine values were up to 463 μmol/liter, and it is conceivable that there could be a maturation defect in the glycine cleavage system.

Dr. Endres: I want to pursue the question of dopamine therapy. L-dopa is mainly decarboxylated in the periphery to dopamine, which cannot enter the brain. Since we require dopa to enter the brain, where its active metabolite forms, we administer at the same time a peripheral decarboxylase inhibitor (e.g., carbidopa). We do this in the severe forms of tetrahydrobiopterin deficiency. I saw on your Table 5 that you use 30 mg/kg·day of L-dopa. In comparison to our children this is a very high dose. As there are some long-term side effects such as nightmares and others, I would like to ask: What is the disadvantage of adding carbidopa to the medication of your patients?

Dr. Mannaerts: If you do not add a peripheral dopa decarboxylase inhibitor, most of the administered dopa will be decarboxylated to dopamine by a first-pass effect in the liver. Dopamine cannot penetrate the brain and can cause a number of serious side effects.

Dr. Casaer: In our present study protocol, we use L-dopa together with a peripheral decarboxylase inhibitor. As to side effects, we have never seen any gastrointestinal side effects. We monitor sleep and wake behavior very carefully and we pay detailed attention during the clinical examination to the possible development of dyskinesia or other "release" symptoms. In contrast to the children with juvenile Parkinson's disease, we have had few or no problems with finding an optimal dose in the children with Segawa syndrome.

Dr. Saudubray: About pyridoxine-responsive disorders, do you keep a difference between the so-called "pyridoxine dependency" and the pyridoxine-responsive convulsions? I remember an old paper with this distinction. Is it true?

Dr. Jaeken: No, it is not relevant. We have several patients with low-CSF GABA who do not respond to pyridoxine and I am sure that there are glutamate decarboxylase–deficient patients who are not responsive to pyridoxine as well, although this has not been yet reported. It is not easy to prove this because glutamate decarboxylase has many isoenzymes and there are different isoenzymes in brain and other tissues. This means that brain tissue is necessary for final diagnosis.

Dr. De Meirleir: In the last Münich meeting there was a presentation of a case of deficiency of L-aromatic decarboxylase, which is an enzyme responsible for the synthesis of serotonin and L-dopa. This is also a new neurotransmitter disease. How can we diagnose this easily?

Dr. Jaeken: This is an interesting disorder recently discovered by K. Hyland and P. Clayton in twins with severe hypotonia and convulsions. They showed decreased CSF and plasma serotonin and increased L-dopa, 5-hydroxytryptophan, and 3-methoxytyrosine, an L-dopa metabolite. A deficiency of aromatic L-amino acid decarboxylase was found, providing evidence that the decarboxylation of L-dopa and 5-hydroxytryptophan is catalyzed by a single enzyme in the human. Treatment with a monoamine oxidase inhibitor clearly improved the symptomatology.

Dr. De Meirleir: Would it be sufficient to measure serotonin levels in CSF or plasma?

Dr. Jaeken: I don't think so; you have to measure dopa itself.

Dr. Schaub: My question is: Can you use urine instead of plasma or cerebrospinal fluid for the diagnosis of deficiencies?

Dr. Jaeken: It depends on the disorder; for example, in GABA transaminase deficiency,

GABA is not increased in the urine and only slightly in the plasma. Therefore, CSF analysis is necessary for diagnosis.

Dr. Mannaerts: It might be possible to follow neurotransmitter release or turnover in the brain by following the urinary excretion of some specific metabolites.

Dr. Endres: I think in measuring urinary metabolites the problem is that we don't know whether they are coming from the brain or from the liver. So only in cases where we have a distinct disease (e.g., tetrahydrobiopterin deficiency) does it make sense to measure, for example, 5-hydroxyindole acetic acid and homovanillic acid in the urine. But, of course, it would be better to measure dopamine and serotonin in the CSF. However, it is clearly easier to obtain urine than CSF.

Dr. Dhondt: In your patients with L-dopa responsive dystonia, have you checked prolactin levels?

Dr. Jaeken: These levels were normal.

REFERENCES

1. Draye J, Vamecq JP. Interactions between the omega and beta oxidation of fatty acids. *J Biochem* [Tokyo] 1987;102:225–42.
2. Luder AS, Davidson A, Goodman SI, Greene CL. Transient nonketotic hyperglycinemia in neonates. *J Pediatr* 1989;114:1013–5.
3. Gitzelmann R, et al. Nonketotic hyperglycinemia treated with strychnine, a glycine receptor antagonist. *Helv Paediatr Acta* 1977;32:517–25.
4. Gitzelmann R, et al. Strychnine treatment attempted in newborn twins with severe nonketotic hyperglycinemia. *Helv Paediatr Acta* 1979;34:589–99.

Inborn Errors of Metabolism, edited by
J. Schaub, F. Van Hoof, and H. L. Vis.
Nestlé Nutrition Workshop Series, Vol. 24.
Nestec Ltd., Vevey/Raven Press, Ltd.,
New York © 1991.

Galactosemia

John B. Holton

Department of Clinical Chemistry, Southmead General Hospital, Westbury-on-Trym, Bristol, BS10 5NB, United Kingdom

Galactosemia, caused by a deficiency of galactose-1-phosphate uridyl transferase (EC 2.7.7.10), was the first clearly defined and is the most commonly occurring of the disorders of galactose metabolism. Although it has been proposed that galactosemia should be used as a collective term to describe all the forms of galactose disorder (1), this chapter is concerned only with galactose-1-phosphate uridyl transferase (transferase) deficiency, and galactosemia will refer specifically to this abnormality.

The term "classical galactosemia" is used to describe the most severe, neonatally presenting form of galactosemia and might be expected to result from a complete enzyme deficiency. In fact, patients described as transferase deficient may have a few percent of normal enzyme activity in red cells (2), and some who have an acute neonatal presentation are variants with as much as 10% of normal liver transferase activity (3). Although the early presentation may be similar to patients with quite varying amounts of transferase activity, those with significantly higher enzyme levels appear to have a better long-term outlook, at least in respect of the development of primary ovarian failure (4).

CLINICAL ASPECTS

The clinical picture of galactosemia is widely known and well described (1). The outcome of subjects with the classical form, given normal milk feeds, was usually neonatal death. Some patients survived into adult life because, fortuitously, galactose was restricted in their diet. The full, acute clinical picture is rarely seen if neonatal screening is introduced; and early diagnosis, with few clinical sequelae, is possible by maintaining a high index of suspicion, without screening. In a recent UK-based study of patients diagnosed clinically (Table 1), the most frequent presenting sign was prolonged neonatal jaundice, and a few babies developed severe signs, such as hepatosplenomegaly. This contrasts markedly with earlier data on neonatal presentation (5).

The long-term outcome of patients on the usual galactose-restricted diet causes

TABLE 1. *Frequency of clinical features in galactosemia diagnosed by clinical suspicion*

Clinical feature	UK survey[a] [Number (% of total)]	USA survey[b] [Number (% of total)]
Jaundice	13 (81)	34 (79)
Failure to thrive	5 (31)	23 (53)
Septicemia	1 (6) ⎫	
Urinary tract infection	1 (6) ⎬	5 (12)
Hepatomegaly	3 (18) ⎫	
Splenomegaly	1 (6) ⎬	39 (90)
"Hepatitis"	3 (18) ⎭	
Vomiting	2 (12)	17 (39)
Cataracts	2 (12)	19 (44)
	n = 16	*n* = 43

[a] 1988 data by Honeyman HM, Green A, Holton JB, Leonard JV, unpublished observations.
[b] Data collected from 1949 to 1978 by Donnell GN, et al. (5).

TABLE 2. *Survey of long-term outcome in 340 cases of diet-treated galactosemia*

	Method of diagnosis		
	Clinical symptoms	Newborn screening	Known relative
Total number in group	149	147	44
Median age and range (years)	10 (0–38)	3.5 (0–21)	13 (0–32)
Median age starting diet and range (days)	25 (3–550)	9 (2–45)	1 (1–7)

Late onset complications (age at assessment)	Percentage showing complications[a] (total number assessed)		
Developmental delay (≥6 years)	45 (95)	36 (36)	32 (25)
Speech abnormality (≥4 years)	53 (105)	57 (63)	70 (27)
Ovarian dysfunction (≥12 years)	87 (38)	80 (5)	80 (15)
Growth retardation (≥1.5 years)	21 (126)	14 (106)	12 (28)

[a] None of the differences between diagnostic groups reach significance.
From Buist N, et al. (6).

much concern, however. A survey of a large group of patients (Table 2) has indicated the full extent of the problems in mental development, growth, and speech, and the recently recognized complication in females, ovarian failure. It should be noted that the incidence of the clinical abnormalities does not appear to vary with the time of starting diet, and therefore the implication is that the problems may originate prenatally or may be caused because of inadequate or unsuitable treatment.

Two unusual complications should be mentioned. First, pseudotumor cerebri (cerebral edema) has occurred in sufficient cases neonatally to suggest that it is a direct consequence of the disease (7). Its possible pathogenesis will be discussed later. Second, a few patients have developed severe neurological degeneration despite dietary treatment (8). Features include profound mental retardation, hypotonia, tremor, and ataxia. These cases may be regarded as a separate subgroup of the condition, in which case a specific cause for the complications has to be postulated. Otherwise, they may be seen as the extreme of a continuous range of the usual neurological signs, which include mild mental retardation and abnormal speech.

BIOCHEMISTRY

Figure 1 shows the main pathways of galactose metabolism and the principal enzymes involved. Transferase is an essential requirement for the production of glc-1-P from galactose, via galactose-1-P and UDPgal. This pathway is particularly important in the infant, whose principal carbohydrate source is lactose. As discussed later, and contrary to earlier understanding, transferase also appears necessary for the optimal production of UDPgal, the cofactor for incorporation of galactose into galactosides.

A deficiency of transferase leads to three important metabolic perturbations. First,

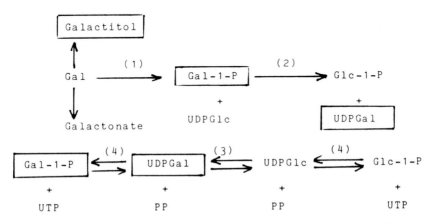

FIG. 1. Pathways of galactose metabolism: The boxed metabolites are those thought to be most concerned in the pathogenesis of galactosemia. Enzymes; *1,* galactokinase; *2,* galactose-1-phosphate uridyl transferase; *3,* UDP galactose-4-epimerase; *4,* pyrophosphorylase.

increased concentrations of galactitol are formed from galactose and accumulate in plasma, urine, and tissues (9). Brain and muscle of galactosemic patients have particularly high levels of galactitol, but the concentration in the lens of the eye is fairly moderate in comparison. This is contrary to the findings in experimental galactosemia in rats fed high-galactose diets, in which the highest concentrations of galactitol were in the lens (9). Although the plasma and urine concentrations of galactitol in galactose-restricted galactosemic patients are very significantly reduced, they remain above the normal range.

The second metabolic abnormality in galactosemia is a large accumulation of gal-1-P in tissues and erythrocytes. The levels of gal-1-P also decline on a galactose-restricted diet, but certainly red cell levels continue to be significantly elevated. This has been described as a "self-intoxication" (10), due to endogenous synthesis of gal-1-P from glc-1-P involving pyrophosphorylase and epimerase (Fig. 1). Some doubt has to be placed on this explanation in view of the foregoing discussion on UDPgal depletion in treated galactosemics. An alternative explanation is that the small amount of galactose which remains in the diet, and which is released from the turnover of glycoproteins, is trapped by efficient conversion to gal-1-P (11).

The final and most recently recognized metabolic abnormality is a low concentration of UDPgal demonstrated in treated galactosemics in erythrocytes (12), and additionally, in cultured skin fibroblasts and liver (13). Ng et al. (13) have argued that UDPgal cannot be generated in sufficient quantities from Glc-1-P, via the pyrophosphorylase and epimerase reactions (Fig. 1), and transferase is essential to maintain normal UDPgal levels. On the other hand, patients with as little as 1% of normal transferase activity can maintain UDPgal levels (Table 3). As mentioned in the preceding paragraph, the apparent inability to maintain normal UDPgal levels in treated

TABLE 3. *Erythrocyte gal-1-P, UDPglc, and UDPgal levels[a] in control subjects, classical galactosemia, and low-activity transferase variant patients[b]*

	Galactosemia patients		
	Classical (n = 26)	Low-activity variants (n = 3)	Control subjects
Gal-1-P (mg/100 ml RBC)	2.66 ± 0.53	2.25 ± 0.47	0
UDPglc (μmol/100 g Hb)	38.9 ± 14.6	44.1 ± 10.2	38.1 ± 7.1
UDPgal (μmol/100 g Hb)	3.88 ± 1.79	9.4 ± 3.53	10.3 ± 3.5

[a] Level are mean ± SEM.
[b] Transferase activities (μmol/g Hb/h) were control subjects, greater than 7; classical galactosemia patients, zero; low-activity variant patients, 0.15, 0.018, and 0.004.
From Kaufman FR, et al. (4).

galactosemic patients would suggest that the high gal-1-P concentrations in them are unlikely to arise from the pyrophosphorylation of UDPgal.

PATHOGENESIS

Three pathogenic mechanisms have been postulated to explain the clinical manifestations of galactosemia, and each is connected to one of the main biochemical changes discussed in the preceding section. The accumulation of galactitol in the lens of the eye has been linked to the formation of cataracts (1), particularly since an abnormality of this metabolite is the principal biochemical finding in galactokinase deficiency, and cataracts are the only established clinical sign of this disorder. The actual process of cataract formation consequent upon galactitol accumulation and osmotic swelling of the lens has received a great deal of attention, particularly because the problem seems analogous to that in diabetic cataract in which the polyol, sorbitol, is involved. One proposal is that increased lens polyols cause, secondarily, a depletion in myoinositol levels, and this is the key mediator in cataract formation (14).

Polyol accumulation, myoinositol depletion, and consequently, deranged phosphatidylinositol turnover have also be postulated to constitute a mechanism of diabetic peripheral neuropathy (15). This hypothesis has been extended to implicate galactitol in the pathogenesis of mental retardation in galactosemia. Synaptosomes prepared from the cerebra of galactose-intoxicated rats show an impairment of phosphatidylinositol turnover linked to stimulation with acetylcholine (16). Despite these interesting experiments, their relevance to the cause of mental retardation in galactosemic patients has to be questioned because this clinical abnormality does not complicate galactokinase deficiency despite the same tendency to accumulate galactitol.

Galactitol accumulation has been implicated in pseudotumor cerebri, which was mentioned earlier (7). The high concentration of galactitol in brain, its osmotic effect, and the fact that this clinical complication has been described in galactokinase deficiency make the connection plausible. The question that has to be addressed is why the abnormality occurs only in rare instances.

The earliest hypothesis on the pathogenesis of galactosemia involved gal-1-P, and this arose mainly because the rapid fall in gal-1-P levels subsequent to dietary treatment precede the resolution of the acute toxic signs of the disorder, and because neither this biochemical sign nor the early clinical signs are features of galactokinase deficiency. However, direct evidence for the hypothesis, or for the exact mechanism, is lacking. Experimentally, gal-1-P is an inhibitor of various enzymes in the glycolytic and pentose phosphate pathways *in vitro* (17), but there is no indication that inhibition occurs in galactose-intoxicated animals. The idea that trapping of ATP in gal-1-P causes a general depletion of high-energy compounds is a more plausible mechanism and is supported by observations on the toxicity of galactose analogs in animals, in which liver damage is a feature (18). In addition, reduced liver ATP and erythrocyte

TABLE 4. *Carbohydrate composition of transferase deficient and control cell lines grown on a galactose-depleted medium[a]*

Cell type	$\dfrac{\mu\text{g mannose}}{\text{mg protein}}$	$\dfrac{\mu\text{g galactose}}{\text{mg protein}}$	$\dfrac{\mu\text{g(sialic acid + galactose)}}{\mu\text{g mannose}}$	$\dfrac{\mu\text{g galactose}}{\mu\text{g mannose}}$
Controls ($n = 8$)	0.85 ± 0.25	0.83 ± 0.21	1.46 ± 0.37	1.00 ± 0.22
Transferase-deficient ($n = 6$)	0.78 ± 0.37	0.60 ± 0.32	$1.08^b \pm 0.13$	$0.77^b \pm 0.08$

[a] Skin biopsies were cultured and stored by standard techniques. In the experiments, cells were grown for at least three passages in TC 199 culture medium supplemented with 10% (v/v) fetal calf serum that had been dialyzed against three changes of 50 volumes of isotonic saline to remove uncombined galactose. The cells were then washed in three changes of phosphate buffer saline and harvested with trypsin/EDTA solution. The cell suspension was centrifuged and the supernatant discarded. The cells were resuspended in water, an aliquot removed for protein estimation, and the remainder was freeze-dried after freezing in liquid nitrogen. The carbohydrate composition of the freeze-dried cells was determined by gas-liquid chromatography.
[b] Difference control and transferase-deficient cell lines, $p < 0.05$.

UTP levels have been found in galactosemic patients (19). This may be a model for liver damage in galactosemia, but there is no clear indication of other clinical signs that may be due to the gal-1-P mechanism.

One original concern about the future of galactosemic patients regarded whether they could incorporate galactose normally into complex molecules, particularly when dietary galactose was restricted. It was argued, however, that a failure in galactoside synthesis would have a profound effect on a child's development, perhaps being incompatible with life, and the apparent health of treated patients seemed to rule out this worrying possibility. Moreover, a biochemical pathway for the endogenous production of UDPgal, the cofactor for galactoside synthesis, appeared to be available, as discussed earlier.

The recent demonstration of UDPgal depletion in galactosemia reintroduced the possibility of defective galactoside synthesis. A close correlation between low UDPgal levels in erythrocytes and the presence of ovarian failure (4) suggested an involvement of UDPgal in the pathogenesis of this clinical complication, through an effect on galactoside synthesis. The extremely high concentration of galactosides in the ovary seems to lend support for this hypothesis.

As with all the proposed pathogenic mechanisms, direct evidence for the foregoing hypothesis is lacking. Recently, however, it has been shown that skin fibroblasts from galactosemic patients, grown on a low galactose medium, have a significantly reduced amount of galactose in glycoprotein compared to normal fibroblasts under the same conditions (Table 4). The essential role of galactosides in many tissues (e.g., the central nervous system) suggests a possibly wider implication for this pathogenic mechanism than simply ovarian failure.

TREATMENT

The mainstay of the present treatment is removing milk and milk products from the diet. The need for restricting galactoside-containing foods as a source of free galactose is debatable (20). Recent data, albeit on a limited number of patients, suggest that the introduction of legumes and pulses causes a rise in gal-1-P levels (Table 5), although it is not known whether this is significant in terms of outcome.

The long-term outcome of galactosemic patients is a cause for concern. Many questions need to be answered to plan a logical strategy to achieve a satisfactory improvement in outcome. First, is damage caused in the fetus which is irreversible and affects prognosis? It is known that the metabolic disorder is well established in the midterm fetus. Second, is the present level of galactose restriction satisfactory since it allows slightly raised levels of galactitol and gal-1-P to persist? Third, if UDPgal depletion is a pathogenic factor, can measures be taken to stimulate UDPgal synthesis and improve outcome? There is already some work which suggests that orotic acid administration might have a beneficial effect (21,22).

Since the preceding questions may take many years to answer, empirical approaches to new therapies may be justified provided that they are carried out in a systematic way. These trials could include attempts to stimulate transferase activity, particularly in patients with some initial amount of enzyme (23), administration of inositol to counteract the effects of persistent galactitol accumulation and consequent inositol depletion, attempts to control gal-1-P levels by dietary or other measures, and treatment with uridine, or orotic acid, to stimulate UDPgal synthesis. The answer to the question regarding possible intrauterine origin of damage is paramount, however, since if this occurs, successful prevention, if it is possible, holds the key to achieving better outcome.

TABLE 5. *Effect of incorporating pulses and legumes into the diet of galactosemic children*

Diet group	Mean gal-1-P (μmol/liter packed RBC) (number of observations)		% Change
	Jan 1978 to Dec 1982	Jan 1983 to Dec 1988	
Supplemented			
Patient 1	59 (9)	118 (9)	+100
2	78 (9)	118 (11)	+51
3	86 (12)	104 (11)	+21
4	65 (10)	103 (7)	+58
Unsupplemented			
Patient 1	211 (12)	175 (36)	−17
2	72 (10)	99 (18)	+37
3	46 (11)	37 (9)	−19
4	146 (3)	112 (4)	−23

DIAGNOSIS

The presumptive diagnosis of galactosemia can be made from newborn population screening or can rely on clinical suspicion of the disease. There is considerable division of opinion on the need for screening. All the evidence suggests that early diagnosis and treatment is not a factor in influencing long-term outcome (Table 2), and therefore the principal reason for screening is not fulfilled. Screening at an early age, with efficient production of results, will however prevent the death of some galactosemic infants whose diagnosis is missed, or made too late, by the clinician. The proportion of babies in this category is not known accurately but may not exceed 10% of living cases. In a situation in which the health budget is strictly controlled, the limited benefits of galactosemia screening may not justify its introduction.

A definitive diagnosis should always be made using a quantitative erythrocyte transferase assay, and in view of the work discussed linking outcome with very small differences in the level of enzyme activity, a sensitive method that can distinguish these differences in activity is advisable (2).

Prenatal diagnosis is rarely requested at the present time, but it is possible to perform it by the direct assay of transferase in chorionic villi, or in cultured amniotic fluid cells, and by galactitol estimations in amniotic fluid supernatant (24). Despite the availability of a cDNA gene probe for transferase, it has not yet been found possible to track the galactosemia gene (25).

REFERENCES

1. Segal S. Disorders of galactose metabolism. In: Stanbury JB, Wyngaarden JB, Fredrickson DS, Goldstein JL, Brown MS, eds. *The metabolic basis of inherited disease*. New York: McGraw-Hill Book Co., 1983; 167–91.
2. Ng WG, Kline F, Lin J, Koch R, Donnell GN. Biochemical studies of a human low activity galactose-1-phosphate uridyl transferase variant. *J Inher Metab Dis* 1978;1:145–51.
3. Segal S, Rogers S, Holtzapple PG. Liver galactose-1-phosphate uridyl transferase. Activity in normal and galactosemic subjects. *J Clin Invest* 1971;50:500–6.
4. Kaufman FR, Xu YK, Ng WG, Donnell GN. Correlation of ovarian function with galactose-1-phosphate uridyl transferase level in galactosemia. *J Pediatr* 1988;112:754–6.
5. Donnell GN, Koch R, Fishler K, Ng WG. Clinical aspects of galactosaemia. In: Burman D, Holton JB, Pennock CA, eds. *Inherited disorders of carbohydrate metabolism*. Lancaster, UK: MTP Press Ltd, 1980;103–15.
6. Buist N, Waggoner D, Donnell GN, Levy H. The effect of newborn screening in galactosemia: results of the international survey. *Abstracts of the 26th Annual Symposium of the Society for the Study of Inborn Errors of Metabolism*. SSIEM, 1988;53.
7. Huttenlocher PR, Hillman RE, Hsia YE. Pseudotumor cerebri in galactosemia. *J Pediatr* 1970;76: 902–5.
8. Lo W, Packman S, Nash S, *et al*. Curious neurologic sequelae in galactosemia. *Pediatrics* 1984;73: 309–12.
9. Quan-Ma R, Wells H, Wells W, Sherman F, Egan T. Galactitol in the tissues of a galactosemic child. *Am J Dis Child* 1966;112:477–8.
10. Gitzelmann R, Hansen RG. Galactose metabolism, hereditary defects and their clinical significance. In: Burman D, Holton JB, Pennock CA, eds. *Inherited disorders of carbohydrate metabolism*. Lancaster, UK: MTP Press Ltd. 1980;61–101.
11. Pourci ML, Mangeot M, Lammonier A. Origin of the galactose-1-phosphate present in erythrocytes and fibroblasts of treated galactosemic patients. *IRCS Med Sci* 1985;13:1232–3.

12. Shin YS, Rieth M, Hoyer S, Endres W. Uridine diphosphogalactose, galactose-1-phosphate and galactitol concentration in patients with classical galactosemia. *Abstracts of the 23rd Annual Symposium of the Society for the Study of Inborn Errors of Metabolism.* SSIEM, 1985;35.

13. Ng WG, Xu YK, Kaufman F, Donnell GN. Deficit of urine diphosphate galactose (UDPgal) in galactosemia (abstract). *Am J Hum Genet* 1987;41(Suppl):A12.

14. Broekhuyse R. Changes in myo-inositol permeability in the lens due to cataractous condition. *Biochim Biophys Acta* 1968;163:269–72.

15. Finegold D, Lattimer SA, Nolle S, Bernstein M, Greene DA. Polyol pathway activity and myo-inositol metabolism: a suggested relationship in the pathogenesis of diabetic neuropathy. *Diabetes* 1983;32: 988–92.

16. Berry G, Yandrasitz JR, Segal S. Experimental galactose toxicity: effects on synaptosomal phosphatidylinositol metabolism. *J Neurochem* 1981;37:888–91.

17. Sidbury JB. The role of galactose-1-phosphate in the pathogenesis of galactosemia. In: Gardner LI, ed. *Molecular genetics and human disease.* Springfield, IL: Charles Thomas, 1961;61–82.

18. Starling JJ, Kepler DOR. Metabolism of 2-deoxy-*d*-galactose in liver induces phosphate and uridylate trapping. *Eur J Biochem* 1977;80:373–9.

19. Forster J, Schuchmann L, Hans C, Niederhoff H, Künzer W, Keppler D. Increased serum urate in galactosaemia patients after a galactose load: a possible role of nucleotide deficiency in galactosaemic liver injury. *Klin Wochenschr* 1975;53:1169–70.

20. Anon. Clouds over galactosaemia. *Lancet* 1982;ii:1379–80.

21. Tada K, Kudo Z, Ohno T, Akabane J, Chica R. Congenital galactosemia and orotic acid therapy with promising results. *Tohoku J Exp Med* 1962;77:340–2.

22. Keppler D, Rudiquier J, Reutter W. Orotate prevents galactosamine hepatitis. *Hoppe Saylers Z Physiol Chem* 1970;351:102–4.

23. Pesch LA, Segal S, Topper Y. Progesterone effects on galactose metabolism in prepubertal patients with congenital galactosaemia and in rats maintained on high galactose diets. *J Clin Invest* 1960;39:178–84.

24. Holton JB, Allen JT, Gillett MG. Prenatal diagnosis of disorders of galactose metabolism. *J Inher Metab Dis* 1989;12(Suppl 1):202–6.

25. Reichardt JKV, Berg P. Cloning and characterization of a cDNA encoding human galactose-1-phosphate uridyl transferase. *Mol Biol Med* 1988;5:107–22.

DISCUSSION

Dr. Schaub: Can galactitol pass the placenta from the fetus to the mother? And has galactitol ever been detected in the urine of a pregnant heterozygote mother of a homozygote fetus?

Dr. Holton: I don't think there is any evidence that the galactitol passes the placenta from the fetus to the mother. It would probably be very small amounts if it did. We have measured galactitol in the pregnant mothers carrying a homozygote galactosemic fetus and it was not increased. Galactitol accumulates in very large amounts in the fetus. Concentrations in the liver and fluids of the fetus are equivalent to the postnatal levels, or very close to postnatal levels. So if it is cleared it is not cleared very efficiently by the mother.

Dr. Odièvre: We recently followed a homozygous mother on a galactose-free diet during her pregnancy (1). We measured galactose-1-phosphate in the red blood cells and urinary lactose excretion. She excreted large amounts of lactose in the urine during the last weeks before parturition, while the concentration of gal-1-P in RBC and galactitol in urine was increased. The fetus was heterozygous and the level of galactose-1-phosphate in his blood cord was very high. Urinary galactose in the mother resulted from *de novo* synthesis of lactose. It would be interesting to see if similar findings are also present in heterozygous mothers. Can we hope to prevent lactose synthesis by the mother before parturation using some kind of hormonal treatment?

Dr. Endres: I would like to try to answer this question concerning the neurological abnormalities in treated galactosemics. Until some years ago we believed that treatment of galactosemia was very easy and there were no grounds for prenatal diagnosis. Then we heard from two groups, one in Erlangen, Germany, and the other in Los Angeles, that some patients with neurological abnormalities had been observed despite of good dietary treatment. Then we had the international survey, in which we participated too. I would like to show you some data concerning the German patients. We correlated mental development to the start of therapy. In patients where the dietary treatment was started before 2 weeks of age there were two patients who were severely retarded. If you correlate the neurological abnormalities to the start of diet, there were five patients who developed neurological abnormalities despite the fact that the therapy was started at an early stage. In 17 of 64 patients (i.e., 27%) mental retardation and neurological abnormalities have been observed, and in two of these 17 patients early diagnosis and treatment was established. In the remaining 15 patients either the diagnosis was too late or the dietary control was bad or unknown. In several cases we had no information about galactose-1-phosphate levels in red blood cells. We need to perform an international prospective study to discover whether it is really true that in about one third of the well-treated patients there is a delay in development.

Dr. Van Hoof: I agree with Dr. Endres' proposal about an international prospective study on galactosemia. The data we collected in Belgium are also much less alarming than those of Dr. Holton. The current disappointment of physicians about the outcome of galactosemia patients reminds me of the situation, a decade ago, about phenylketonuria. People had expected a complete remission of the metabolic disorder from the dietary treatment. They were thus frustrated to see that the therapy had been only 70–90% efficient! The fact that we have heard of so many galactosemic patients is to credit the publication by Eggermont and Hers (2) of a very efficient technique to measure galactose oxidation in erythrocytes. This test has been used in 82 patients, and in recent times primarily to confirm the results of the systematic newborn screening program. Satisfactory answers about mental status and clinical symptoms have been obtained in an inquiry on 42 patients born before 1975. All these patients have been on dietary treatment since the diagnosis. Only five of them (12%) present significant mental retardation; they were unable to complete schooling and/or to find any job. Slight retardation was reported in seven patients (17%), and this coincides largely with speech abnormalities. Growth retardation exists or was reported only in five patients and none suffers from cataracts, which we tend to consider as a sign of poorly monitored dietary treatment. Another interesting fact revealed by this inquiry is that 12 siblings of our 82 patients died from septicemia, at ages between 5 and 27 days. Probably, these infants also suffered from the disease and this reminds us that systematic screening of galactosemia in newborns has to be done very quickly after birth (it can be performed on cord blood).

Dr. Holton: These are interesting data. It is unfortunate that all the data are not being put together because this would give us a complete picture and maybe answer some of the questions about what is really determining the outcome. I am interested in the number of siblings dying, because it is very close to the original figure that was produced in Los Angeles that says that about 20% of the siblings died.

Dr. Hobbs: Changing the phagocytes and red blood cells to normal by a displacement bone marrow transplant (DBMT) could protect a galactosemia patient from hypoglycemia and circulating toxic byproducts, and might permit adequate galactoside synthesis. Provided that brain damage had not occurred *in utero,* a DBMT from a normal compatible sibling is nowadays a relatively low risk procedure with 95% success expected. It might prevent the sad neurological damage which seems to be occurring from present conservative managements. As a bone marrow team we would be delighted to cooperate with a galactosemia team for some pilot studies in their patients. If that present treatment is not as good as was thought, such studies now seem justifiable on ethical grounds.

Dr. Holton: I can't comment on the ataxia, but I tend to feel that most of the other manifestations are caused by postnatal events. I am not absolutely convinced about the possibility of prenatal damage occurring and I think we have to be quite sure about that. I think we need to look particularly at UDPgal levels in the fetus and also in the period between birth and diet restriction. I wonder whether low UDPgal levels are in fact a result of galactose restriction, and UDPgal levels may be normal in the fetus and in the first 3 days of life, because they have high gal-1-P levels and gal-1-P is converted to UDP galactose. There is some evidence that this could be so. I think it is things like this that we need to be looking at at the present time.

Dr. Harms: You might remember that Keppler did his work with galactosamine, not with galactose. And he showed that after giving a rat galactosamine this was followed by a depletion of uridine phosphates and after birth the animal developed hepatitis. I want to mention that if you give galactose before you give galactosamine, no hepatitis will occur in these animals. So I don't think it is clear that UDP depletion is connected with the hepatic damage. The other question I want to add is: Has anybody measured UDP or uridine phosphate in galactosemic patients?

Dr. Holton: Yes, they have. Keppler showed that orotic acid prevented the damage caused by galactosamine, which fits very nicely with what we are doing here, because orotic acid is converted to uridine.

Dr. Odièvre: I wish to come back to the clinical presentation of galactosemia. In our experience one typical situation is the association of jaundice and hemorrhagic diathesis between the age of 7 and 12 days of life. Another situation is the existence of septicemia due to *E. coli:* galactosemic infants are very susceptible to this organism. In a small town in the southern part of France three or four cases of galactosemia have been recognized within 10 years because all babies presenting with this type of infection are screened for it. I have a further comment concerning detection of the developmental delay. Sensitive tests for detecting early delay before the school age are still lacking. So a correct evaluation of the mental development is very difficult during the two first years of life.

Dr. Vis: I want to come back to this point because it is a very important matter also for the guidance of patients with other metabolic diseases, such as phenylketonuria or hypothyroidism. A number of evaluation methods are available which are much more sensitive than the ones used to determine developmental or intelligence quotients (IQs). These techniques enable us to detect minor abnormalities very early in life, before primary school. It is a pity that these techniques are not utilized in most cases. The IQ tests used with children between 6 and 12 years of age (primary school) are usually easier to perform than the ones used in older children. Thus the difficulties seem to increase for the children, although their intellectual development remains at the same level. I would like to address a question to Dr. Van Hoof: How does the psychomotor development of children with galactosemia in your series compare with the development of their healthy siblings? In PKU patients, each time this has been examined their IQs, although in the normal range, were below those of their siblings.

Dr. Van Hoof: A precise answer to such a question is always difficult. In our inquiry we asked the parents and sometimes the patients themselves a series of questions about schooling, what occurred after schooltime, how quickly a job was found, and so on. We also evaluated the galactosemic child in comparison with siblings and this revealed, mostly when the parents were of a high educational level, that galactosemics tend to get less qualified jobs than those obtained by their siblings. Whether this can be attributed to minimal brain damage or to other organic causes, such as speech problems or psychological causes caused for example by overprotection by the parents, is difficult to assess.

Dr. Mowat: From the point of view of early diagnosis one feature I have seen in all the cases of galactosemia has been an unusually higher unconjugated bilirubin in the first week of life, often before the patient became septicemic, and I think that could be a clue to pediatricians to make the diagnosis by finding galactosuria at that time. On the question of the IQ of these children, Komrower many years ago in Manchester showed that the IQ of patients with galactosemia was significantly lower than that of their siblings. On the question of the galactosamine liver damage, this is a cause of experimental liver injury only in the presence of endotoxins. If endotoxins are excluded by doing a colectomy or giving antibiotics, liver damage does not occur. Finally, is there any evidence of the biochemical heterogeneity of galactosemia having an influence on the outcome?

Dr. Holton: The answer to that is yes, because, whatever the reason, there is a difference between the classical galactosemics and the variants in respect of ovarian dysfunction.

REFERENCES

1. Brivet M, Raymond JP, Konopka P, Odièvre M, Lemonnier A. Effect of lactation in a mother with galactosemia. *J Pediatr* 1989;115:280–2.
2. Eggermont E, Hers HG. Une nouvelle méthode de détection de la galactosémie congénitale. *Clin Chim Acta* 1962;7:437–42.

Inborn Errors of Metabolism, edited by
J. Schaub, F. Van Hoof, and H. L. Vis.
Nestlé Nutrition Workshop Series, Vol. 24.
Nestec Ltd., Vevey/Raven Press, Ltd.,
New York © 1991.

Hereditary Fructose Intolerance

Georges Van den Berghe

Laboratory of Physiological Chemistry, International Institute of Cellular and Molecular Pathology, Avenue Hippocrate 75, B-1200 Brussels; and Department of Pediatrics, University Hospital Gasthuisberg, Herestraat 49, B-3000 Leuven, Belgium

Fructose "idiosyncrasy" was first reported in 1956 by Chambers and Pratt (1) in a single adult patient. In 1957, Froesch et al. (2) described hereditary fructose intolerance as an inborn error of metabolism in four children, including a brother and sister pair, and suspected a deficiency of a fructose-metabolizing enzyme as its cause. The enzyme defect was characterized in 1961 by Hers and Joassin (3), who demonstrated that the patients' liver aldolase had lost the ability to split fructose 1-phosphate. Since then, a few hundred cases, mainly from Europe and North America, have been reported in the literature. The inheritance of the disorder is autosomal recessive. Its frequency is estimated at approximately 1:20,000, but as discussed below, the true incidence may be higher. In this chapter the clinical symptoms, diagnostic tests, enzyme defect, pathophysiology, and treatment of hereditary fructose intolerance are reviewed. The toxicity of fructose for normal subjects is also discussed, owing to its general medical importance and because its study has contributed substantially to the understanding of the pathophysiology of hereditary fructose intolerance. For a more extensive review on fructose metabolism and its disorders, the reader is referred to ref. 4.

CLINICAL PICTURE

Subjects with hereditary fructose intolerance do not present any symptoms of the enzyme defect as long as they do not ingest foods containing fructose. Typically, babies do well during breast feeding. Symptoms appear on introduction of cow's milk formulas sweetened with sucrose (composed of a molecule of fructose linked to a molecule of glucose) or at weaning, when fruits and vegetables are given (5). In infants and small children, the first signs are those of gastrointestinal discomfort and hypoglycemia following meals containing fructose. Nausea, vomiting, pallor, sweating, trembling, lethargy, and eventually jerks and convulsions may be observed. If the condition is not recognized and fructose excluded from the diet, failure to thrive, liver disease manifested by hepatomegaly, jaundice, bleeding tendency, eventually edema and ascites, and proximal renal tubular dysfunction appear. The younger the child and the higher the intake of fructose, the more severe the clinical picture, which when its cause it not recognized, may lead to liver and kidney failure and eventually to death.

In some cases, hereditary fructose intolerance is recognized and adequately treated by suppression of fructose-containing nutrients, although not medically diagnosed. Certain mothers quickly learn that their baby does not tolerate certain foods and suppress these from the diet, so that the infant develops normally. Older children acquire a distinct aversion toward foods containing fructose. This aversion protects them, but is at times considered anomalous behavior.

Although hereditary fructose intolerance is a rare inborn error of metabolism, it should always be considered a diagnostic possibility in an infant with the clinical signs and symptoms listed above. Occasionally, diagnosis is established during preschool or school age, following the finding of hepatomegaly of growth delay. Other cases are diagnosed only after life-threatening perfusions with fructose (6) or sorbitol. Because approximately half of the adults with hereditary fructose intolerance are completely free of caries, diagnoses have also been made by dentists. All these observations indicate that subjects with hereditary fructose intolerance remain undiagnosed in the general population.

DIAGNOSTIC TESTS

When hereditary fructose intolerance is suspected, an intravenous fructose tolerance test should be performed after some weeks of fructose withdrawal. Oral loading tests are not recommended because they provoke more ill effects and are less reliable. Fructose should be administered as a 20% solution, at the dose of 200 mg/kg body weight (7). Blood glucose and serum phosphate should be measured, preferably at two 1-min time intervals before the administration of fructose, and 10, 20, 30, and 45 min thereafter (Fig. 1). In normal children, a slight, 5–20 mg/dl increase in blood glucose is recorded, with little change in serum phosphate. In affected children, glucose diminishes progressively, by 30–50 mg/dl over 30–45 min, whereas phosphate decreases more rapidly, by 1–2 mg/dl over 10–20 min. It is thus useful to include serum phosphate among the variables measured during a fructose tolerance test. Other modifications that can be measured during the test include an increase in serum magnesium (Mg^{2+}), which is not observed in normal children, and an increase in serum urate, which is more pronounced in patients than in normal children (Fig. 1).

Other laboratory findings in patients with hereditary fructose intolerance, in whom fructose intake has not been suppressed, are those of liver disease (elevations of serum transaminases and bilirubin, depletion of blood clotting factors) and of proximal tubular dysfunction (proteinuria, melituria, generalized hyperaminoaciduria, metabolic acidosis).

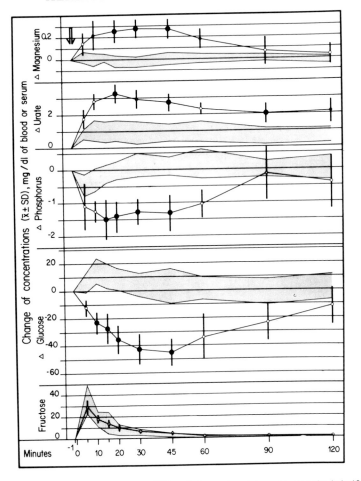

FIG. 1. Fructose tolerance tests. Fructose (200 mg/kg) was given intravenously at 0 min in 10 children with hereditary fructose intolerance and in 16 control children. The shaded areas depict mean ± 1 SD of the controls. Bars represent mean ± 1 SD of the patients. Open symbols indicate overlap between the two groups. From Gitzelmann R, et al. (4).

ENZYMES OF FRUCTOSE METABOLISM

Fructose is metabolized predominantly in liver, kidney cortex, and small intestinal mucosa, owing to the existence in these tissues of a specialized pathway, discovered by Hers (8), and composed of three enzymes: fructokinase, aldolase type B, and triokinase (reviewed in refs. 4 and 9). This enzyme sequence converts fructose into intermediates of the glycolytic-gluconeogenic pathway (Fig. 2). Fructokinase catalyzes the phosphorylation of fructose to fructose-1-phosphate. Adenosine triphosphate (ATP) is the main phosphoryl donor, but as recently demonstrated (10), gua-

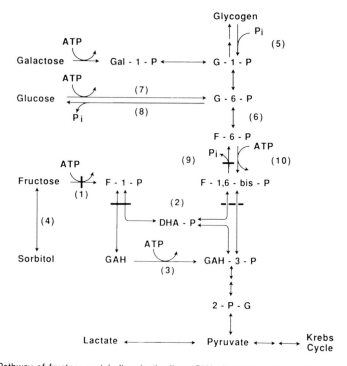

FIG. 2. Pathway of fructose metabolism in the liver. *DHA*, dihydroxyacetone; *G*, glucose; *GAH*, D-glyceraldehyde; *F*, fructose; *P*, phosphate; *P*ᵢ, inorganic phosphate; *2-P-G*, 2-phosphoglycerate. (*1*) fructokinase, (*2*) aldolase B, (*3*) triokinase, (*4*) sorbitol dehydrogenase, (*5*) glycogen phosphorylase, (*6*) phosphohexose isomerase, (*7*) glucokinase (and hexokinase), (*8*) glucose-6-phosphatase, (*9*) fructose-1,6-bisphosphatase, (*10*) phosphofructokinase. The aldolase B defect is depicted by both the solid and the dotted bar. Also shown are fructokinase deficiency and fructose-1,6-bisphosphatase deficiency.

nosine triphosphate (GTP) can also be utilized. Fructokinase has a high affinity for fructose (K_m is around 0.5 mM) and a particularly high V_{max} (about 10 μmol/min per g of liver at 37°C). Aldolase B catalyzes the splitting of both fructose-1-phosphate into D-glyceraldehyde and dihydroxyacetone phosphate, and that of fructose-1,6-bisphosphate into dihydroxyacetone phosphate and D-glyceraldehyde-3-phosphate. Aldolase B also has a high V_{max} of about 10 μmol/min per g of liver, which is about the same with fructose-1-phosphate and with fructose-1,6-bisphosphate. This is in contrast with the isozymes aldolase A (found in muscle) and aldolase C (found in brain), which have a 50- and 10-fold lower V_{max} with fructose-1-phosphate than with fructose-1,6-bisphosphate. Triokinase converts D-glyceraldehyde into D-glyceraldehyde-3-phosphate, thereby allowing the nonphosphorylated product of the cleavage of fructose-1-phosphate to reach the glycolytic-gluconeogenic pathway. Triokinase utilizes ATP preferentially as phosphoryl donor, but other nucleoside triphosphates, such as GTP, can also be used. The maximal activity of triokinase reaches around 1.5 μmol/min per g of liver and is thus markedly lower than that of fructokinase and aldolase B.

Alternative pathways in the metabolism of fructose have been proposed (reviewed in ref. 11). These include utilization of D-glyceraldehyde by two possible enzyme sequences: (i) reduction to glycerol by alcohol dehydrogenase or aldose reductase, followed by phosphorylation to glycerol-3-phosphate, and oxidation to dihydroxy-acetone phosphate; and (ii) oxidation to D-glycerate and phosphorylation to 2-phos-phoglycerate. Both pathways have been ruled out by kinetic studies of the glycer-aldehyde-metabolizing enzymes and by isotope studies *in vivo*. Recently, it has been claimed that fructose-1-phosphate can be directly converted into fructose-1,6-bis-phosphate, without being split by aldolase (12). This proposal is based on studies performed with uniformly labeled [^{13}C]fructose. These have shown that about 50% of infused [^{13}C] fructose was recovered as uniformly labeled [^{13}C]glucose in blood. Owing to the cleavage of the fructose molecule by aldolase and its recombination with unlabeled triose molecules, one would have expected only C1-C2-C3- and C4-C5-C6-labeled glucose to be found. Conversion of fructose into blood glucose by way of phosphorylation to fructose-6-phosphate by hexokinase, followed by iso-merisation to glucose-6-phosphate, was ruled out because conversion of uniformly labeled [^{13}C]fructose into uniformly labeled [^{13}C]glucose did not occur in patients with fructose-1,6-bisphosphatase deficiency (13). Although challenging, these studies are, nevertheless, difficult to interpret, because at the amounts used, [^{13}C]fructose cannot any more be considered as a tracer.

In recent years, the molecular biology of the aldolases has been investigated ex-tensively, particularly because it offers the opportunity to study the genetic mech-anisms that regulate the expression of isozymes (reviewed in ref. 4). The human aldolase B gene is located on chromosome 9 and has been sequenced (14). It is 14,500 base pairs long and contains nine exons. The corresponding cDNA has also been sequenced and encodes a 364-amino-acid protein (15).

ENZYME DEFECT

In patients with hereditary fructose intolerance, the capacity of aldolase B to split fructose-1-phosphate is reduced, on average to a few percent of normal (3,7). There is also a distinct but less marked reduction of the activity of the enzyme toward fructose-1,6-bisphosphate. As a consequence, the ratio of the V_{max} toward fructose-1,6-bisphosphate versus the V_{max} toward fructose-1-phosphate, which is approxi-mately 1 in control liver, is increased to 2 to ∞ in patients. Kinetic studies have shown that the mutant aldolase B has an abnormally high K_m for both fructose-1-phosphate and fructose-1,6-bisphosphate (16). The defect of aldolase B has been most extensively investigated in the liver of the patients, but can also be demon-strated in their kidney cortex (7) and jejunal mucosa (17). The activities of aldolase A and C are normal.

Hereditary fructose intolerance is genetically heterogeneous. This is evidenced by several observations: (i) clinically, certain patients are very sensitive to fructose, whereas others can tolerate moderate intakes of fructose (up to 250 mg/kg·day, compared to an average intake of 1–2 g/kg·day in Western societies); (ii) the activity of adolase B toward fructose-1-phosphate may vary from undetectable to 15% (7) and even 30% of normal (6); and (iii) immunologically reactive aldolase B is detectable in all affected tissues, but the amount of cross-reacting material found may vary from less than 3% to 100% of controls (18). However, up to now, only one molecular lesion of the aldolase B gene has been identified (19). The mutation is a G to C base change in exon 5, which results in the substitution of an alanine by a proline residue at position 149 of the protein. The mutation also creates a new recognition site for the restriction enzyme Ahall,which renders it easily detectable. The same mutation was found in four unrelated subjects with hereditary fructose intolerance. Obviously, more patients will have to be analyzed to verify if this genetic lesion is the prevailing one in hereditary fructose intolerance or if, as observed for instance in the deficiency of hypoxanthine-guanine phosphoribosyltransferase (20), the heterogeneity of the clinical syndrome can be explained by a variety of mutations.

PATHOPHYSIOLOGY

All the manifestations of hereditary fructose intolerance can be traced back to the buildup, upon ingestion or infusion of fructose, of fructose-1-phosphate in the tissues that possess the specialized fructose pathway. The accumulation of fructose-1-phosphate results from its formation by fructokinase, combined with the inability of aldolase B to catalyze its splitting. In turn, the accumulation of fructose-1-phosphate provokes depletion of ATP, GTP, and inorganic phosphate. The loss of ATP and GTP is caused by their utilization as phosphoryl donors in the fructokinase reaction. The depletion of inorganic phosphate is due to its consumption in the mitochondria to regenerate ATP (Fig. 2). These modifications, which were first demonstrated in studies of the effects of fructose loads in animals, reviewed in the next section, were for a long time only indirectly documented in patients. The loss of ATP is manifested by an elevation of serum and urinary uric acid, and of serum Mg^{2+} (Fig. 1). The depletion of inorganic phosphate is reflected by a decrease of serum phosphate. In recent years, however, noninvasive ^{31}P nuclear magnetic resonance spectroscopy has allowed the demonstration of the accumulation of fructose-1-phosphate and of the depletion of ATP and inorganic phosphate, in the liver of patients *in vivo* (21).

The characteristic rapidly progressive hypoglycemia induced by fructose in hereditary fructose intolerance can be explained by the combined operation of three mechanisms: (i) a block of glycogenolysis; (ii) an inhibition of gluconeogenesis; and (iii) probably also a stimulation of the uptake of glucose, as evidenced by recent studies of glucokinase. The block of glycogenolysis is evidenced both by the absence of dilution of infused radioactive glucose by endogenous glucose (22) and by the inability of glucagon to raise blood glucose during fructose-induced hypoglycemia (23). Detailed investigations of the effects of fructose on the glycogenolytic mechanism (24, reviewed in ref. 25) have shown that fructose administration (i) decreases the capacity of the liver to form cyclic AMP; and (ii) provokes an inhibition of the activity of phosphorylase *a*. The decreased capacity to form cyclic AMP is explained by the loss of ATP, the substrate of adenylate cyclase, and evidenced by a marked reduction of the glucagon-induced urinary excretion of cyclic AMP. The decreased formation of cyclic AMP is, however, not sufficient to explain the absence of response to glucagon since the fructose-induced hypoglycemia can also not be corrected by dibutyryl cyclic AMP. The explanation for the block of glycogenolysis was found to be an inhibition of liver phosphorylase *a*, caused by the accumulation of fructose-1-phosphate, combined with the depletion of inorganic phosphate, one of the substrates of the enzyme.

The decreased activity of aldolase B toward fructose-1,6-bisphosphate in hereditary fructose intolerance has no clinical consequences on gluconeogenesis in the sense that patients do not display fasting hypoglycemia in the same way as patients with defects of gluconeogenesis (e.g., fructose-1,6-bisphosphatase deficiency). During fructose-induced hypoglycemia an inhibition of gluconeogenesis is, nevertheless, evidenced by the fact that glycemia cannot be corrected by dihydroxyacetone, which enters the glycolytic-gluconeogenic pathway by way of triokinase. The inhibition of gluconeogenesis is explained by the inhibitory effect of fructose-1-phosphate on glucose-6-phosphate isomerase (26), and on the condensation of the triose phosphates to fructose-1,6-bisphosphate by aldolase (Bally C, Leuthardt F, unpublished data cited in ref. 4). Inhibition of gluconeogenesis probably plays a determining role in the hypoglycemic effect of fructose in the fasting state.

Recent studies of the phosphorylation of glucose by isolated rat hepatocytes (27) have shown that it is stimulated by low concentrations of fructose. At 200 µM concentration, fructose stimulates the phosphorylation of a physiological concentration of glucose, namely 5 mM, two- to fourfold. Fructose acts by increasing the apparent affinity for glucose of glucokinase, the only glucose phosphorylating enzyme in liver parenchymal cells. V_{max} is not modified. Further studies (28) have led to the discovery of a protein regulator of glucokinase, which inhibits the enzyme by decreasing its affinity for glucose. The inhibitory effect is greatly potentiated by the presence of micromolar concentrations of fructose-6-phosphate. It is, however, antagonized by similar concentrations of fructose-1-phosphate. The accumulation of fructose-1-phosphate, resulting from the intake of fructose, may thus contribute to the hypoglycemia of hereditary fructose intolerance, by relieving the inhibition exerted on glucokinase by the synergic action of its protein regulator and fructose-6-phosphate. In addition to its importance for the pathophysiology of hereditary fructose intolerance, this effect of fructose-1-phosphate may also explain the repeat observation that fructose stimulates the synthesis of glycogen from glucose (reviewed in ref. 9), and the long-standing belief that small amounts of fructose may be beneficial to diabetic patients.

The other toxic effects of fructose recorded in hereditary fructose intolerance— the hepatic and renal dysfunction and the gastrointestinal discomfort—are most likely explained by the loss of ATP and GTP in the fructose-metabolizing tissues.

ATP and GTP, ''energy currencies'' of the cell, are indeed required for many cellular functions, and their depletion causes several disturbances, as reviewed in the next section.

TOXICITY OF FRUCTOSE IN NORMAL ORGANISMS

After the discovery of hereditary fructose intolerance, fructose toxicity was first thought to be restricted to individuals with a deficiency of aldolase B. However, the development of parenteral nutrition led to the recognition, in the late 1960s of deleterious effects of intravenous fructose in normal humans. The main findings were lactic acidosis (29) and hyperuricemia (30, reviewed in refs. 4, 9, and 11).

Intravenous infusion of fructose may increase blood lactate by two- to fivefold, whereas intravenous glucose on the average does not increase blood lactate more than twofold. The more rapid conversion of fructose into lactate, as compared to glucose is explained by several factors: (i) the approximately 10-fold higher V_{max} of fructokinase as compared to the maximal glucose phosphorylating capacity of glucokinase; (ii) the fact that fructolysis bypasses phosphofructokinase, the principal regulatory enzyme of glycolysis; and (iii) the stimulation by fructose-1-phosphate of pyruvate kinase, another regulatory enzyme of the glycolytic pathway. In addition, fructose may, under certain conditions (31), increase the concentration of fructose-2,6-bisphosphate, the main stimulator of liver glycolysis (32), and thereby increase the production of lactate from glucose. The fructose-induced increase in lactic acid may provoke metabolic acidosis, which may become life threatening, particularly in liver failure (33).

Hyperuricemia and hyperuricosuria following the intravenous administration of fructose have been repeatedly documented, not only in subjects with hereditary fructose intolerance, but also in patients without the aldolase B defect. In the latter, they become generally apparent at infusion rates above 1.0 to 1.5 g/kg·h. Explanation of the increased production of uric acid induced by intravenous fructose in normal organisms requires an understanding of the factors that determine the velocity of the metabolism of fructose in normal liver. As said before, the V_{max} of both fructokinase and aldolase reaches about 10 μmol/min per g of liver. This is severalfold more than the V_{max} of triokinase, which reaches only 1.5 μmol/min·g, or those of the fluxes through the glycolytic and gluconeogenic pathways, which do not exceed 2 μmol of C6 units/min·g. Fructose-1-phosphate can thus easily accumulate, owing to the fact that the velocity of its formation can markedly surpass the rate of its further metabolism. The formation of fructose-1-phosphate is, however, determined not only by the kinetic characteristics of fructokinase. It is also dependent on the transport of fructose inside the hepatocyte. This transport system has a K_m value that reaches around 100 mM (as compared to about 0.5 mM for fructokinase) and a V_{max} equal to about 30 μmol/min·g of liver (34). After an oral load of fructose, the concentration of fructose in the portal vein reaches maximally about 2.5 mM. During intravenous infusion of fructose at the rates 0.5, 1.0, and 1.5 g/kg·h, fructosemia

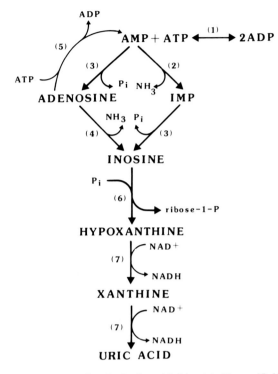

FIG. 3. Pathways of purine catabolism in the liver. (*1*) Adenylate kinase, (*2*) AMP deaminase, (*3*) cytosolic 5'-nucleotidase, (*4*) adenosine deaminase, (*5*) adenosine kinase, (*6*) purine nucleoside phosphorylase, (*7*) xanthine dehydrogenase (also named oxidase). From Gitzelmann R, et al. (4).

reaches 2.3, 4.8, and 7 mM, respectively (35). Intravenous fructose thus results in a higher rate of entry of fructose in the liver, which allows fructose-1-phosphate to accumulate to toxic levels. These can be defined as those that result in depletion of ATP, GTP, and inorganic phosphate.

The decrease in ATP induced by fructose is not accompanied by a commensurate increase in AMP, as observed, for example, in anoxia, but by a loss of adenine nucleotides as a whole. This loss can be explained as follows. The catabolism of the adenine nucleotides ATP, ADP, and AMP, which are maintained in equilibrium by adenylate kinase (Fig. 3), originates from AMP. The catabolism of AMP can, in theory, be initiated by two different reactions: either deamination by AMP deaminase, or dephosphorylation by cytosolic 5'-nucleotidase(s). Studies of the catabolism of the adenine nucleotides in isolated rat hepatocytes have shown that the initial catabolism of AMP, leading to the formation of uric acid and/or allantoin (the terminal purine catabolite in lower mammals), proceeds exclusively by way of AMP deaminase (36, reviewed in ref. 9). Dephosphorylation of AMP takes place but does not contribute to the production of allantoin, because the resulting adenosine is continuously recycled by adenosine kinase (37). Liver AMP deaminase has complex kinetic properties and is strongly influenced by various metabolites: ATP is a potent stimulator, whereas inorganic phosphate and GTP are inhibitors. At physiologic concentrations of substrate and effectors, the enzyme is 95% inhibited (38). The accumulation of fructose-1-phosphate, by decreasing not only ATP but also GTP and inorganic phosphate, thus causes deinhibition of AMP deaminase. This results in a loss of the adenine nucleotide pool as a whole, which is manifested by hyperuricemia and hyperuricosuria. The increased production of uric acid induced by fructose is thus not a harmless phenomenon, but an indication of the degradation of ATP, the main "energy currency" of the cell. Owing to the potent Mg^{2+} chelating effect of ATP, its loss results in a decrease of Mg^{2+} in the liver, and in an increase of plasma Mg^{2+} (Fig. 1). In the fructose-metabolizing tissues, depletion of ATP results in a series of disturbances. These include inhibition of the synthesis of RNA and protein, disaggregation of ribosomes, and ultrastructural lesions (reviewed in refs. 4, 9, and 11).

From the above it appears that fructose is a potentially dangerous compound in parenteral nutrition, not only for undiagnosed fructose-intolerant children and adults, but also for patients with normal aldolase B. The same holds true for the mixtures of glucose and fructose, known as invert sugar, and for sorbitol, which is converted into fructose in the liver by sorbitol dehydrogenase (Fig. 2). The use of fructose and related compounds as substitutes for glucose in parenteral nutrition has therefore been strongly discouraged by several authors (4,33,39).

TREATMENT

Treatment of hereditary fructose intolerance consists in the elimination of all sources of fructose from the diet. This involves suppression of all foods in which fructose and/or sucrose and sorbitol occur naturally or have been added intentionally. The major natural sources of fructose are fruits, particularly apples, pears, grapes, and sweet cherries, and certain vegetables, such as beets and carrots. Lists of the fructose content of various foodstuffs are available (40). The presence of fructose in medications and in infant formulas, although declining, should also be checked. A fructose-free diet should be instituted as soon as hereditary fructose intolerance is suspected. The beneficial effect of the diet is usually seen within days of its initiation and provides a first clue to the diagnosis. Fructose tolerance tests and the assay of aldolase B in a biopsy of liver or, alternatively, of small intestine, should only be performed when the clinical status has improved.

Despite adequate treatment, small children with hereditary fructose intolerance usually display hepatomegaly for months and even years (41). The reason for this is unclear and has been linked to a too strict, as well as to an insufficiently stringent, limitation of fructose intake. An insufficient restriction of fructose was apparently the cause of the isolated growth retardation recorded in two boys aged 5 and 4 years who displayed no symptoms of fructose toxicity on a self-imposed diet, resulting in an average intake of fructose of approximately 160 mg/kg body weight per day (42).

Indeed, when a stricter diet was prescribed, providing them with only 20 to 40 mg of fructose/kg body weight per day, catch-up growth was recorded. The intake of fructose should thus, at least in childhood, not be determined by its subjective tolerance, but a diet should be prescribed composed of foodstuffs with no or very low fructose content. Needless to say, patients (and their parents) should be made aware of the fact that infusions containing fructose, sorbitol, or invert sugar are life threatening for them, and they should report fructose intolerance on any hospital admission.

REFERENCES

1. Chambers RA, Pratt RTC. Idiosyncrasy to fructose. *Lancet* 1956;ii:340.
2. Froesch ER, Prader A, Labhart A, Stuber HW, Wolf HP. Die hereditäre Fructoseintoleranz, eine bisher nicht bekannte kongenitale Stoffwechselstörung. *Schweiz Med Wochenschr* 1957;87:1168–71.
3. Hers HG, Joassin G. Anomalie de l'aldolase hépatique dans l'intolérance au fructose. *Enzymol Biol Clin* 1961;1:4–14.
4. Gitzelmann R, Steinmann B, Van den Berghe G. Disorders of fructose metabolism. In: Scriver CR, Beaudet AL, Sly WS, Valle D, eds. *The metabolic basis of inherited disease*, 6th ed. New York: McGraw-Hill, 1989:399–424.
5. Baerlocher K, Gitzelmann R, Steinmann B, Gitzelmann-Cumarasamy N. Hereditary fructose intolerance in early childhood: a major diagnostic challenge. Survey of 20 symptomatic cases. *Helv Paediatr Acta* 1978;33:465–87.
6. Lameire N, Mussche M, Baele G, Kint J, Ringoir S. Hereditary fructose intolerance: a difficult diagnosis in the adult. *Am J Med* 1978;65:416–23.
7. Steinmann B, Gitzelmann R. The diagnosis of hereditary fructose intolerance. *Helv Paediatr Acta* 1981;36:297–316.
8. Hers HG. *Le métabolisme du fructose*. Brussels: Arscia, 1957:200 pp.
9. Van den Berghe G. Fructose: metabolism and short-term effects on carbohydrate and purine metabolic pathways. *Prog Biochem Pharmacol* 1986;21:1–32.
10. Phillips MI, Davies DR. The mechanism of guanosine triphosphate depletion in the liver after a fructose load. The role of fructokinase. *Biochem J* 1985;228:667–71.
11. Van den Berghe G. Metabolic effects of fructose in the liver. *Curr Top Cell Regul* 1978;13:97–135.
12. Lapidot A, Gopher A, Vaisman N. Fructose metabolism in hereditary fructose intolerance and control children using [U-^{13}C]fructose and ^{13}C NMR. Development of a diagnostic test. Presented at the *Eighth Annual Meeting of the Society of Magnetic Resonance in Medicine*, Amsterdam, August 12–18, 1989.
13. Lapidot A, Gopher A, Gutman A. Metabolic studies in patients with fructose-1,6-diphosphatase deficiency by [U-^{13}C]fructose and ^{13}C NMR. Development of a diagnostic test. Presented at the *Eighth Annual Meeting of the Society of Magnetic Resonance in Medicine*, Amsterdam, August 12–18, 1989.
14. Tolan DR, Penhoet EE. Characterization of the human aldolase B gene. *Mol Biol Med* 1986;3:245–64.
15. Rottmann WH, Tolan DR, Penhoet EE. Complete amino acid sequence for human aldolase B derived from cDNA and genomic clones. *Proc Natl Acad Sci USA* 1984;81:2738–42.
16. Koster JF, Slee RG, Fernandes J. On the biochemical basis of hereditary fructose intolerance. *Biochem Biophys Res Comm* 1975;64:289–94.
17. Streb H, Posselt HG, Wolter K, Bender SW. Aldolase activities of the small intestinal mucosa in malabsorption states and hereditary fructose intolerance. *Eur J Pediatr* 1981;137:5–10.
18. Grégori C, Schapira F, Kahn A, Delpech M, Dreyfus JC. Molecular studies of liver aldolase B in hereditary fructose intolerance using blotting and immunological techniques. *Ann Hum Genet* 1982;46:281–92.
19. Cross NCP, Tolan DR, Cox TM. Catalytic deficiency of human aldolase B in hereditary fructose intolerance caused by a common missense mutation. *Cell* 1988;53:881–5.
20. Wilson JM, Stout JT, Palella TD, Davidson BL, Kelley WN, Caskey T. A molecular survey of hypoxanthine-guanine phosphoribosyl transferase deficiency in man. *J Clin Invest* 1986;77:188–95.
21. Oberhaensli RD, Rajagopalan B, Taylor DJ, et al. Study of hereditary fructose intolerance by use of ^{31}P magnetic resonance spectroscopy. *Lancet* 1987;ii:931–4.

22. Dubois R, Loeb H, Ooms HA, Gillet P, Bartman J, Champenois A. Etude d'un cas d'hypoglycémie fonctionelle par intolérance au fructose. *Helv Paediatr Acta* 1961;16:90–6.
23. Cornblath M, Rosenthal IM, Reisner SH, Wybregt SH, Crane RK. Hereditary fructose intolerance. *N Engl J Med* 1963;269:1271–8.
24. Van den Berghe G, Hue L, Hers HG. Effect of the administration of fructose on the glycogenolytic action of glucagon. An investigation of the pathogeny of hereditary fructose intolerance. *Biochem J* 1973;134:637–45.
25. Van den Berghe G. Biochemical aspects of hereditary fructose intolerance. In: Hommes FA, Van den Berg CJ, eds. *Normal and pathological development of energy metabolism*. London: Academic Press, 1975;211–26.
26. Zalitis J, Oliver IT. Inhibition of glucose phosphate isomerase by metabolic intermediates of fructose. *Biochem J* 1967;102:753–9.
27. Van Schaftingen E, Vandercammen A. Stimulation of glucose phosphorylation by fructose in isolated rat hepatocytes. *Eur J Biochem* 1989;179:173–7.
28. Van Schaftingen E. A protein from rat liver confers to glucokinase the property of being antagonistically regulated by fructose 6-phosphate and fructose 1-phosphate. *Eur J Biochem* 1989;179:179–84.
29. Bergström J, Hultman E, Roch-Norlund AE. Lactic acid accumulation in connection with fructose infusion. *Acta Med Scand* 1968;184:359–64.
30. Perheentupa J, Raivio K. Fructose-induced hyperuricaemia. *Lancet* 1967;ii:528–31.
31. Hue L, Bartrons R. Role of fructose 2,6-bisphosphate in the control by glucagon of gluconeogenesis from various precursors in isolated rat hepatocytes. *Biochem J* 1984;218:165–70.
32. Hers HG, Van Schaftingen E. Fructose 2,6-bisphosphate 2 years after its discovery. *Biochem J* 1982;206:1–12.
33. Woods HF, Alberti KGMM. Dangers of intravenous fructose. *Lancet* 1972;ii:1354–7.
34. Sestoft L, Fleron P. Determination of the kinetic constants of fructose transport and phosphorylation in the perfused rat liver. *Biochim Biophys Acta* 1974;345:27–38.
35. Smith LH Jr, Ettinger RH, Seligson DA. Comparison of the metabolism of fructose and glucose in hepatic disease and diabetes mellitus. *J Clin Invest* 1953;32:273–82.
36. Van den Berghe G, Bontemps F, Hers HG. Purine catabolism in isolated rat hepatocytes. Influence of coformycin. *Biochem J* 1980;188:913–20.
37. Bontemps F, Van den Berghe G, Hers HG. Evidence for a substrate cycle between AMP and adenosine in isolated hepatocytes. *Proc Natl Acad Sci USA* 1983;80:2829–33.
38. Van den Berghe G, Bronfman M, Vanneste R, Hers HG. The mechanism of adenosine triphosphate depletion in the liver after a load of fructose. A kinetic study of liver adenylate deaminase. *Biochem J* 1977;162:601–9.
39. Van den Berghe G, Hers HG. Dangers of intravenous fructose and sorbitol. *Acta Paediatr Belg* 1978;31:115–23.
40. Hardinge MG, Swarner JB, Crooks H. Carbohydrates in foods. *J Am Diet Assoc* 1965;46:197–204.
41. Odièvre M, Gentil C, Gautier M, Alagille D. Hereditary fructose intolerance in childhood. Diagnosis, management and course in 55 patients. *Am J Dis Child* 1978;132:605–8.
42. Mock DM, Perman JA, Thaler MM, Morris RC Jr. Chronic fructose intoxication after infancy in children with hereditary fructose intolerance. A cause of growth retardtion. *N Engl J Med* 1983;309:764–70.

DISCUSSION

Dr. Mannaerts: You said that the K_m for the hepatic fructose transport system is 100 mM and that during an intravenous fructose infusion portal concentrations of 7 mM are reached. This would mean that the transport system is operating at less than 7% of its V_{max}, which would be less than the V_{max} of the gluconeogenic pathway, or is it possible that under certain circumstances you would reach higher fructose concentrations, which would then become dangerous?

Dr. Van den Berghe: I agree with you. Figures for V_{max} (30 μmol/min · g) and K_m (approximately 100 mM) of fructose transport were taken from data obtained by Sestoft and Fleron (1) in perfused rat liver. Parameters of fructose transport are, however, difficult to measure, owing to its very rapid metabolism. More recent investigations of fructose transport into isolated rat hepatocytes (2) have given a value of 291 mmol/min per ml of cell water for V_{max}, and of 212 mM for K_m. With these figures, one can calculate that the rate of transport of fructose will be higher than the capacity of the glycolytic-gluconeogenic pathway.

Dr. Endres: I found some different figures concerning the self imposed fructose restrictions in adults. Newbrun et al. (3) reported some adults with hereditary fructose intolerance (HFI) who did not know that they had this disease and who had a daily intake of about 2.5 g sucrose (i.e., 1.25 g of fructose) and with an average weight of 60–70 kg that is about 15–20 mg/kg. In a retrospective study in Germany we investigated 56 patients. Interestingly, the first exposure to fructose in 45 of 56 patients was below 6 weeks of age and you could conclude from these figures that a high proportion of patients will never be detected because there must be many more newborns who will not receive fructose or sucrose within these first weeks of life. Concerning the clinical symptoms observed in our patients, there is one symptom that has not been reported in the literature, and that is diarrhea. This has been reported in 80% of our patients. Concerning routine laboratory investigations, it became evident that hypophosphatemia, hyperuricemia, and hypoglycemia are found mainly during the fructose loading test rather than in the chronic state. Between patients who received fructose immediately after birth and those who received it later, there was a statistically significant difference in the development of cirrhosis, while no correlation was found between the *amount* of fructose ingested and the development of liver cirrhosis. Hence it is not important how much they received, but it is very important how early they received it. Nine of 10 patients who developed liver cirrhosis received fructose-containing formulas immediately after birth; however, there are other infants who had also been fed fructose who did not develop cirrhosis. In summary it can be said that fructose-containing formulas already fed in the neonatal period lead to cirrhosis of the liver in one third of all HFI patients regardless of the amount ingested, and among patients with HFI receiving small amounts of fructose a mild clinical course can be observed five times more often than a severe one. Two of 10 patients suffering from cirrhosis due to HFI died soon after diagnosis during the first months of life.

This is my recommendation: Don't use fructose-containing formulas in any infant below 3 months of age. There is no advantage of giving fructose or sucrose in comparison to lactose, glucose, or its polymers. The intake of fructose should be restricted to amounts less than 1 g per day.

Dr. Van den Berghe: With respect to the sensitivity to fructose, I would like to comment that it has been well documented that some patients are ignorant of their hereditary fructose intolerance until a sometimes dramatic incident occurs. For example, Lameire et al. (4) have reported a 21-year-old Belgian patient in whom hereditary fructose intolerance was only diagnosed following the infusion of invert sugar as part of the treatment of viral meningitis. This was followed by life-threatening acute icterus, complicated by severe gastrointestinal bleeding, hypoglycemia, and proximal renal tubular acidosis. Analysis of a liver biopsy showed that aldolase B activity was 30% of normal. This high residual activity probably explains why hereditary fructose intolerance had remained undiagnosed.

Dr. Vis: I suppose that everybody will agree that we should not give fructose to an infant before 3 months of age. Indeed, commercially available infant formulas do not contain fructose. But what about drugs? Some syrups contain fructose; sorbitol is present in some suppositories. We should ask, in all countries, as is already the case in some, that fructose be withdrawn from drug preparations for young infants.

Dr. Schaub: Fatty infiltration of the liver cell is a common feature of fructose intolerance, even in well-treated patients. Do you have any explanation for this formation of fat in the liver cells? We have a family with two children, where the second child was diagnosed in the first week of life; after 14 months of fructose- and saccharose-free treatment this child had mild steatosis of the liver cells.

Dr. Van den Berghe: To my knowledge there is no satisfactory explanation for the fatty acid infiltration in the liver of patients with hereditary fructose intolerance. Fructose is known to favor triglyceride synthesis, most likely because it increases glycerol-3-phosphate, which is formed from dihydroxyacetone phosphate and is the cosubstrate of long chain fatty acyl-CoA in the synthesis of triglycerides. However, when aldolase B is deficient there is no conversion of fructose into dihydroxyacetone phosphate.

Dr. Schaub: Is it possible that this fat formation in the liver cell is independent of fructose intake?

Dr. Odièvre: This is a difficult problem. In our experience liver steatosis remains present in all patients until 6–7 years of age despite good compliance to the restricted diet. The steatosis seems to disappear when the child is placed on a self-imposed diet, possibly less restricted than the previous one. I know several patients in whom the fructose intolerance was only diagnosed at 7 or 8 years after several years of self-imposed diet; these patients had no steatosis at the time of diagnosis. The amount of fat contained in the fructose-free diet is from a caloric point of view relatively high; in some patients about 50% of their energy intake is represented by fat. A last, somewhat provocative remark can be made: When we perform a liver biopsy in young babies not intolerant of fructose and who are receiving only human milk there is some discrete degree of steatosis in the liver. This finding raises the question as to whether fructose could possibly be an essential carbohydrate for human beings; in that case, an overrestricted diet in fructose intolerance might favor the persistence of steatosis.

Dr. Van den Berghe: Perhaps I might add that fructose remains a very active and exciting field of investigation. Fructose-2,6-bisphosphate was only discovered in 1980, and the finding of regulatory effects of fructose esters on glucokinase opens additional perspectives.

Dr. Saudubray: I have a general question on physiology. Fructose is classically considered as a carbohydrate that does not induce insulin secretion. Is this true, and why?

Dr. Van den Berghe: The classical theory is that fructose by itself does not stimulate the secretion of insulin, but that it potentiates the effect of low concentrations of glucose. Since the pancreatic β cell also contains glucokinase, the regulatory effects of the fructose esters on the latter enzyme might play a role in this potentiation.

Dr. Mowat: Is there any evidence that the liver disease progresses when patients are on a fructose-free diet? Do they, for example, develop malignancy in the liver?

Dr. Van den Berghe: I am not aware of a tendency to develop malignancy. On the other hand, several people with hereditary fructose intolerance are known to have reached very old age, and with excellent teeth!

Dr. Odièvre: One adult patient, who probably had fructose intolerance because he presented typical manifestations when he was young and had complete aversion to sweets throughout his life, died at 49 years with a hepatoma. I think it would be interesting to ask our colleagues for a history of aversion to sweets when they see hepatoma in adults. I have a second comment. If you give fructose intravenously in normal patients you observe a peak of insulin during the first minutes after injection; this early peak is not seen in patients with fructose intolerance given a fructose load.

Dr. Van den Berghe: This may be due to the fact that in normal individuals fructose is converted into glucose, but not in patients with hereditary fructose intolerance.

Dr. Eggermont: When H. G. Hers discovered the aldolase defect in a patient with fructose intolerance, he also measured the enzymes involved in the degradation of glycogen and found glucose-6-phosphatase to be very high. Subsequently, he measured the aldolase activity in liver biopsy specimens with high glucose-6-phosphatase activities and was able to detect several other patients with fructose intolerance.

Dr. Van den Berghe: The high glucose-6-phosphatase activity in livers of patients with hereditary fructose intolerance has been attributed to the stabilizing effect of their elevated glycogen content (6). The high glycogen is explained by the inhibition of the glycogenolytic mechanism.

Dr. Odièvre: Do you think that a block of glycogenolysis and neoglucogenesis associated with a stimulation of glucose uptake by the liver can explain the abrupt character of hypoglycemia induced by fructose?

Dr. Van den Berghe: The rapidity and the degree of hypoglycemia will depend both on the amount of fructose administered and on the metabolic state of the patient: a low glycogen reserve and a low rate of gluconeogenesis would increase the sensitivity to fructose.

Dr. Saudubray: A general statement in the classical textbooks is that one should not use fructose in cases of hepatocullular insufficiency, not merely in fructose intolerance, but in general. I am not sure that this statement has a real foundation. I have investigated three or four patients with very severe hepatocellular dysfunction of unknown origin in neonatal period, presenting with lactic acidemia and severe hypoglycemia after 2, 3, or 4 h of fast. I tried investigating the hypoglycemia by giving various gluconeogenic substrates—lactate, alanine, dihydroxyacetone and fructose after 2–3 h of fasting. To my surprise with fructose we got a marvelous increase in blood glucose, each time, contrasting with the very severe hepatocellular dysfunction and with a complete absence of response with alanine and lactate. My feeling is that the toxic effect of fructose is very specific for fructose intolerance in the hereditary fructose intolerance, but I am not sure whether in a nonspecific sense it is true.

Dr. Van den Berghe: Fructose is normally rapidly converted to glucose. In fact, it is one of the best gluconeogenic precursors because it enters the gluconeogenic pathway above the limiting steps which are found at the level of the so-called "pyruvate crossroads," through which lactate and alanine have to go. That fructose is very rapidly converted into glucose does not mean that it cannot have toxic effects. First, it is also very quickly converted to lactate and may thus contribute to lactic acidosis. The other toxic effects of intravenous fructose can be related to the decrease in ATP it induces. That these effects on liver ATP often do not seem to impress clinicians may be explained by the fact that ATP cannot be measured by routine clinical chemistry. The introduction of (expensive) NMR equipment could change this. I also would like to warn against overextrapolation of experimental, *in vitro*, data on clinical situations. For example, in liver perfused in the absence of oxygen, fructose but not glucose was found to be protective against cell damage (6). This may be explained because anaerobic fructolysis is more rapid than glycolysis, and thus allows some preservation of ATP. These are, however, short-term experiments performed in extreme conditions which are difficult to compare with clinical situations.

Dr. Vis: What is the real incidence of disease? Is one out of 20,000 newborns not an optimistic figure? Is it not more than that?

Dr. Van den Berghe: The frequency of 1:20,000 is the one that is classically given by Gitzelmann and his co-workers for Switzerland. I have been told that it may be lower in North America and in England.

Dr. Odièvre: The figure is probably higher; many cases are not diagnosed because patients die from apparently unexplained hepatic failure after birth. I disagree with Professor Saudubray because fructose intolerance is a classic cause of acute liver insufficiency, so that we have to be very cautious about fructose administration until fructose intolerance is excluded.

Dr. Saudubray: Yes, I agree with you.

Dr. Odièvre: We saw several cases of fructose intolerance many years ago when the babies were fed with milk containing sucrose. Since they are now fed milk without sucrose, fructose intolerance seems less frequent. In fact, the symptoms appear later and are more discrete, but the frequency of the disease remains the same.

Dr. Van den Berghe: Maybe we could obtain figures by asking school children if they like sweets. . . .

REFERENCES

1. Sestoft L, Fleron P. Determination of the kinetic constants of fructose transport and phosphorylation in the perfused rat liver. *Biochim Biophys Acta* 1974;345:27–38.
2. Craik JD, Elliott KRF. Transport of D-fructose and D-galactose into isolated rat hepatocytes. *Biochem J* 1980;192:373–5.
3. (from Dr Endres)
4. Lameire N,Mussche M, Baele G, Kint J, Ringoir S. Hereditary fructose intolerance: a difficult diagnosis in the adult. *Am J Med* 1978;65:416–23.
5. Cain ARR, Ryman BE. High liver glycogen in hereditary fructose intolerance. *Gut* 1971;12:929–32.
6. Anundi I, King J, Owen DA, Schneider H, Lemasters JL, Thurman RG. Fructose prevents hypoxic cell death in liver. *Am J Physiol* 1987;253:G390–6.

Inborn Errors of Metabolism, edited by
J. Schaub, F. Van Hoof, and H. L. Vis.
Nestlé Nutrition Workshop Series, Vol. 24.
Nestec Ltd., Vevey/Raven Press, Ltd.,
New York © 1991.

Problems of Transfer of Carbohydrates at the Level of the Intestinal Mucosa

Ephrem Eggermont

*Department of Pediatrics, University of Leuven, University Hospital Gasthuisberg,
Herestraat 49, B-3000 Leuven, Belgium*

In humans, about half the daily energy is ingested as carbohydrates. Most have to be hydrolyzed by the salivary and pancreatic α-amylases and/or the brush border glycosidases of the enterocytes. The end products of the intestinal digestion of the dietary carbohydrates are glucose, galactose, and fructose (1,2). The resorption of the end products and not the hydrolysis of the oligosaccharides is the limiting step for all disaccharides except lactose and the α-1,6-oligosaccharides. Hydrolysis of oligomers larger than maltohexaose is rate limiting for glucose absorption in the absence of luminal α-amylase activity (3). Although most of the hexoses are absorbed in the small intestine, the colon has some salvage function (4).

In this chapter I shall review (1) some aspects of normal and abnormal absorption of glucose, galactose, and fructose; (2) the molecular basis of the absorption of glucose; and (3) the genetic control of the glucose carrier.

NORMAL AND ABNORMAL ABSORPTION OF HEXOSES IN THE SMALL INTESTINE

From 1960 on, Robert Crane and co-workers presented increasing evidence that the small intestine is able to absorb glucose and galactose, but not fructose, against a concentration gradient (5,6). At about the same time, Lindquist & Meeuwisse (7) and Laplane et al. (8) independently described infant patients with profuse watery diarrhea from birth following the ingestion of milk. Because the diarrhea ceased if carbohydrate-free feeds were offered or if fructose was substituted for glucose and galactose in the diet, the authors proposed that the affected infants suffered from a specific abnormality of glucose and galactose absorption. For these reasons the normal and abnormal absorption of glucose and galactose and of fructose is discussed separately.

TABLE 1. *Study of active transport in small intestinal biopsy specimens in normal and glucose-galactose-intolerant children*[a]

	Relative tissue concentration (C_t/C_m)		
	Glucose		Leucine
	Na^+	K^+	Na^+
Control subjects			
Mean ± 1 SD	6.35 ± 2.33	0.76 ± 0.30	7.19 ± 2.30
(Number of subjects)	(n = 12)	(n = 8)	(n = 11)
Glucose-galactose-intolerant patients			
Mean ± 1 SD	0.83 ± 0.42	0.68	7.24 ± 3.37
(Number of subjects)	(n = 5)	(n = 2)	(n = 5)

[a] The active transport has been studied according to the technique described by E. Eggermont and H. Loeb (45). Active transport is found whenever the biopsy specimen is able to achieve higher concentrations of the substrate (C_t) than present in the incubation medium (C_m). Glucose is studied in the presence of Na^+ or in the absence of Na^+ replaced by K^+. The accumulation of leucine, in the presence of Na^+, is studied as a control.

Absorption and Malabsorption of Glucose and Galactose

In the adult, the absorption of monosaccharides from the jejunum has been studied by perfusion techniques (9). It has been shown that as the concentration of glucose or galactose in the perfusion fluid is increased, the absorption rate of glucose and galactose approaches a maximum. An apparent maximum velocity (V_{max}) and half-saturation concentration (K_m, Michaelis constant) can be calculated. These are for glucose V_{max} 0.73 g/cm·min, K_m 220 mM (4 g/dl), and for galactose V_{max} 1 g/30 cm·min, K_m 330 mM or 5.9 g/dl. In the young infant, we found an absorption of approximately 0.235 g glucose per 30 cm·min at a glucose concentration of 550 mM or 10 g/dl (10). The development of D-glucose absorption in the perinatal period has been studied by McNeish et al. (11).

In infants with glucose-galactose malabsorption, the reduced uptake of glucose (0.080 g/30 cm·min) together with the normal absorption of fructose (0.261 g/30 cm·min) could directly be demonstrated by disappearance of the monosaccharides from a 10% solution continuously infused into the lumen (10). Quantitative investigations on the residual capacity of glucose and galactose absorption in patients with glucose-galactose malabsorption were performed by several authors using the perfusion technique. Although glucose concentrations differed widely in the infusion solutions (between 11 and 556 mM), the absorption ratios were similarly low, 6–15% of the intake (12). The residual absorption of glucose and galactose in these patients is similar to the uptake of mannitol and may, therefore, be attributed to a passive process based on diffusion. With the use of radioactive sugars, Linneweh et al. demonstrated that the uptake of glucose or galactose did not exceed 10% of the administered dose, whereas the normal child resorbed over 90% (13).

Patients with glucose-galactose malabsorption also have a renal tubular transport maximum for glucose ($T_mG/1.73$ m^2) of no more than 25% of adult normal values, with an apparent inability to maintain this low level of function with prolonged increase in the filtered load (14). Although there are several indications that glucose can be absorbed from the lumen of the fetal lung by active mechanisms, glucose-galactose malabsorption seems to have no clinical expression during fetal life (15).

Infants and children suffering from glucose-galactose malabsorption can be treated effectively with a diet free of these monosaccharides (16,17). As only about 50 patients have been described in published reports, good follow-up studies are lacking. However, some clinical remission seems to occur with increased age even though active jejunal glucose transport remains absent. The intestinal absorptive surface area and intraluminal volume probably increase with increasing age, thereby reducing the effects of malabsorbed glucose on water secretion and intestinal motility (18).

Absorption and Malabsorption of Fructose

The absorption rate of fructose, on the other hand, is directly proportional to its concentration in the infused fluid. If the rate of glucose absorption is taken as 100%, then from 1 g/100 ml sugar solution the relative rate of fructose absorption is 64%, while from 5 g/100 ml solution it is as high as 89% (9). For these reasons, fructose absorption in humans seems to take place by energy-independent facilitated transport, although an active transport has been found in the rat small intestine (19). Recently, intestinal D-fructose absorption has been investigated using measurements of breath hydrogen, and was frequently found to be incomplete both in children (20) and in adults (21–23). Incomplete absorption may be associated with symptoms of cramps and diarrhea and may occur after the ingestion of as little as 5 g of fructose, even in the adult (22).

Glucose, however, which stimulates fructose uptake in a dose-dependent fashion, may abolish the intolerance, although apple juice, which contains fructose in excess of glucose, might induce abdominal symptoms in susceptible children (20). Barnes et al. reported on a patient aged 12 years, in whom challenge with as little as 1 g of fructose was followed by watery bowel movements and some abdominal discomfort (24).

Secondary Monosaccharide Intolerance

This condition occurs only in young infants and despite its temporary state, may be life threatening. The diarrhea stops only with the removal of all sugars, including fructose, from the diet. The jejunal morphology and the enzymic activities may either be normal or disturbed. Secondary monosaccharide intolerance is tentatively attributed to a "contaminated small bowel." Therefore, the condition is frequently associated with small intestinal obstruction or protracted gastroenteritis (25).

GLUCOSE-GALACTOSE CARRIER

As almost no information is available on the fructose carrier, the present discussion will be limited to the properties of the glucose-galactose carrier operating in the brush border membrane of the small intestine.

In 1958, Riklis and Quastel made the observation that the intestinal movement of glucose is dependent on the presence of Na^+ in the medium (26). In 1962, Bihler et al. showed that reduction in tissue energy supplies eliminates the accumulation of glucose against a concentration gradient but not the Na^+-dependent equilibration of glucose (27). They postulated that the sugar carrier possesses a binding site for cations and later demonstrated that in the presence of Na^+, the carrier manifests about 100 times more affinity for its substrate than in the presence of K^+ (28,29). Since the carrier is assumed to be exposed alternately to the luminal content, rich in Na^+, and to the cytoplasm, low in Na^+ and rich in K^+, the sugar can be transported against its concentration gradient because of ionic differences. The perpetuation of the active transport of glucose will, however, depend on the continuous extrusion of Na^+ by the (Na^+/K^+) -activated ATPase located in the serosa facing membranes (30).

In recent years, the D-glucose transport system has been studied extensively *in vitro* with the use of intact small intestinal tissue preparations or isolated brush border membrane vesicles. The state of the art can be found in two review articles written by Giorgio Semenza who has made major progress in this field (31,32). At present, there is evidence that, apart from the capacity for diffusion (33), the brush border membrane is endowed with two Na^+, D-glucose cotransporters (31,34). The two systems are already operating in the jejunum and ileum of 17- to 20-week-old human fetuses (35). With the use of brush border membrane vesicles from guinea pig jejunum and with D-glucose as substrate, Alvarado et al. could demonstrate that at low glucose concentrations (1 mM or less) most of the uptake occurs through cotransporter-1; this system saturates rapidly and becomes practically constant at about 4 mM glucose (34). Although cotransporter-2 has a much lower affinity (25 mM versus 0.5 mM), its V_{max} is much larger (2300 pmol/mg protein·s versus 340). Hence, starting at about 4 mM glucose, the contribution of the cotransporter-2 to the total uptake increases steadily and a plateau is reached only around 100 mM glucose. Therefore, the two systems function as a tandem: cotransporter-2 takes care of the initial, rapid processing of the sugar load and cotransporter-1 takes over later so that no free sugar remains in the lumen during periods of fast. As concerns simple diffusion, this is negligible at low substrate concentrations but increases rapidly, so that at concentrations of 75 mM or higher (34) its contribution to total glucose uptake exceeds that of cotransporter-1.

The Na^+, D-glucose cotransporter is inserted asymmetrically in the brush border membrane and has asymmetric functional properties. The transport agency does show kinetic asymmetric gated channel characteristics, and its function is probably related to protein structure fluctuation (35,36). The D-glucose transport is stimulated by Na^+ only, and other monovalent cations have no effect (37). The positive charge associated with Na^+ is not compensated by the co-movement of an anion or the countermovement of a cation via the glucose carrier (38). At the moment, a Na^+/ D-glucose stoichiometric ratio of 2:1 is a real possibility (31). Na^+ binds to the glucose carrier of the intestinal brush border and induces a rapid conformation change in the transporter which increases its affinity for glucose (39,40).

The active transport of glucose is significantly greater in the jejunum than in the mid-ileum, whereas the terminal ileum does not exhibit Na^+-dependent D-glucose transport (41). It has also been shown that the Na^+-glucose cotransporter activity decreases with age (42). In the rat, fish oil as compared to the butter fat dietary regimen increases the *n*-3 fatty acids of the brush border membrane, decreases lipid fluidity, and concomitantly, increases Na^+-dependent D-glucose transport (43).

The biochemical studies on the intestinal mucosa from patients with glucose-galactose malabsorption are in agreement with a defect at the level of the brush border sodium-dependent D-glucose transporter. This information has been obtained by different techniques: quantitative radioautography of sugar transport in intestinal biopsies (44), Na^+-dependent accumulation of glucose in intact small intestinal biopsy specimens (45) (see Table 1), sodium-dependent glucose transport in jejunal brush border membrane vesicles (46), and the measurement of short-circuit current as a function of D-glucose concentration in the bathing solution (47,48). One out of four patients with glucose-galactose malabsorption was reported to have no mutarotase activity in the intestinal mucosa (49). More observations are needed before this finding can be interpreted.

GENETIC CONTROL OF THE GLUCOSE CARRIER

From the study of the pedigree of six cases, Meeuwisse and Melin were able to conclude that glucose-galactose malabsorption is an autosomal recessive metabolic disorder (50). Recently, Hediger et al. were able to localize the human intestinal Na^+-glucose cotransporter gene at the q 11.2 → q ter region of chromosome 22; the genes for facilitated glucose carriers, on the other hand, have been mapped to chromosomes 1 and 3 (51). As the Na^+-glucose cotransporter makes up less than 0.2% of the membrane proteins, Hediger et al. preferred to clone and sequence the gene (52). RNA synthesized from the clone and injected into *Xenopus laevis* oocytes increased Na^+-dependent sugar uptake more than 1000-fold, and had no effect on the rate of Na^+-independent uptake. The isolated DNA sequence codes for 662 amino acid residues with a relative molecular mass of 73,080, which is consistent with the Mr of the brush border Na^+-glucose cotransporter (75,000). The proposed model contains 11 membrane-spanning sequences, and the Na^+-active site seems to be 30–40 Å away from the glucose site. Furthermore, there is no detectable homology between the Na^+-glucose cotransporter and either the facilitated glucose carrier or the *E. coli* sugar transporters. This suggests that the mammalian Na^+-driven glucose transporter has no evolutionary relationship to the other sugar transporters (52).

CONCLUSION

In the last 30 years major contributions to the active intestinal transport of glucose and its genetic control have been achieved. The study of patients suffering from glucose-galactose malabsorption has greatly stimulated basic research in the field. On the other hand, comprehension of the function of the glucose-Na$^+$ transport system greatly changed our insights in the understanding and treatment of acute diarrhea. It is hoped that in the near future the same advances will be obtained in the elucidation of the mechanisms of fructose absorption.

ACKNOWLEDGMENTS

The scientific part of the study was supported by Grant 3.0047.89 of the National Fund of Scientific Research of Belgium. We gratefully thank Mrs. W. Coen for typing the manuscript.

REFERENCES

1. Eggermont E. The genetics of intestinal carbohydrate intolerance. In: Steinberg AG, Bearn AG, eds. *Progress in medical genetics*, vol 6. New York and London: Grune & Stratton, 1969;241–79.
2. Eggermont E. Biochemical basis of gastrointestinal intolerance to alpha-D-glucosides. In: Lebenthal E, ed. *Textbook of gastroenterology and nutrition in infancy*. New York: Raven Press, 1981;961–78.
3. Jones BJM, Higgins BE, Silk DBA. Glucose absorption from maltotriose and glucose oligomers in the human jejunum. *Clin Sci* 1987;72:409–14.
4. Caspary WF. Verdauung und Resorption von Kohlenhydraten. *Ernährungs-Umschau* 1989;36:91–6.
5. Crane RK. Hypothesis for mechanism of intestinal active transport of sugars. *Fed Proc* 1962;21:891–5.
6. Crane RK. Na$^+$-dependent transport in the intestine and other animal tissues. *Fed Proc* 1965;24:1000–63.
7. Lindquist B, Meeuwisse GW. Chronic diarrhea caused by monosaccharide malabsorption. *Acta Paediatr Scand* 1962;51:674–85.
8. Laplane R, Polonovski C, Etienne M, Debray P, Lods JC, Pissarro B. L'intolérance aux sucres à transfert intestinal actif. Ses rapports avec l'intolérance au lactose et le syndrome coeliaque. *Arch Fr Pediatr* 1962;19:895–944.
9. Holdsworth CD, Dawson AM. The absorption of monosaccharides in man. *Clin Sci* 1964;27:371–9.
10. Dubois R, Loeb H, Eggermont E, Mainguet P. Etude clinique et biochimique d'un cas de malabsorption congénitale du glucose et du galactose. *Helv Paediatr Acta* 1966;21:577–87.
11. McNeish AS, Mayne A, Ducker DA, Hughes CA. Development of D-glucose absorption in the perinatal period. *J Pediatr Gastroenterol Nutr* 1983;2(suppl 1):S222–6.
12. Beyreiss K, Hoepffner W, Scheerschmidt G, Mueller F. Digestion and absorption rates of lactose, glucose, galactose, and fructose in three infants with congenital glucose-galactose malabsorption: perfusion studies. *J Pediatr Gastroenterol Nutr* 1985;4:887–92.
13. Linneweh F, Schaumloeffel E, Barthelmai W. Angeborene Glucose- und Galactose-Malabsorption. *Klin Wochenschr* 1965;43:405–9.
14. Liu HY, Anderson GJ, Tsao MU, Moore BF, Giday Z. Tm glucose in 2 cases of congenital intestinal and renal malabsorption of monosaccharides. *Pediatr Res* 1967;1:386–94.
15. Strang LB. Solute and water transport across the pulmonary epithelium: a new chapter in long physiology inaugurated by Alfred Jost. *Biol Neonate* 1989;55:355–65.
16. Laplane R, Polonovski C. Directives diététiques pratiques de l'intolérance congénitale aux sucres à transfert intestinal actif. *Rev Practicien* 1965;15:1887–97.
17. Francis D. *Diets for sick children*. Oxford: Blackwell Scientific Publications, 1987;26–7.

18. Elsas LJ, Lambe DW. Familial glucose-galactose malabsorption: remission of glucose-intolerance. *J Pediatr* 1973;83:226–32.
19. Macrae AR, Neudoerffer TS. Support for the existence of an active transport mechanism of fructose in the rat. *Biochim Biophys Acta* 1972;288:137–44.
20. Kneepkens CMF, Vonk RJ. Fernandes J. Incomplete intestinal absorption of fructose. *Arch Dis Child* 1984;59:735–8.
21. Ravich WJ, Bayless TM, Thomas M. Fructose: incomplete intestinal absorption in humans. *Gastroenterology* 1983;84:26–9.
22. Rumessen JJ, Gudmand-Hoyer EG. Absorption capacity of fructose in healthy adults. Comparison with sucrose and its constituent monosaccharides. *Gut* 1986;27:1161–8.
23. Truswell AS, Seach JM, Thornburn AW. Incomplete absorption of pure fructose in healthy subjects and the facilitating effect of glucose. *Am J Clin Nutr* 1988;48:1424–30.
24. Barnes G, McKellar W, Lawrance S. Detection of fructose malabsorption by breath hydrogen test in a child with diarrhea. *J Pediatr* 1983;103:575–7.
25. Anderson CM, Burke V, Gracey M. *Paediatric gastroenterology.* Melbourne: Blackwell Scientific Publications, 1987;369–70.
26. Riklis E,Quastel JH. Effects of cations on sugar absorption by isolated surviving guinea pig intestine. *Can J Biochem Physiol* 1958;36:347–62.
27. Bihler J, Hawkins KA, Crane RK. Studies on the mechanism of intestinal absorption of sugars. *Biochim Biophys Acta* 1962;59:94–102.
28. Crane RK, Forstner G, Eichholz A. Studies on the mechanism of the intestinal absorption of sugars. *Biochim Biophys Acta* 1965;109:467–77.
29. Crane RK. Uphill outflow of sugar from intestinal epithelial cells induced by reversal of the Na^+-gradient: its significance for the mechanism of Na^+-dependent active transport. *Biochem Biophys Res Commun* 1964;17:481–5.
30. Czáky TZ, Hara Y. Inhibition of active intestinal sugar transport by digitalis. *Am J Physiol* 1965;209:467–72.
31. Semenza G, Kessler M, Hosang M, Weber J, Schmidt U. Biochemistry of the Na^+, D-glucose cotransporter of the small intestinal brush border membrane. *Biochim Biophys Acta* 1984;779:343–79.
32. Semenza G, Kessler M, Schmidt U, Venter JC, Fraser CM. The small intestinal sodium-glucose cotransporter(s). *Ann NY Acad Sci* 1985;456:83–96.
33. Dawson DJ, Burrows PC, Lobley RW, Holmes R. The kinetics of monosaccharide absorption by human jejunal biopsies: evidence for active and passive processes. *Digestion* 1987;38:124–32.
34. Alvarado F, Brot-Laroche E, Delhomme B, Serrano MA, Supplisson S. Heterogeneity of sodium-activated D-glucose transport systems in the intestinal brush border membrane: physiological implications. *Boll Soc Ital Biol Sper* 1986;62:110–32.
35. Malo C. Kinetic evidence for heterogeneity in Na^+-D-glucose cotransport systems in the normal human fetal small intestine. *Biochim Biophys Acta* 1988;938:181–8.
36. Kessler M, Semenza G. The small intestinal Na^+, D-glucose cotransporter: an asymmetric gated channel (or pore) responsive to $\Delta \Psi$. *J Membr Biol* 1983;76:27–56.
37. Luecke H, Berner W, Menge H, Murer H. Sugar transport by brush border membrane vesicles isolated from human small intestine. *Pflugers Arch* 1978;373:243–8.
38. Murer H, Hopfer U. Demonstration of electrogenic Na^+-dependent D-glucose transport in intestinal brush border membranes. *Proc Natl Acad Sci USA* 1974;71:484–8.
39. Peerce BE, Wright EM. Sodium-induced conformational changes in the glucose transporter of intestinal brush borders. *J Biol Chem* 1984;259:14015–12.
40. Peerce BE, Wright EM. Examination of Na^+-induced conformational change in the intestinal brush border sodium/glucose symporter using fluorescent probes. *Biochemistry* 1987;26:4272–9.
41. Bluett MK, Abumrad NN, Arab N, Ghishan FK. Aboral changes in D-glucose transport by human intestinal brush border membrane vesicles. *Biochem J* 1986;237:229–34.
42. Vincenzini MT, Jantomasi T, Stio M, Favilli F, Vanni P, Tonelli F, Treves C. Glucose transport during ageing by human intestinal brush border membrane vesicles. *Mech Ageing Dev* 1989;48:33–41.
43. Brasitus TA, Dudeja PK, Bolt MJG, Sitrin MD, Baum C. Dietary triacylglycerol modulates sodium-dependent D-glucose transport, fluidity and fatty acid composition of rat small intestinal brush border membrane. *Biochim Biophys Acta* 1989;979:177–86.
44. Stirling CE, Schneider AJ, Wong MD, Kinter WB. Quantitative radioautography of sugar transport in intestinal biopsies from normal humans and a patient with glucose-galactose malabsorption. *J Clin Invest* 1972;51:438–51.

45. Eggermont E, Loeb H. Glucose-galactose intolerance. *Lancet* 1966;ii:343.
46. Booth JW, Patel PB, Sula D, Brown GA, Buick R, Beyriss K. Glucose-galactose malabsorption: demonstration of specific jejunal brush border membrane defect. *Gut* 1988;29:1661–5.
47. Grasset E, Heyman M, Dumontier AM, Lestradet H, Desjeux JF. Possible sodium and D-glucose cotransport in isolated jejunal epithelium of children. *Pediatr Res* 1979;13:1240–6.
48. Grasset E, Evans LAR, Dumontier AM, Heyman M, Faverge B, Beau JP, Desjeux JF. La malabsorption intestinale du glucose et du galactose. *Arch Fr Pediatr* 1982;39:729–33.
49. Keston AS, Meeuwisse GW, Fredrikzon B. Evidence for participation of mutarotase in sugar transport: absence of the enzyme in a case of glucose-galactose malabsorption. *Biochem Biophys Res Commun* 1982;108:1574–80.
50. Meeuwisse GW, Melin K. Studies in glucose-galactose malabsorption. A clinical study of 6 cases and a genetic study. *Acta Paediatr Scand* 1968;Suppl 188:1–24.
51. Hediger MA, Budarf ML, Emanuel BS, Mohandas TK, Wright EM. Assignment of the human intestinal Na$^+$/glucose cotransporter gene (SGLT 1) to the q 11.2 → q ter region of chromosome 22. *Genomics* 1989;4:297–300.
52. Hediger MA, Coady MJ, Ikeda TS, Wright EM. Expression cloning and c-DNA sequencing of the Na$^+$/glucose cotransporter. *Nature* 1987;330:379–81.

DISCUSSION

Dr. Brodehl: Tubular glucose reabsorption is also defective in glucose-galactose malabsorption. Do you know whether this is controlled by the same genetic system? Are the renal and intestinal glucose carriers comparable?

Dr. Eggermont: This has been suggested, but the information we have for the moment is only clinical evidence and there are no biochemical data that the renal and intestinal glucose carriers are related to each other. The glucose-galactose carrier has also recently been described in the fetal lung. Up to now, we are not aware of clinical manifestations during fetal life in children affected by glucose-galactose intolerance.

Dr. Hobbs: If you infuse glucose in your patients with a defective carrier do you get glycosuria?

Dr. Eggermont: Yes, and the more glucose you infuse, the more pronounced is the glycosuria.

Dr. Schaub: Concerning the discussion on fructose intolerance I want to ask if there are any side effects if fructose is the sole carbohydrate in the diet of these children.

Dr. Eggermont: I think fructose in the diet must be limited; otherwise, the child develops osmotic diarrhea. On the other hand, the simultaneous administration of glucose enhances fructose absorption.

Dr. Schaub: Is fructose phosphorylated in the gut?

Dr. Eggermont: Yes, Ginsburg & Hers (1) showed that fructose is phosphorylated in the small intestinal mucosa as well as in the liver.

Dr. Schaub: So the osmotic effect cannot be high.

Dr. Eggermont: No, the osmotic effect within the gut lumen *is* high because you have a system of dose-dependent resorption; on the other hand, active transport is the ideal system for efficient resorption at low concentrations.

Dr. Baerlocher: You said that in your experience monosaccharide intolerance is no more of any clinical importance, since it has disappeared in recent years. What is your explanation for this? Personally, I have the impression that there are still many discussions about secondary monosaccharide intolerance in clinical practice.

Dr. Eggermont: My opinion is very clear. In the past we have exaggerated the problem of sugar intolerance. The best argument for this is that glucose is now used in oral rehydration solutions for treatment of acute diarrhea in many countries.

Dr. Vis: Glucose-electrolyte solutions remain effective, even in case of jejunal atrophy, such as in extreme cases of cow's milk protein intolerance. Thus the glucose-coupled sodium transport still occurs in these circumstances. Do we know where this transport takes place? Where do we locate the carriers? Over whole of the mucosal surface or only in the crypts?

Dr. Eggermont: The glucose-galactose carrier is localized in the brush border membrane but we have no information where the maximum activity of the carrier is localized, whether on the top or at the base of the villus.

Dr. Vis: How does chloride absorption occur? Where are the chloride transport mechanisms located?

Dr. Eggermont: There is no combined transport of sodium, glucose and chloride. Chloride is absorbed by an independent system.

Dr. Saudubray: Do you know how the transcription of the gene is regulated? Is it regulated by glucose-galactose itself?

Dr. Eggermont: At present we don't know. It is amazing, however, that this important carrier in the brush border makes up only about 0.2% of the total protein content. In comparison, the sucrase-isomaltase enzyme makes up about 25% of the total proteins of the brush border membrane.

Dr. Hobbs: We used to do experiments with yeasts, where if you cultured them in a glucose medium free of galactose they became very good at taking up and utilizing glucose but very bad at taking up galactose. If you then cultured them in a galactose medium free of glucose, exactly the opposite occurred. From these adaptation experiments it seems likely that in the yeasts there are distinctive carriers for glucose and galactose, rather than a common glucose-galactose carrier. Do you know if this has been studied?

Dr. Eggermont: Yes, certainly; it is well known that the facilitative glucose transporters are different from the Na+/glucose cotransporter. More information can be found in the paper by Gould and Bell (2).

REFERENCES

1. Ginsburg V, Hers HG. On the conversion of fructose to glucose by guinea pig intestine. *Biochim Biophys Acta* 1960;38:427–34.
2. Gould GW, Bell GI. Facilitative glucose transporters: an expanding family. *TIBS* 1990;15:18–23.

Inborn Errors of Metabolism, edited by
J. Schaub, F. Van Hoof, and H. L. Vis.
Nestlé Nutrition Workshop Series, Vol. 24.
Nestec Ltd., Vevey/Raven Press, Ltd.,
New York © 1991.

Development of New Therapeutic Strategies for Inborn Errors of Metabolism Involving the Liver

Alex P. Mowat

King's College School of Medicine and Dentistry, Department of Child Health, Variety Club Children's Hospital, Bessemer Road, London SE5 9PJ, United Kingdom

In only a small percentage of genetic disorders or inborn errors of metabolism can the clinical features be ameliorated by manipulating the metabolic pathway by dietary measures, drugs, vitamins, cofactor supplementation, enzyme induction, or end-product replacement (1). Even if such intervention has dramatically beneficial effects in the short term, the long-term outcome may be less than ideal; for example, the 40% incidence of developmental delay and 80% incidence of ovarian failure in patients with galactosemia treated with a galactose-free diet (2). The development of improved modes of treatment applicable to a much wider range of disorders is imperative.

In view of the key role of the liver in metabolism, much attention has been directed toward the functioning of this organ. Brief consideration is necessary of some microanatomical and physiological features which are required for effective hepatic function. A major task of the liver is the uptake of substrates, exogenous (absorbed from the intestine) and endogenous (the metabolic products of various organs) (3). These are metabolized, stored, and distributed as required to other organs. The liver in health is able to maintain in the hepatic vein blood a mixture of solutes and macromolecules within finely regulated concentration limits, adjusted both for the metabolic demands of the body at that time and for recent dietary intake. These functions are modulated by regulatory factors which are mainly humoral. They induce great variation in the phenotypic expression of the organ. The liver has a unique structure that facilitates these tasks. It is worth emphasizing that there are at least three types of cells involved in maintaining metabolic homeostasis. The prime cell is, of course, the hepatocyte, with over 5,000 identified metabolic pathways expressed within each cell. Hepatocytes show considerable functional heterogeneity. Those near the portal tract frequently express very different metabolic activity from those near the portal vein.

A second unique cell is the specialized endothelial cell which lines the sinusoid, separating the circulating blood from the space of Disse. These cells have, in their cytoplasm, fenestrae occurring in small patches, called sieve plates, which provide channels of variable diameter. Thus solutes and macromolecules can pass readily from the plasma space to the space of Disse, into which abut the microvilli on the hepatocyte cell surface. Partially metabolized chylomicrons can pass through these channels. The other function of the sinusoidal cell is receptor-mediated uptake of a wide range of macromolecules.

The third cell is another specialized endothelial cell, the Kupffer cell, which has a unique surface membrane which facilitates adherence, pinocytosis, and phago-cytosis. Like other macrophages, these cells are engaged in antigen processing and antigen presentation. It has become increasingly clear that these three types of cells interact physiologically and pathophysiologically in important ways. Kupffer cells, for example, can be stimulated to release a factor which decreases cytochrome P450 activity in hepatocytes. They can also be stimulated to produce a factor that inhibits protein synthesis within the hepatocyte. Substances taken up by Kupffer cells or endothelial cells may subsequently be transferred to hepatocytes.

The fourth cell, the fat storage cell or Ito cell, may also influence hepatic function by producing extracellular matrix components (EMCs). These may have a direct effect on hepatocyte function by interacting with specific receptors (e.g., for laminin or fibronectin) on the hepatocyte surface. The metabolism of these cells is influenced by the other liver cells and by cytokines from migratory cells of the reticuloen-dothelial system. In chronic liver disease the rate of synthesis exceeds that of deg-radation of EMCs which accumulate and impair circulation and cell-to-cell transfer. In bone marrow transplantation the replacement of host Kupffer cells by that of the donor may have an adverse effect on intracellular interactions and may stimulate formation of ECM.

With respect to treatment in the infant, it should be remembered that at birth hepatocyte plates are usually two cells thick. It is not until the age of 5 that the plates are one cell thick, maximizing contact between blood and hepatocytes. He-patic function is, of course, dependent on parenchymal blood flow. It depends on the gradient between the pressure in the terminal portal vein, estimated at 50 ml H_2O, and in the initial hepatic vein branch, approximately 10 ml H_2O. It should be appreciated that the biotransformation systems which are most active and best stud-ied in the liver may be present in other organs, such as the kidney, small intestine, and endocrine organs.

There are at present four ways of modifying hepatocyte metabolism in genetic disorders which require consideration. The first exploits the techniques of genetic engineering to introduce a new function into the hepatocyte. In this Chapter (*this volume*), Dr. Friedman considers the role of hepatotropic viruses as targeting agents to introduce new DNA into the host cell. Another approach has been to use specific receptors such as that for transferrin or asialoglycoproteins, which are found only on hepatocytes. Material bound to these hepatocyte receptors are internalized. Thus if a genetic message is combined with asialoglycoprotein in a plasmid carrier system which includes the required gene and its promotor, and agents that allow binding and integration of DNA in a nondamaging reaction, gene expression is possible. In rats injected intravenously with such a targeted DNA complex, it has been possible to obtain expression of the bacterial enzyme, chloramphenicol acetyl transferase in the hepatocytes. To date, gene expression has not been shown to persist beyond 14 days (4,5).

Another means of replacing deficient enzymatic activity is hepatocyte replacement. Although this has been achieved in the short term in experimental animals (6), major problems remain, including the prevention of the rejection and the provision of hepatotrophic factors which promote hepatocyte engraftment, functioning, and endogenous regeneration. A further obstacle is the identification of a source of hepatocytes and development of means of storage and transportation. *In vitro* hepatocytes are very dependent on the culture matrix (7). *In vivo* they survive, on histological assessment, for 6 months in the pancreas and for 9 months in the spleen. A demonstration of functional survival has been of shorter duration. Detectable albumin synthesis in analbuminemic rats has been achieved (8).

A further and possibly more promising approach has been to utilize auxiliary (heterotopic) liver transplantation in which the patient's liver remains *in situ*, but another liver or part of a liver is placed surgically within the abdomen. Recently, surgeons in Rotterdam have reported encouraging short-term results using this mode of transplantation in patients with advanced chronic liver disease (9). Whether a heterotopic liver would survive if a structurally intact host liver remains *in situ* without the provision of hepatotrophic factors (poorly understood) is a matter for speculation.

Orthotopic liver transplantation is thus now the only established mode of therapy that may offer a good quality of life for children with metabolic disorders that cause liver damage or in whom a deficient metabolic process in the liver causes damage to other vital organs, such as the brain or kidneys (10–12). For some disorders orthotopic liver transplantation will suffice. Others will require transplantation of other organs, such as the kidneys, pancreas, or lung.

THE PRESENT STATUS OF ORTHOTOPIC LIVER TRANSPLANTATION

Liver transplantation, first successfully performed in a child of 18 months in 1968, is now established as a therapeutic option offering long-term survival with a good quality of life in almost all forms of chronic liver disease and fulminant hepatic failure (10,13,14). Liver transplantation remains a formidable surgical procedure. The recipient is likely to have one or more life-threatening complications in the operative or immediately postoperative period. Primary graft failure, vascular thrombosis, and the prevention of rejection without causing toxicity such as renal damage or increasing susceptibility to infection are major problems (15). Cytomegalovirus infection is strongly associated with chronic rejection, with disappearance of bile ducts (vanishing bile duct syndrome) (16).

Most difficulties occur in the first months after transplantation, resulting in a 1-year graft survival that is usually less than 60%. Supply of donors of suitable size and blood group remains a major limiting factor in developing liver transplantation in children. Two recent developments have improved donor availability. Children can be successfully engrafted using part of a liver from a much larger donor, with results comparable to those obtained with whole organ grafting (17,18). Extended *in vitro* preservation of the liver using a solution developed in the University of Wisconsin has important logistic implications but may also allow time for prospective cross-matching between the donor and the recipient (19). An important limitation with respect to metabolic disease is the finding that donor Kupffer and endothelial cells are replaced by recipient cells early in the post-transplantation period (20). Thus liver transplantation is ineffective for disorders affecting primarily Kupffer cells, such as Niemann-Pick type C (white blood cell sphingomyelinase activity normal) (21).

Starzl and co-workers, reporting their experience in the first 1,000 liver transplants performed since cyclosporin became available as an immunosuppressant, recorded a 1-year actuarial survival of 74%, with a 5-year survival of 64% (10). It should be noted, however, that the 5-year survival of children under 1 year of age, the age at which some of the most severe metabolic disorders would benefit from transplantation, was only 37%, significantly lower than that of older children or adults. Long-term problems following liver transplantation include chronic rejection, opportunistic infection, lymphoproliferative disease associated with Epstein-Barr virus infection, bile duct stenosis, both anastomotic and nonanastomotic, and the development of malignancy. A recent estimate of cost of liver transplantation, with an average hospital stay of 41 days, was greater than $140,000. Long-term costs are likely to remain high, with cyclosporin costing approximately $5,000 per year (14).

Patients who avoid major complications have a good quality of life with catch-up growth and normal development (22). The longest survivor to date remains well 17 years after transplant. A more enthusiastic attitude toward donor procurement by pediatricians and other health care professionals will be necessary to make sufficient livers available to fully utilize the potential of this technique unless legislative changes are made to facilitate donor retrieval (23).

Note: For the discussion, see the next chapter.

REFERENCES

1. Scriver CR, Beaudet AL, Sly WS, Valle D, eds. *The metabolic basis of inherited disorders*, 6th ed. New York: McGraw-Hill, 1989.
2. Buist N. Internationsl survey of galactosemia. *Abstracts of the 27th Annual Symposium of the Society for the Study of Inborn Errors of Metabolism.* SSIEM, 1989;9.
3. Arias IM, Jakoby WB, Popper H, Schachter D, Shafritz DA. *The liver: biology and pathobiology*, 2nd ed. New York: Raven Press, 1987.
4. Wu GY. Targeting in diagnosis and therapy. In Arias IM, Jakoby WB, Popper H, Schachter D, Shafritz DA, eds. *The liver: biology and pathobiology*, 2nd ed. New York: Raven Press, 1987;1303–13.
5. Wu GY, Wilson JM, Wu CH. Targeting genes: delivery and expression of a foreign gene driven by an albumen promoter in vivo. *Hepatology* 1988;8:1251.
6. Goulet F, Normand C, Morin O. Cellular interactions promote tissue specific function, biomatrix deposition and junctional communication of primary cultured hepatocytes. *Hepatology* 1988;8:1010–8.
7. Bumgardner GL, Fasola C, Sutherland DER. Prospects for hepatocyte transplantation. *Hepatology* 1988;8:1158–61.

8. Demetriou AA, Reisner A, Sanchez J, et al. Transplantation of micro carrier-attached hepatocytes into 90% partially hepatectomised rats. *Hepatology* 1988;8:1006–9.
9. Terpstra OT, Reuvers CB, Schall SW. Auxiliary heterotopic liver transplantation. *Transplantation* 1988;45:1003–7.
10. Iwatsuki S, Starzl T, Todo S, et al. Experience in 1000 liver transplants under cyclosporin-steroid therapy: a survival report. *Transplant Proc* 1988;20s:498–504.
11. Mowat AP. Liver disorders in childhood: the indications for liver replacement in parenchymal and metabolic diseases. *Transplant Proc* 1987;19:3236–41.
12. Esquivel CO, Marino IR, Fiioravanti V, Van Thiel DH. Liver transplantation for metabolic disease of the liver. *Gastroenterol Clin N Am* 1988;17:165–75.
13. Shaw BW, Wood RP, Kaufman SS, et al. Liver transplant therapy for children (2 parts). *J Pediatr Gastroenterol Nutr* 1988;7:157–66, and 797–815.
14. Paradis KJG, Freese DK, Sharp HL. A pediatric perspective on liver transplantation. *Pediatr Clin N Am* 1988;35:409–33.
15. Rubin RH. Infectious disease problems. In: Maddrey WC, ed. *Transplantation of the liver* (Current topics in Gastroenterology Series) New York: Elsevier 1988;279–308.
16. O'Grady JG, Alexander GJM, Sutherland SS, et al. Cytomegalovirus infection and donor-recepient HLA antigens: interdependent co-factors in pathogenesis of vanishing bile duct syndrome after liver transplantation. *Lancet* 1988;ii:302–5.
17. Broelsch CE, Emond JC, Thistlethwaite JR, et al. Liver transplantation, including the concept of reduced-size liver transplants in children. *Ann Surg* 1988;208:410–20.
18. Otte JB, Yandza T, De Ville De Goyet J, Tan KC, Salizzoni M, De Hemptinne B. Pediatric liver transplantation: report on 52 patients with a 2-year survival of 86%. *J Pediatr Surg* 1988;23:250–3.
19. Kalayoglu M, Sollinger HW, Stratta RJ, et al. Extended preservation of the liver for clinical transplantation. *Lancet* 1988;ii:617–9.
20. Gouw ASH, Houthoff HJ, Hintema J, et al. Expression of major histocompatibility complex antigens and replacement of donor cells by recipient ones in human liver grant. *Transplantation* 1987;43:291–7.
21. Gartner JC, Bergman I, Malatak JJ, et al. Orthotopic liver transplantation in children *Pediatrics* 1986;77:104–9.
22. Mowat AP. Liver transplantation—a role for all paediatricians. *Arch Dis Child* 1987;62:325–6.
23. Stewart SM, Uauy R, Waller DA, Kennard BD, Benser M, Andrews WS. Mental and motor development, social competence and growth one year after successful pediatric liver transplantation. *J Pediatr* 1989;114:574–81.

DISCUSSION

Note: The discussion relative to this chapter is to be found at the end of the chapter that follows.

Inborn Errors of Metabolism, edited by
J. Schaub, F. Van Hoof, and H. L. Vis.
Nestlé Nutrition Workshop Series, Vol. 24.
Nestec Ltd., Vevey/Raven Press, Ltd.,
New York © 1991.

Liver Transplantation for Inborn Errors of Metabolism and Genetic Disorders[1]

A. T. Cohen, *Alex P. Mowat, **B. H. Bhaduri,
*G. Noble-Jamieson, Roger Williams, †N. Barnes,
and ‡R. Y. Calne

*Liver Unit, King's College Hospital, London SE5 9RS; * Department of Child Health, King's College Hospital, London SE5 9RS; ** Paediatric Liver Transplantation Service, King's College Hospital, London SE5 9RS; † Department of Child Health, University of Cambridge, Addenbrooke's Hospital, Cambridge CB2 2QQ; and ‡ Department of Surgery, University of Cambridge, Addenbrooke's Hospital, Cambridge CB2 2QQ, United Kingdon*

Inborn errors of metabolism or genetic disorders comprise 22% of referrals to the pediatric liver service at King's College Hospital, London (1). In the Cambridge/King's College Hospital liver transplantation program, 23% of children and 6% of adults receiving orthotopic liver transplantation have such liver disease (2). For such patients liver transplantation is now a very promising form of therapy (3). In this chapter we concentrate on aspects of the natural history and the effects of other forms of therapy, as well as on our experience of liver transplantation in three disorders: liver disease associated with α-1-antitrypsin deficiency, Wilson's disease, and tyrosinemia (fumaryl acetoacetate hydrolase deficiency) (Table 1). The role of liver and/or kidney transplantation in primary hyperoxaluria will also discussed. It will thus complement other chapters in this volume.

α-1-ANTITRYPSIN DEFICIENCY (GENOTYPE PIZZ)

α-1-Antitrypsin deficiency, coded for by a variant of a single polymorphic gene on chromosome 14, is inherited in an autosomal codominant fashion (4). It is one of the more common single-gene defects, occurring in about 1 in 2,000 to 1 in 7,000 newborns of European origin. The plasma deficiency of the glycoprotein is due to a block in secretion from the endoplasmic reticulum rather than a defect in the synthesis of the Z polypeptide.

The clinical features associated with the deficiency state are very variable, with

---

[1] Experience in the King's College Hospital, London, and Addenbrooke's Hospital, Cambridge, Program.

TABLE 1. *Liver transplantation for metabolic disorders*

Cambridge/King's series	Children	Adults
α-1-Antitrypsin deficiency	15	4
Wilson's disease	3	11
Primary oxaluria	2	6
Tyrosinemia	4	—
Hemochromatosis	—	2
Protoporphyria	1	—
Crigler-Najjar syndrome	1	—
Galactosemia	1	—
Total	27	23

some having no overt disease, up to 20% developing liver disease of variable severity, and up to 60% developing emphysema. Although over 50% of infants with the deficiency state have abnormal biochemical tests of liver function and these remain abnormal in over 30% throughout the first 12 years of life, only 10 to 15% develop symptomatic liver disease (5). In 90% this takes the form of a conjugated hyperbilirubinemia with hepatosplenomegaly and disturbed biochemical tests of liver function presenting in the first 4 months of life. In 10% of these infants, a serious bleeding diathesis due to vitamin K malabsorption is an important component of their illness, frequently leading to permanent neurological abnormality (6). One to 2% present in later childhood or adult life with cirrhosis, with no history of prior jaundice in infancy (7). Emphysema usually has its onset in early adult life.

What causes the liver disease or determines its severity is unknown (8,9). α-1-Antitrypsin is a small monomeric glycoprotein (molecular weight 52,000) with three complex carbohydrate side chains. Circulating α-1-antitrypsin is only one of several antiproteases in the blood. It pervades tissue and is found in secretions. Its concentration increases with other acute-phase proteins under appropriate stress. In PiZZ individuals a single amino acid substitution in the polypeptide core is associated with the retention in the endoplasmic reticulum of α-1-antitrypsin deficient in carbohydrate side chains. Circulating concentrations of α-1-antitrypsin are only between 10 and 15% of normal but may rise to the lower limit of normal in stress, making phenotyping essential for diagnosis in the presence of liver disease. The physiological role of α-1-antitrypsin is unknown. *In vitro,* it inhibits elastase, collagenase, and leukocyte and bacterial proteases, including many that are critical in initiating or perpetuating components of the inflammatory response, such as complement activation, coagulation, and fibrinolysis. α-1-Antitrypsin is also formed by circulating mononuclear cells but not in sufficient concentration to affect the circulating concentrations. Whether these contribute to tissue concentrations is unknown (10). The accepted dogma is that emphysema is caused by the uninhibited action of proteases, activated particularly by cigarette smoking. The storage of α-1-antitrypsin within the endoplasmic reticulum of liver cells is not the cause of liver damage, since it is found in PiZZ subjects with otherwise normal livers. A more likely hypothesis is that a tissue damage by proteases, however initiated, continues uninhibited because of lack of antiproteases. The situation may be aggravated by the production of oxidants by myeloperoxidase. Oxidants inactivate α-1-antitrypsin, further limiting its inhibitory capacity.

Liver transplantation in this disorder increases the serum α-1-antitrypsin concentration to the normal range and changes the phenotype to that of the donor (11). The features of end-stage cirrhosis are reversed. It is yet to be shown that liver transplantation will prevent the development of emphysema. The genesis of this may already be present, with over 10% of our patients having increased lung volumes in the first decade (12). Recombinant DNA technology using retroviruses has allowed the insertion of the normal α-1-antitrypsin gene into bacteria, yeasts, and bone marrow cells, but the glycoprotein produced is deficient in some of the carbohydrate side chains. The Piz polypeptide has positively charged lysine replacing negatively charged glutamate at position 342. By inserting a second gene mutation which changes the amino acid at point 290 in the polypeptide chain from lysine to glutamate, the configuration of the peptide is restored to one that can be excreted in an experimental cell line (13).

To date α-1-antitrypsin for administration has been limited to plasma-derived material. It has a half-life of only 6 days. It has not been used in children with acute or chronic liver disease. Trials have been performed in adults with emphysema, confirming that it is possible to raise the serum concentration. Perhaps its use in infants with acute liver injury would inhibit the tissue-damaging cascade initiated by white cell protease, which activates coagulation, complement, and kallikrein production. Other possible antiproteases would include eglin C, aprotinin variants, and antioxidants such vitamin E. We are currently involved in a controlled trial of the use of colchicine as an anti-inflammatory, antifibrotic agent in this disorder. None of these therapies have an established role at present. There is thus no treatment for end-stage liver disease other than liver transplantation. The question is: When should this be done? In a few instances the liver disease in infancy is so severe that decompensated cirrhosis develops rapidly, with death as early as a few weeks of age. For such infants, should transplantation be considered?

The majority of patients recover from the acute hepatitis, the jaundice clears, and nutrition improves. A period of well-being follows. There is, however, persistent hepatomegaly with or without splenomegaly, and standard biochemical tests of liver function remain abnormal. In the course of the first decade, these will return to the normal range in approximately 25% of patients. Survival into the third decade without features of cirrhosis has been recorded in such patients. Approximately 25% die of cirrhosis, usually by 10 years of age. Features of decompensation appear up to 4 years prior to death; that is, the jaundice may return, the serum albumin drop, and diuretics may be required in controlling ascites. A further 25% with histologically confirmed cirrhosis remain in a compensated state with good growth and development throughout childhood despite persistently abnormal biochemical tests of liver function. In general, the prognosis of liver diseases is related to the severity and duration of the acute hepatitis in early infancy, but in the individual patient the liver biopsy in the first 6 months of life is the best guide to prognosis. Those with the prospect of early death or cirrhosis can be identified by the changes seen in liver biopsies (i.e., marked portal tract changes with increased fibrosis, edema, or established cirrhosis). Such infants require reappraisal at regular intervals throughout childhood.

An important development in cirrhosis associated with α-1-antitrypsin deficiency is evidence of renal involvement, with a variety of glomerulonephropathies (14,15). Renal involvement may cause hematuria and/or proteinuria and contribute to hypoalbuminemia. The development of this renal complication does add to the difficulties after liver transplantation, particularly severe hypertension. It would seem desirable to proceed to liver transplantation before features of renal involvement are manifest.

We suggest that evaluation for liver transplantation should occur in infants with severe hepatic fibrosis in whom the cholestasis does not recede, and on the recurrence of jaundice, deteriorating coagulation studies, and/or falling serum albumin. Eleven of 15 children transplanted because of decompensated cirrhosis in 14 instances and severe growth failure in the other case are alive up to 5 years later. These required re-transplantation. After transplantation the serum α-1-antitrypsin phenotype is that of the donor, with concentrations in the normal range. The risk of future lung disease is unknown. No evidence of emphysema was found in four cases followed for more than 6 years after transplantation (11).

WILSON'S DISEASE

Wilson's disease, an autosomal recessive disorder occurring worldwide with an estimated frequency of 1 in 50,000, is due to a defective gene on chromosome 13 (16). An abnormality in the transport and storage of copper results in copper accumulation and tissue damage. The exact pathogenesis is unclear. There is a defect in ceruloplasmin production, diminished biliary copper excretion with low concentrations of a high-molecular-weight copper-binding protein in bile (17). It has been postulated that this protein may inhibit copper reabsorption from the gut.

Early symptoms are frequently nonspecific and unless clinical signs of liver disease, or less commonly neurological abnormalities, are carefully sought for or abnormal liver function tests obtained, diagnosis is delayed for many months until jaundice or features of decompensated cirrhosis appear.

The initial presentation may be hemolysis or an apparent nephrotic syndrome. Symptomatic liver involvement in Wilson's disease may mimic any form of acute or chronic liver disease. It is invariably fatal unless treated. Except in the four categories detailed below, D-penicillamine or other chelating agents, such as triethylene tetraamine, together with a low copper diet, should adequately control liver damage, creating a stable compensated cirrhosis compatible with a good long-term prognosis. Oral zinc sulfate may also stabilize liver disease if the toxic side effects of these

TABLE 2. *Hepatic prognosis in Wilson's disease at institution of therapy*

Score	Bilirubin (μmol/liter)	AST (IU/liter)	Prolongation of prothrombin time
0	<100	<100	<4
1	101–150	101–150	4–8
2	151–200	151–200	9–12
3	201–300	201–300	13–20
4	>300	>300	>20

Total score: 6 or less, chelation and dietary therapy; >6, arrange transplantation.

drugs cause their withdrawal. Zinc has an antagonistic action against copper in many metabolic processes. Its inhibitory effect on copper absorption has been used to maintain a negative copper balance and to reverse abnormal biochemical and pathological abnormalities in patients already treated with penicillamine. These are reports in neurological literature of zinc being used as the sole mode of therapy.

Patients presenting with fulminant hepatic failure die, as do those with decompensated cirrhosis (18,19). If encephalopathy or severe hepatic decompensation occurs, hemofiltration or plasmapheresis may keep the patient alive until grafting is possible. For those with less severe liver disease we have developed a prognostic index (Table 2) based on the degree of abnormality of the prothrombin time, serum aspartate aminotransferase, and bilirubin concentration at the time of instituting therapy in 27 patients, 13 of whom died within 56 days of initiating treatment. It has correctly predicted the response to treatment in all but one subsequent case (see below). Patients with a prognostic index of 7 or greater should be referred for liver transplantation.

In one 12-year-old with decompensated cirrhosis and a prognostic index score of 9 we prescribed zinc sulfate 100 mg every 12 h, giving penicillamine in standard doses at the intervening 6 h. Gradually over the course of 2 months the liver function improved and subsequently returned to complete normality with a remission of all clinical features of liver disease. This has not occurred in other cases and we would not advocate this other than as a measure to be taken while waiting for an organ to become available.

Liver transplantation must also be considered for those who relapse because therapy has been stopped against medical advice. Hepatic decompensation occurs within 6 to 18 months and rarely (if ever) is it controlled by reinstituting penicillamine. Will such patients take immunosuppressants indefinitely? Following transplantation, serum ceruloplasmin levels return to normal over the course of 1–2 months. Radiolabeled copper studies show normal copper uptake by the liver graft with prompt biliary excretion. Kayser-Fleischer rings may be present for up to 2.5 years. Neurological abnormalities may improve rapidly, but some improvement may occur over the course of the next 4 years even in those with very advanced disease (20). Eight of 14 patients transplanted at a mean age of 20 years (range 5.6 to 38.5 years) survived 6 months to 5 years after transplantation. Four were transplanted having had a fulminant presentation, the remainder having decompensated cirrhosis.

HEREDITARY TYROSINEMIA

The biochemical and diagnostic features and dietary treatment of hereditary tyrosinemia are considered elsewhere in this volume. Some clinical features should be emphasized. The acute form presents in the first 12 weeks of life with failure to thrive, vomiting, diarrhea, a cabbage-like odor, hepatomegaly, edema, ascites, splenomegaly, and a bleeding diathesis. Death from liver failure usually occurs by 8 months of age, with less than 10% surviving to 1 year (21,22). Such patients should be considered for transplantation if, despite conventional dietary and drug treatment, features of liver failure are not ameliorated or growth arrest occurs.

The chronic form may evolve from the acute or present with cirrhosis, renal tubular dysfunction, and hypophosphatemic rickets. Hepatocellular carcinoma develops on the basis of a macronodular cirrhosis in over 30% surviving beyond 2 years of age and is presumably likely to develop in all. Neither serum α-fetoprotein concentrations nor scanning by ultrasound, CAT, or NMR distinguish malignant transformation from regenerating nodules. It has been suggested that a "window of opportunity" for transplantation exists between 24 and 36 months of age. Although occasional survival into adult life has been described, there seems to be little reason to delay transplantation after the child weighs 10 kg or after 24 months of age if no extrahepatic metastasis has been identified. Our experience is limited to four patients, one of whom died of metastatic disease having received a transplant at 5.4 years, while those receiving transplants at 1.6, 2.1, and 7.4 years survive 1.5–2.5 years later.

PRIMARY HYPEROXALURIA TYPE I

Primary hyperoxaluria type I is an autosomal recessive disorder with a defect in hepatic metabolism leading to renal and cardiovascular damage. There is deficiency of peroxisomal alanine:glyoxylate aminotransferase (EC 2.1.44) in liver, kidney, and spleen. Glyoxylate accumulates and is metabolized to oxalate and glycolate. The oxalate is excreted in the urine, causing calcium oxalate nephrolithiasis, nephrocalcinosis, and renal failure (23).

Initially, renal transplantation was attempted for this disorder, but calcium oxalate causes early graft failure. This led to the introduction of liver and kidney grafting, which has proved successful. Another approach is to perform a liver trasplantation, then to proceed to renal transplantation when the oxalate pool is diminished, so as to avoid renal allograft failure. It is important that transplantation be performed before severe cardiovascular disease arises due to systemic oxalosis. Eight patients with a median age of 19 years (range 10–28) have been transplanted in this program with five long-term survivors. The youngest had a combined kidney–liver transplant with excellent renal and hepatic status 18 months later, although he continued to pass renal calculi for 9 months after the procedure. It particularly important to maintain a very high urinary output for the first few days post-transplant when the renal oxalate load is still very high (24).

CYSTIC FIBROSIS

With increasing long-term survival in cystic fibrosis, it has become recognized that between 10 and 20% of young adults develop features of cirrhosis. The major problems are alimentary bleeding from esophageal varices and massive splenomegaly with features of hypersplenism. Liver transplantation has been reported, with 50% surviving with a very good quality of life, without evident deterioration of pulmonary function (25). In at least one instance, combined liver–heart–lung transplant has been performed. In the United Kingdom, heart–lung transplant has been performed in over 60 patients with cystic fibrosis with 1-year survival rate of 60%. The majority of deaths are due to technical problems in the immediate post-transplant period, although some late deaths occur from an obliterative bronchiolitis. Cirrhosis may be well complicated in cystic fibrosis and its presence may only come to light after transplantation. The role of organ transplantation in this condition is at present less well defined than in other disorders, where there is less multisystem involvement.

CONCLUSION

Liver transplantation at present has a well-defined role in giving a good quality of life to patients with in an increasing range of metabolic disorders. It also gives new insight into the basic metabolic defects in many disorders and defines the hepatic contribution to their pathophysiology. Its place in management will require constant review as new forms of therapy evolve and as techniques of liver transplantation change.

REFERENCES

1. Mowat AP. Liver disorders in children: indication for liver replacement in pharenchymal and metabolic diseases. *Transplantation proc* 1987;19:3236–41.
2. Polson RJ, Williams R. Application to inborn errors of metabolism in liver transplantation. Cambridge–King's College Hospital experience. In: Calne R, ed. *Liver transplantation*, 2nd ed. London: Grune & Stratton, 1987.
3. Esquivel CO, Marino IR, Fioravanti V, Van Thiel PH. Liver transplantation for metabolic disease of the liver. *Gastroenterol Clin N Am* 1988;17:167–75.
4. Schroeder WT, Miller MTE, Woo SLC, Saunders GF. Chromosomal localisation of the human alpha-1-antitrypsin gene (Pi) to 14 Q 31-32. *Am J Hum Genet* 1985;37:868–72.
5. Sveger T. The natural history of liver disease in alpha-1-antitrypsin deficient children. *Acta Paediatr Scand* 1988;77:847–51.
6. Psacharopoulos HT, Mowat AP, Cook PJL, et al. Outcome of liver disease associated with alpha-1-antitrypsin deficiency (PiZ). *Arch Dis Child* 1983;58:882–7.

7. Eriksson S, Carlson J, Velez R. The risk of cirrhosis and primary liver cancer in alpha-1-antitrypsin deficiency. *N Engl J Med* 1986;314:736–9.
8. Povey S. The genetics of alpha-1-antitrypsin deficiency in relation to neonatal liver disease. *Mol Biol Med* 1990;7:161–72.
9. Mieli-Vergani G, Doherty DG, Donaldson PT, et al. HLA status in children with alpha-1-antitrypsin deficiency (PiZ) and chronic liver disease. *Pediatr Res* 1987;22:98.
10. Krivit W, Miller J, Nowicki M, Freier E. Contribution of monocyte-macrophage system to serum alpha-1-antitrypsin. *J Lab Clin Med* 1988;112:437–42.
11. Shaw BW, Wood RP, Kaufman SS, et al. Liver transplant therapy for children [two parts]. *J Pediatr Gastroenterol Nutr* 1988;7:157–66, 797–815.
12. Greenough A, Pool JB, Ball C, Mieli-Vergani G, Mowat AP. Functional residual capacity related to hepatitic disease. *Arch Dis Child* 1988;63:850–2.
13. Brantly M, Courtney M, Crystal RG. Repair of the secretion defect in the Z form of alpha-1-antitrypsin by the addition of a second mutation. *Science* 1988;242:1700–2.
14. Levy M. Severe deficiency of alpha-1-antitrypsin associated with cutaneous vasculitis, rapidly progressive glomerular nephritis and colitis. *Am J Med* 1986;81:363–4.
15. Strife CF, Hug G, Chuck G, et al. Membranoproliferative glomerulonephritis and alpha-1-antitrypsin deficiency in children. *Pediatrics* 1983;71:88–92.
16. Yuzbasiyan-Gurkan V, Brewer GJ, Boerwinkle E, Venta PJ. Linkage of the Wilson's disease gene to chromosome 13 in North-American pedigrees. *Am J Hum Genet* 1988;42:825–9.
17. Iyengar V, Brewer GJ, Dick RD, Owyang C. Studies of cholecystokinin-stimulated biliary secretions reveal a high molecular weight copper binding substance in normal subjects that is absent in patients with Wilson's disease. *J Lab Clin Med* 1988;111:267–74.
18. Rakela J, Kurtz SB, McCarthy JT, et al. Fulminant Wilson's disease treated with post dilutional hemofiltration and orthotopic liver transplantation. *Gastroenterology* 1986;90:2004–7.
19. Nazer H, Ede RJ, Mowat AP, Williams R. Wilson's disease: clinical presentation and use of prognostic index. *Gut* 1986;27:1377–81.
20. Polson RJ, Rolles K, Calne RY, Williams R, Marsden D. Reversal of severe neurological manifestations of Wilson's disease following orthotopic liver transplantation. *Q J Med* 1987;64:685–91.
21. Kvittingen EA. Hereditary tyrosinaemia type 1: an overview. *Scand J Clin Lab Invest* 1986;46(s146):27–34.
22. Dehner LP, Snover DC, Sharp HL, et al. Hereditary tyrosinaemia type 1 (chronic form): pathological finding in the liver. *Hum Pathol* 1989;20:149–58.
23. Morgan SH, Watts RW. Perspectives in the assessment and management of patients with primary hyperoxaluria type 1. *Adv Nephrol* 1989;18:95–106.
24. Watts RW, Calne RY, Rolles K, et al. Successful treatment of primary hyperoxaluria type 1 with combined renal and hepatic transplantation. *Lancet* 1987;ii:474–5.
25. Mieles LA, Orenstein D, Teperman L, et al. Liver transplantation in cystic fibrosis. *Lancet* 1989;i:2203–4.

DISCUSSION

Dr. Otte: We have a patient suffering from α-1-antitrypsin deficiency who has hematuria and probably kidney damage. What is the future of the child if he is transplanted? Is it going to be reversible?

Dr. Mowat: We followed four patients who have had albuminuria and two of them had hematuria; over the course of 18 months it cleared.

Dr. Otte: For Wilson's disease presenting as the fulminant form you mentioned that transplant should be done when the score was above 6. We have had a very poor experience with this kind of disease, and we have never been able to save a patient without a transplantation. I wonder how you would define the fulminant form. Is this a patient with neurological disorder or with hemolysis?

Dr. Mowat: The patients we have defined were those with encephalopathy, but any with a score of 7 or over would need a transplant, unless we have some better way of treating it. I think these patients need very active intervention with hemofiltration and plasmapheresis while you try to get a liver. I think they should go right to the top of the list. As I described, we had five children who died within 5 days of admission.

Dr. Otte: Regarding the Crigler-Najjar syndrome, you said, and this is quite obvious, that transplantation should be performed before brain damage occurs. But how can you predict when brain damage is going to occur? If it has occurred it is too late; it is not reversible as far as I know, since there is destruction of the brain tissue. So do you refer to the age of the patient, or how else can you predict it? When are you going to consider having the child transplanted?

Dr. Mowat: I don't think you can predict the brain damage. Our data base for serum bilirubin and brain damage goes back to the late 1940s, where we had a lot of experience with rhesus immunization. Since then there has been little new evidence, so we tend to go along with the belief that if we can keep the serum bilirubin less than 300 μmol/liter or 20 mg/dl, the risk of brain damage is relatively low. Professor Otte is quite right to be concerned about this because the children with Crigler-Najjar type 1 who have not died in infancy but have gone through to early adolescence very frequently develop neurological deterioration, even though the serum bilirubin may not have been higher than perhaps 250 μmol/liter. I try to keep my patients' serum bilirubin below 200 μmol/liter, hoping that they have sufficient reserve to withstand a rise in bilirubin if they get an infection.

Dr. Buts: Do you believe that in Wilson's disease there is a relationship between the blood level of ceruloplasmin and the severity of the disease?

Dr. Mowat: I have no evidence for this. The vast majority of our patients have unmeasurable ceruloplasmin and I am not aware of an association with the severity of liver disease.

Dr. Van Hoof: To avoid mental retardation in Crigler-Najjar disease, I think that weekly measurement of unconjugated bilirubin is insufficient. The rate of bilirubin production (destruction of heme) can be widely variable, and the transport of unconjugated bilirubin depends on the amount of albumin.

Dr. Mowat: A great deal of effort, particularly in the neonatal period, has gone into trying to get some estimate of reserve capacity for safe carriage of bilirubin. As far as I am aware, we have still no other measure that we can use successfully.

Dr. Sokal: I would like to add a comment about Crigler-Najjar disease. Although I am convinced that the only real therapy is liver transplantation, there is another potential way to help these patients. This has been done in neonates with hyperbilirubinemia due to ABO incompatibility. Administration of a heme synthesis inhibitor such as SN-protoporphyrin leads to a significant decrease in serum bilirubin levels. One child currently on our mailing list has been given this drug since he is not well controlled by phototherapy. His bilirubin level fell from 18 mg to 12 mg per 100 ml (308–205 μmol/liter) without additional phototherapy. However, he had photosensitivity and abnormal liver function tests which are possibly due to this drug; for this reason, this compound should not be recommended for general use, although it is likely to help some critical Crigler-Najjar patients on the waiting list for transplantation.

Dr. Mowat: Under these circumstances you don't need to worry about liver damage. Does it have to be given by injection?

Dr. Sokal: No, it can be given orally.

Dr. Hobbs: I would like to make three comments. First, let me support you in that the protein reference units in Great Britain provide a monitoring service for Wilson's disease and there is no correlation between the residual ceruloplasmin level and the clinical severity. I would fully support Professor Mowat's index, which is a sort of thing you need. Second, α-1-antitrypsin deficiency was first described in 1963 by Laurell and Eriksonn and was associated with lung disease. I believe that I was the first to describe it in association with angionecrotic renal disease in 1971. Three patients had to have renal transplants and one relapsed some years later. I must add that the disappearance of proteinuria or hematuria does not mean that the kidney has recovered. It just means that the leaky glomeruli have been fibrosed completely. But I am quite sure that having corrected the α-1-antitrypsin deficiency you are going to prevent further attacks. Third, I think there is a function for α-1-antitrypsin. Phylogenetically, it has evolved along with antithrombin III and has become a protein that is useful for survival. Its real function is the inhibition of white cell elastase, and it is the elastin destruction that results in the angionecrosis in the renal condition and in the destruction of the lung.

Inborn Errors of Metabolism, edited by
J. Schaub, F. Van Hoof, and H. L. Vis.
Nestlé Nutrition Workshop Series, Vol. 24.
Nestec Ltd., Vevey/Raven Press, Ltd.,
New York © 1991.

Displacement Bone Marrow Transplantation Can Correct Some Inborn Errors of Metabolism

John R. Hobbs

Charing Cross & Westminster Medical School, Department of Immunology,
Westminster Hospital, 17 Page Street, London, SW1P 2AR, United Kingdom

The objective of displacement bone marrow transplantation (DBMT) is to obtain 100% healthy donor-type marrow which can correct an inborn error that was expressed in the bone marrow of the recipient, and at the same time endow the recipient with the immunology of the donor so that the healthy gene product will enjoy immune tolerance and not be subjected to humoral or cellular reactions by the host. These could be the major problem when gene transfer is undertaken *in vivo* after birth. DBMT is only applicable to about 7% of understood genetic diseases, where correction has been achieved for over 40 previously fatal genetic diseases, with partial correction for another six, but there has now been failure in at least five diseases. While Good and colleagues (1) were able first to treat a genetic disease, severe combined immune deficiency, by a simple bone marrow transplant with no induction, the need for a displacement induction was demonstrated by work done in 1970–1973 at Westminster, where bone marrow transplant was also extended to include other family (2,3) and volunteer unrelated donors (4) needed for the four out of five patients who do not have a healthy matched sibling. Bone marrow transplantation can correct genetic diseases in two main ways: (a) by replacing genetically deranged or absent blood cells [as when Steinmuller and Motulsky (5) corrected spherocytosis in an animal; or Good's team installed helper T-cells in a boy (1)] and (b) by implanting bone marrow cells that will deliver a normal protein to the tissues of the host, as was discovered by the team of Hobbs in 1970 when they showed that the lymphocytes of a healthy brother could transfer the capacity to produce migration inhibitory factor (MIF) to the cells of an elder brother, achieved both *in vitro* and then *in vivo* by the transplant (6). It was the evolution of the latter work that led to the displacement concept and the proposal by Hobbs in 1978 to a Working Party of the European Bone Marrow Transplant organization that over 30 previously fatal genetic diseases might respond to DBMT. The introduction of busulfan for bone marrow transplant induction in mice by Santos encouraged its successful use in a boy with Hurler's

TABLE 1. *Principles to correct inborn errors by displacement bone marrow transplantation*

1. The inborn error should be expressed in bone marrow stem cells.
2. The patient's abnormal marrow should be displaced.
3. Donor marrow factory produces the normal gene product.
4. The host must be immunologically tolerant to that product.

For enzymes, proteins, etc.
5. Leukocyte production can be 50–300 g/day
6. Leukocytes circulate, release the component, or deliver cell to cell.
7. Defective tissues should be able to accept the component.
8. The component finds its functional site to a degree adequate to correct the defect.

disease, and the proposal was then published (7). Since then, DBMT with immunoprophylaxis has been extensively used and reviewed (8–11). The principles are summarized in Table 1, lists of the treatable diseases in Tables 2 and 3, and optimal conditions for elective DBMT in Table 4. In this chapter I outline the procedures, including immunoprophylaxis, and consider the results, always remembering that the most serious complications of infection and graft-versus-host diseases (GVHD) can cause serious morbidity (8,10) so that DBMT is confined to otherwise fatal inborn errors for which no better treatment has yet been established.

PROCEDURE

If optimal results are to be obtained (see Table 4), it is imperative to assess the patient for referral before irreversible damage has occurred. Such assessment is undertaken by the referring team, our own team, and when the disease is one with which our team is not familiar, by a further expert opinion. Such assessments will indicate any urgency, or permit wider donor search, and even the setting up of *in vitro* assays to test potential transfers and to see if any binding antibodies have been generated in the patient by previous exposures to normal components. Such antibodies can persist postgraft (12) and have been found in nine patients to date.

The final decision with regard to a donor depends on the exact status relevant to the inborn error (normal homozygotes are preferred), and a two-way mixed lymphocyte culture (MLC) result with a transformation index (TI) under 1.64 (13), which has been the most reliable parameter in over 220 of our transplants. Use of such donors has caused <7% fatal GVHD without the use of T-cell depletion [which can cause rejection rates up to 15%, or unstable partial chimerism; without 100% donor-type bone marrow, the graft can be lost any time up to 7 years later (7)]. Appropriate measures (14) are taken for any blood group differences. Full viral studies are undertaken for patient and donor to plan appropriate measures during the procedure (e.g., use of CMV-negative blood products) and experienced psychological and social workers are involved in the consultation and advice to the parents, including a home

TABLE 2. *Inborn errors where displacement bone marrow transplantation can provide normal cells*[a]

Already successfully corrected	Thalassemia major (RBC)
Reticular dysgenesis (leukocytes)	Sickle cell (RBC)
Sex-linked (helper T ± B)	Spherocytosis (RBC)
Swiss-type autosomal recessive (T + B)	Osteopetrosis (osteoclasts)
SCID with cartilage-hair dysplasia (T + B)	
Late adenosine-deaminase (new T + B)	**Possibly correctable**
Late purine nucleoside phosphorylase	Severe elliptocytosis (RBC)
(new T + B)	Erythropoietic porphyria (RBC)
Late Di George (new T)	Severe pyruvate kinase (RBC)
Connatal GVHD (new T)	Other severe hemoglobinopathy (RBC)
Wiskott-Aldrich (new T + B + phagocytes)	Homozygous G6PD deficiency (phagocytes)
Autosomal recessive (helper-T)	Severe myeloperoxidase (phagocytes)
Bare lymphocyte (new class II)	Lysozyme (phagocytes)
Bare lymphocyte (new class I)	Lipochrome histiocytosis (phagocytes)
Bare lymphocyte (new class I + II)	Lactoferrin (phagocytes)
Nezelof/Matsaniotis (T)	Strauss defect (phagocytes)
Interleukin II receptor (T)	Tubulin (phagocytes)
Late onset childhood SCID (T)—not AIDS	Severe myosin (phagocytes)
Nonfunctional B (B ± T)	Severe histiocytosis X (phagocytes)
Adult onset (T + B)—not AIDS	D. Miller's reticuloendotheliosis
Chronic granulomatous disease	(phagocytes)
(phagocytes)	Bruton's (B)
Chediak-Higashi (phagocytes)	Sporadic hypogammaglobulinemia (B)
Kostmann, recessive (neutrophils)	Isolated IgM (B)
Autosomal dominant agranulocytosis	Isolated IgG (B)
(neutrophils)	Severe IgG$_2$ (B)
Lazy phagocyte (phagocytes)	Severe isolated IgA (B)
Cyclic neutropenia (phagocytes)	Duncan's X-linked proliferative (T + B)
Adhesive proteins (phagocytes)	Severe orotic aciduria (T + B)
Diamond-Blackfan (RBC)	

[a] A review (26 papers), *Correction of Certain Genetic Diseases by Transplantation*; is available by sending £22 Sterling payable to Westminster Medical School Research Trust, 17 Horseferry Road, London SW1P 2AR, G.B.

visit. Only after this, at the second interview, are the parents or the child asked to give their final decision about DBMT. The present schedule of induction is outlined in Table 5 and the reasons for it are given elsewhere (10), as are those for avoiding irradiation of children (7).

Immunoprophylaxis

After busulfan, infusion of donor buffy coat allows presentation of any normal antigens to the recipient's immunocompetent lymphocytes, where T-helper function must be available. If exactly 24 hours later cyclophosphamide is given, it results in the deletion of any primary immune responses that might have been made by the recipient. To reduce the risks of GVHD, cyclosporinA (CsA) begins intravenously

TABLE 3. *Inborn errors where displacement bone marrow transplantation can provide* a
transferable component

Already successfully corrected
Chronic mucocutaneous candidiasis (MIF)
Hurlers (α-iduronidase)
Sanfilippo B (acetyl-α-glucosamidase)
Gaucher's Type III Norbottnian
(cerebroside-β-glucosidase)
Gaucher's, onset < 3 years (cerebroside-β-
glucosidase)
Gaucher's, onset 3–16 years (cerebroside-
β-glucosidase)
Fabry's (α-galactosidase)
Refsum's (?)
Immunodeficiency (γ-interferon)
Metachromatic leukodystrophy
(arylsulfatase A)
Wolman's (acid esterase)
Fucosidosis (fucosidase)
(Biotinidase)
Niemann-Pick B (sphingomyelinase)
Fanconi's (DNA-repair enzyme)

Already partially corrected
Hunter's (iduronidate-sulfatase)
Sanfilippo A (heparan-sulfatase)
Morquio B (β-galactosidase)
Maroteaux-Lamy (arylsulfatase-B)
Adrenoleukodystrophy (peroxisomal
enzyme)
Lesch-Nyhan (hypoxanthine-guanine-
phosphoribosyltransferase)
I-cell, mucolipidosis II (mannose
processing enzyme)

Known inadequate correction by 100%
engraftment
GM1 gangliosidosis (acid-β-galactosidase)
Pompe's (acid-α-glucosidase)
Niemann-Pick A (sphingomyelinase)
Krabbe's (galactosylceramidase)
Farber's lipogranlomatosis (acid
ceramidase)

Possibly correctable
Scheie's (α-iduronidase)
Hurler-Scheie compound (α-iduronidase)
Sanfilippo C (α-glucosaminide-
acetyltransferase)
Sanfilippo D (acetyl-α-glucosaminide-6-
sulfatase)
Mannosidosis (mannosidase)
Sialidosis (sialidase)
Mucolipidosis III (? mannose-
phosphorylase)
Niemann-Pick D (?)
Maple syrup urine (leukocyte correctable)
Galactosemia (galactose-1-phosphate-
uridyltransferase)
Ataxia telangiectasia (DNA-repair
enzyme)
Xeroderma pigmentosa (DNA-repair
enzyme)
Morquio A (galactosamine-6-sulfate-
sulfatase)
Batten's (? peroxisomal enzyme)

[a] A review (26 papers), *Correction of Certain Genetic Diseases by Transplantation*; is available by sending £22 Sterling payable to Westminster Medical School Research Trust, 17 Horseferry Road, London SW1P 2AR, G.B.

TABLE 4. *Optimal conditions when referring patients for elective displacement bone
marrow transplant*

1. Before complications have occurred (such as septic foci, transmitted viral diseases, transfusional sensitization, severe bony deformities, irreparable CNS damage).
2. If splenectomy is needed, with immunization planned in advance.
3. If prior enzyme therapy is tried, immunoprophylaxis should have been used (10).
4. In general, the younger the better.
5. Ideally, with a matched sibling who is a normal homozygote.
6. To a center with gnotobiotic facilities, especially for transplants from alternative donors.

TABLE 5. *Induction for displacement bone marrow transplantation*

Day		
−11	To theater for Hickman line and autologous BM harvest; return to sterile laminar flow room.	
−10	Busulfan[a]	4–6 mg/kg
−9	Busulfan	4–6 mg/kg
−8	Busulfan	4–6 mg/kg
−7	Busulfan	4–6 mg/kg
−6	Donor buffy coat *Exactly 24 h later*[b]	
−5	Cyclophosphamide[b,c]	50–75 mg/kg
−4	Cyclophosphamide[b,c]	50–75 mg/kg
−3	Cyclophosphamide[c]	50–75 mg/kg
−2	Cyclophosphamide	50–75 mg/kg
−1	Day of rest	
0	Transplant	

[a] 80 mg/m^2 corrected to not < 4 and not > 6.
[b] 2 g/m^2 mercaptoethane sulfonate and diuresis are used daily with the cyclophosphamide.
[c] T-helper function is needed here, so cyclosporin A or ATG must not be given before day −3.

on day 3, and methotrexate is usually used only where the donor is an unrelated volunteer or where problems can be anticipated. Where there is failure of engraftment, confirmed between days +14 to +21, our usual procedure is to rescue the patient with autologous marrow immediately and not to attempt regraft for at least 3 months, whereafter a second full induction has caused no problems. Should chronic GVHD occur, continuous penicillin is used postgraft until it resolves, as it can be associated with autosplenectomy.

Where possible, we routinely use intravenous CsA, carefully monitoring the free plasma level (plasma being separated at 37° within half an hour of the blood collection) and have found that a window of 70–180 ng/ml is helpful and does not cause too much hypertension or renal failure. Such intravenous CsA continues until day +20 or later if the gut has not recovered to a normal xylose absorption allowing oral doses. If a matched sibling DBMT is followed by no GVH, CsA is abandoned at 3 months but where GVHD above grade 2 has occurred, or in all transplants from mismatched or unrelated donors, CsA is continued for 1 year at least, if possible (15). Prophylactic IgG can be used but live vaccines are not permitted until full immunological recovery has been verified. The splenectomy situation is considered more fully under Gaucher's disease. In general, we expect the majority of our patients to be off all treatment within 1 year of the transplant and this is the case in >90% of our patients.

RESULTS FOR SPECIFIC DISEASES

These are listed in Tables 3 and 4, and the type of donor is indicated as MS (matched sibling), VUD (volunteer matched unrelated donor), or HS (a family donor sharing at least one full genetic haplotype).

Reticular Dysgenesis

In a known family the birth was conducted under aseptic conditions and an MS bone marrow transplant undertaken without any conditioning, to achieve full correction (16). If diagnosed after birth, it would be important to eradicate any infection (e.g., using irradiated leukocytes from one parent so that the other could be an HS donor).

Severe Combined Immune Deficiency (SCID)

The first MS bone marrow transplant, without conditioning (1), has resulted in a healthy chimera, now stable for 21 years. The donor female helper T-cells fortunately cooperate with the recipient's remaining B-cells. In some patients this has not occurred, so where there is any doubt, it would be advisable to use DBMT to achieve all-donor cooperating cells (17). T-helper deficiency is the commonest form of SCID, and simple bone marrow transplant from HS donors, while possible, has often failed to achieve complete correction (18).

Non-Sex-Linked SCID (Swiss Type)

Bone marrow transplant without conditioning has been successful (19), but it is important to deal with existing infection, with antibiotics, intravenous IgG, and even irradiated immune T-cells (e.g., from one parent), to improve the chances of success. Emergency bone marrow transplant has produced good results in less than 60%. Of 12 patients with disseminated BCG, the only two survivors had immune T-cells immediately. Presentation with acute GVHD, transplacental or from unirradiated blood products, is serious: the graft might be possible after rescue by antilymphocyte globulin (ALG), and so on.

SCID with Cartilage Hair Dysplasia

The SCID and hair have been corrected by bone marrow transplant without conditioning (18,20). Today it is felt the cartilage disorder might have responded better to DBMT.

T-cell Deficiencies Diagnosed after Age 3 Months

Today it is important to exclude HIV infection, where reliance cannot be placed on serology: detection of the HIV genome can be achieved within 2 hours (21). At present there is no justification for the use of bone marrow transplantation to treat HIV as growing T-cells propagate the virus and over 40 failures are known. Deficiencies of adenosine deaminase, purine nucleoside phosphorylase, or of the thymus can be corrected by substitution therapy begun within 6–8 weeks of birth, but after the age of 3 months transient responses are more the rule. Since the common form of adenosinedeaminase deficiency arises by deletion of a large part of the genome (22), the normal enzyme generates antibody production to its own inactivation. DBMT is the treatment of choice, preferably correcting infection, prolonged malnutrition, treatable viral infections (HSV, etc.) and even using thymic therapy where indicated, although this can generate GVHD. If enzymes or cells are infused before DBMT, it would be important to practice immunoprophylaxis (10) to abrogate a primary immune response.

Wiskott-Aldrich Syndrome

The underlying membrane protein defect (23) indicates early DBMT (7). Immunomodulation failed to prevent bleeds and malignant transformation (24).

Autosomal Recessive Helper T-Cell Defect

The OKT4 hapten can be absent with completely normal helper function (25). Where malfunction is proven, DBMT is essential to achieve cooperating T- and B-cells, unless the donor is a perfect MS.

Bare Lymphocyte Syndrome

Defects of class I and class II expression (26) require DBMT for full correction. Donor selection can be complicated by failure to stimulate in the MLC. It is hoped molecular biology methods may be developed to assist matching.

Nonfunctional Lymphocytes

Since secondary T-cell deficiency is so common (27), total absence of the suspected cytokine deficiency and failure to induce it with immunomodulators (27) must be shown before undertaking DBMT. Our first patient (6) with candidiasis since birth did not produce migration inhibitory factor (MIF) to all immunogens tested and it was not inducible *in vitro:* five similar patients not given bone marrow transplants all died, confirming the seriousness. Deficiency of gamma interferon can also be so serious (28) that the only treatment seems to be DBMT. More patients with normal numbers of T- and B-subsets are being found with serious malfunction (18). Improving knowledge and assays for cytokines and their receptors may better identify them and the best treatments. The provision of lymphocytes delivering cytokines at short range seems preferable to the complications of lifelong systemic therapies, where malaise, growth failure, and even amyloidogenesis may result. In older patients it is possible that autoimmune mechanisms are active, and where life becomes intolerable, intervention with total body irradiation (TBI) could eradicate the autoimmune process with an MS bone marrow transplant establishing normal immune function and good health.

Errors Intrinsic to Phagocytes

Bone marrow transplantation intended to replace abnormal by normal phagocytes was first undertaken in April 1973 (4) (for chronic granulomatous disease) and from it arose the concept of DBMT. The traditional use of TBI in animals by serendipity deleted the abnormal phagocyte stem cells of mice to cure Chediak-Higashi syndrome (29) and of dogs to correct cyclic neutropenia (30), and in the latter condition, recombinant human granulocyte colony stimulating factor (GM CSF) therapy has had successful initial responses and long-term results are awaited. In contrast, ordinary bone marrow transplant failed for lazy leukocyte syndrome (31) and though achieved after TBI, the subsequent pneumonitis killed the child (31). Kostman's syndrome was corrected by bone marrow transplant after TBI (32) but today may be corrected by treatment with GM CSF (33), avoiding the risks of bone marrow transplant. Cyclophosphamide induction alone achieved only 30% engraftment in another form of congenital neutropenia (34), but today a trial of GM CSF should perhaps first be made before proceeding to proper DBMT. Adhesive protein deficiency also failed to respond to ordinary bone marrow transplant (35) but was successful after total body irradiation. The same sequence occurred for human Chediak-Higashi syndrome (36).

Severe Genetic Anemia

While explaining why previous failures had occurred when only cyclophosphamide was used to try to correct such conditions, it was predicted that DBMT should be successful (7), so it was a pleasure to read that thalassemia major was first successfully corrected using dimethyl busulfan added to the induction (37). The use of Bu/Cy now in over 300 children for MS DBMT has been successful in some 90% of children under 5 years, and in around 80% from 6 to 16 years (38). The alternative of continuous transfusion, despite the use of chelates to reduce iron overload, has had a mortality of 37% within 10 years (39) together with the risks of transmission of CMV, viral hepatites, and worst of all, HIV (36 children who have contracted HIV by blood transfusion for thalassemia are known to the author). Experience has shown that tentative dosages of Bu/Cy result in unstable chimeras with regression to the disease state (40), so that full doses are indicated (41); the risk of veno-occlusive disease has been overestimated, for it rarely occurs (42). The DBMT option seems preferable to conservative management (43) and where parents have to bear the cost is much more effective. In older children who have been less well maintained the risks are higher for either DBMT or continuance, but pregraft high-dose intravenous chelate can remove much iron, and complex isoimmunization can be treated by giving Thymostimulin Serono 1 mg/kg with the buffy coat in our protocol; this recruits many of the secondary memory B-cells and encourages them to commit suicide. For such patients the choice between DBMT and continuing transfusions will be an individual decision.

Congenital spherocytosis in animals was corrected by DBMT serendipitously because total body irradiation was used (5), and now that we know the ongoing risk of splenectomy under 5 years of age (some 30% will die), a MS DBMT seems attractive. Similarly, irradiation intended for leukemia also achieved a DBMT to correct sickle cell anemia (44), which has since been treated successfully with DBMT (45). Blackfan-Diamond syndrome has also been completely corrected by DBMT (46) but may respond to cytokine treatment, where, again, long-term results are awaited. With improving characterization to identify the severe forms of elliptocytosis, pyruvate kinase deficiency, and so on, these might also be best treated by DBMT.

Osteopetrosis

There appear to be four different errors in animals giving rise to this syndrome, but as yet in humans only two major varieties have been identified; the infantile form (which, however, varies in rate of progress between families), which is due, at the time of writing, to an unidentified error in osteoclasts; and the late onset or benign form, due to an absence of carbonic anhydrase type II (47). It is the infantile form which justifies DBMT because bone overgrowth crushes the cranial nerves to cause the blindness and deafness and other paralyses and eventually obliterates the bone marrow to cause death. Successful parabiosis led Walker to the more practical use of bone marrow, but with spleen, to restore bone resorption in microphthalmic mice (48). In 1977 it was shown that bone marrow alone would do, and in mice displacement was not needed (49). Alas, this experiment could not be transferred to the human situation for simple bone marrow transplant (50) failed, as did a heavy induction (51). In 1979, Lamendin (52) recorded success after adding total body irradiation, a practice confirmed in Minnesota (53), but today Bu/Cy is preferred (18, 41). Mobilization of the bone postgraft demands control of the hypercalcemia. In some late patients, the bone is so dense that even with DBMT the marrow cannot get established so, ideally, it DBMT should be undertaken as early as possible, even inducing at 36 weeks of gestation; in this way the cranial nerves can usually be saved. Vitamin D (calcitriol) can delay petrosis (54) during a donor search and brave surgeons can enlarge the optic foramina to buy time. At diagnosis it is important to establish whether the child is blind and/or deaf, so that the parents can be fully informed and may decline a graft option. Current evidence does suggest that the osteoclast may have its own precursor in human bone marrow (55), which is fortunately transferred during the transplant. Alas, at present there is no way of transferring the osteoblast, which, of course, might correct quite a few other diseases.

Mucopolysaccharidoses

Infants presenting with swollen abdomens or hernia (56) should be screened for storage diseases, including mucopolysaccharidoses (MPS), so that diagnosis can be made before damage becomes irreversible. Where the CNS is involved with deposits, clearance beginning under the age of 2 years would permit 1 year of normally continued dendrite growth, and new connections are possible until the age of 3 years. Thereafter, rehabilitation would depend on residual pathways. Nine years' experience has shown that under elective conditions, MS DBMT can achieve over 90% good survival, except that some bone abnormalities cannot be reversed. Normal enzyme has to be delivered across the blood-brain and cartilage barriers in adequate amounts to correct the defect, and this may not always occur. While much transfer of free protein enzyme seems unlikely, in a child iduronidase rose from 0 to 4% of normal (57), and this has been confirmed in dogs, with up to 10% normal (58). Donor cells do cross the blood-brain barrier and become part of the microglia both in mice (59) and in humans (Krivit et al.; to be published). A review (57) of available evidence showed that other enzymes, such as α-*N*-acetylglucosamidase (Sanfilippo B), and arylsulfatase A (metachromatic leukodystrophy) are transferred in amounts adequate to reverse neurologic lesions in the young. Some enzymes such as β-glucuronidase, catalase, and arylsulfatase B are not transferred, and the enzymes for Niemann-Pick A and GM1-gangliosidosis are not transferred in amounts adequate to reverse human disease. Sulfamidase (Sanfilippo A) can reverse early lesions, but so far, iduronate sulfatase (Hunter's syndrome) has not had good results, although the survivors were all older children. For each disease, separate studies and maneuvers will have to be undertaken, and sometimes a comparable animal model does not always transfer to the human situation [e.g., young Twitcher mice get better (59), whereas Krabbe's disease does not improve] (Krivit, personal communication). New cases would best have MS DBMT from a donor with the full normal level of circulating missing enzyme. Certainly, the IQ of many survivors is very pleasing and may be adequate for them to lead a normal life, although none have yet reached the age of 12 years.

Hurler's Disease

Hurler's disease was first treated by the Westminster team (60) and today 5 of 6 MS transplants, 3 of 3 VUD grafts, and 4 of 15 HS attempts have produced survivors who have done well. Eight of the survivors are beyond 3 years postgraft and are attending normal schools. Those whose donors had full normal levels of enzyme showed rapid normalization of liver and spleen, clearing of corneal clouding by 3 months, and marked improvement in heart failure, so that the soft tissue results were excellent. With regard to the bones, the children stand up straight and walk normally, but the beaked vertebra at the main point of the original lumbar gibbus does not change and, so far, three of our patients have had spinal fusion across this lumbar vertebra; the growth of the spine lags somewhat behind the growth of the limbs. All retain enlarged metacarpal bones, but lose their claw hands and are able to undertake fine skilled movements. Some can flatten their fingers together in the prayer position but others (mostly whose donors were heterozygotes) cannot. Postgraft, the accelerated skull growth ceased. In a boy who died at 15 months from a pneumococcal septicemia, α-iduronidase was found at 4% of the level in normal brain after correction had been made from the hemoglobin level for the contained blood (control MPS brains from ungrafted children show no enzyme activity at all); in this patient the rib cartilage showed normalization in its pattern. However, now 8–9 years after their grafts, two of the children are suffering pains around their knee joints which is inhibiting the freedom of movement they had enjoyed; one has stopped playing football and the other no longer jumps on trampolines. As the cartilage thickens, further enzyme may not be delivered to the chondrocytes, which then use up their limited supply and revert to Hurler type. It appears that the hips have become unstable in one patient with a heterozygous donor, and another child at 9 years of age has developed a limp in one leg, despite having a homozygous normal donor. These developments some 8 years after the DBMT are a cause for concern and are being closely followed. In contrast, the membrane bones do well and the Hurler facies and nasal sinuses have normalized, apart from some thickening at the top of the nose (a cartilage bone area). Hearing must be continually assessed, using grommets, if needed, to ensure that the children can benefit from their education; most of our patients are maintaining IQs from 85 to 115, the higher values being in those grafted around 1 year of age. By computed axial tomography and magnetic resonance imaging the brains of the treated children seem vastly improved compared to untreated controls (10). Contrasting the results of all 12 survivors with the natural progress of disease in their families (who cannot all have the Scheie variant with normal IQ), DBMT is at present considered well worthwhile, but we are following the progress of the large joints in our older children, and hoping that when the epiphyses fuse the cartilage will be less thick and perhaps those bones may enjoy the benefits seen in the membrane bones.

San Filippo-B Disease

Nonidentical twin sisters who had HS DBMT (61) when just over 2 years of age have not, in the subsequent 7 years, followed the disastrous progress of their two elder brothers who were each severely affected by the age of 4 years. Their donor was heterozygous, and progress was complicated by severe GVHD and leukopenia.

One of the girls appears to have recovered almost completely from chronic GVHD, but the other is still showing effects. Both have led a reasonably normal life and go to school, but require extra assistance in their education. DBMT under the age of 3 years still seems justifiable but, of course, follow-up must continue.

Gaucher's Diseases

The classifications of this group are continually being revised in the light of new molecular biology. As yet, there is no evidence that the infantile acute neuronopathic form can respond to DBMT. For the mainly nonneurological other forms we prefer to adopt a classification as "fast" (symptoms before age 3 years), "medium" (symptoms 3–16 years of age), and "slow" (symptoms only after 16 years of age). This would encompass the Norrbottnian (62) variety which probably has different genetic origins. Enzyme replacement evaluated in old types I and III (63) had very limited success and it has never been clear whether antibody formation occurred against the enzyme as prepared. While gene transfer has been accomplished in the test tube (64) there was no test against the mature immune system of a patient, and as yet we are unaware of any treatments with recombinant enzyme. The classical Gaucher cell is a mononuclear phagocyte, but early attempts (Hammersmith and Philadelphia) did not use displacement and failed to establish successful grafts. While total body irradiation (65) achieved successful engraftment, the response seemed slower, with longer persistence of the Gaucher cells than in our patient (66), where CAT scans (67) show rapid improvement before all the host monocytes could possibly have been replaced. Thus the idea that all that is necessary is to change the Gaucher cell for the normal phagocyte seems wrong and it is much more likely that enzyme is actually transferred from the engrafted phagocytes to their neighbors. For Gaucher cells locked in fibrous cords in the liver clearance is much slower, possibly because of delivery problems, so some Gaucher cells persist up to 2 years, whereas in the bone marrow they clear within 6 months. It is also possible that the nonuse of immunoprophylaxis (62,65) could have generated antibodies, to explain their high enzyme levels (not found in our nine cases) in the phagocytes for some months after the graft; IgG-tagged enzyme would go back into the white cells to be measured by the assay: delivery elsewhere would be impaired. Splenectomy under the age of 5 years is followed by many septicemic deaths (65,68), so we initially tried transplants, leaving spleens intact in two children with neutrophil counts above 1,000 and platelet counts above 75,000 μl^{-1}. These patients required up to 356 units of platelets, and one never achieved a neutrophil count above 50 μl^{-1}, dying subsequently of aspergillosis. The other recovered completely to normalize spleen, liver, and lung function. Three other splenectomized patients had much easier grafts (67), so four subsequent patients had elective splenectomies pregraft. Pre-splenectomy, they can be immunized with pneumococcal, meningococcal, and hemophilus vaccines, to set up memory status in B-lymphocytes and antigen-processing cells. Immunizing their donors pre-bone marrow transplant ensures that immune recipient and donor cells can cooperate postgraft when a booster dose is given and good antibody levels are obtained. The spleen has an important role in initiating responses against capsular antigens (69), then transferred as memory cells to the bone marrow. The spleen may also have a vital role in filtering the blood (70), so that surgeons should be encouraged to try and leave some spleen. If, however, they leave too much, severe neutropenia can cause postgraft deaths, as in two patients after day +56, although donor red cells were well engrafted. Survivors should take penicillin for life, and while some strains of the offending microorganisms do become resistant, this does not seem yet to be the case for the DF2 type organisms common in cats and dogs, which are known to be able to kill post-splenectomy patients. A major problem in Gaucher's diseases, found in all our patients in pregraft liver biopsies, was quite extensive fibrosis. The impaired liver function tests and raised IgA have normalized in all our survivors postgraft, but biopsies up to 2 years later have not shown very much improvement in the degree of fibrosis, although there has been a large amount of clearing of Gaucher cells. Nevertheless, the children have developed a marked increase in well-being ("new children" say their parents) and achieved active lifestyles. A 16-year-old girl abandoned her 2-year-old leg irons at 3 months, gave up her crutches at 4 months, and now regularly rides a bicycle. Two other girls who had pregraft hip damage now behave as if it did not exist and our orthopedic surgeon is not going to intervene until there is a better indication than a bad X-ray. This is a most rewarding disease to treat by DBMT, although long-term liver results are awaited.

Fabry's Disease

Small increases in α-galactosidase A level achieved by fetal liver transplantation benefited three patients (71). DBMT could do better and confer tolerance to the enzyme for the lifetime of the patient.

Refsum's Disease

Similar benefit followed fetal liver transplantation (71), so DBMT could work even from a heterozygous donor. Current treatments with aphereses and difficult dietary regimes are not satisfactory for all patients.

Metachromatic Leukodystrophy

The first patient to receive DBMT died before the heterozygous enzyme level could affect her progress (72), and another patient continued to progress after ordinary bone marrow transplantation (73) but did improve when DBMT was done. A further patient (74), and two others have also shown measurable improvements in their CNS functions.

Wolman's Disease

The severe form of acid esterase deficiency shows storage visible within leukocytes, and the biochemical abnormalities were fully corrected by DBMT, but alas, the infant died on day +80 from aspergillosis (75).

Fucosidosis

Because affected fibroblasts could be cleared of deposits by adding normal leukocytes to a culture, DBMT was proposed for this disease (76). Hopefully, the human blood-brain barrier can be crossed as easily as in the dog. In dogs, DBMT achieved fucosidase brain levels as high as 48% of normal, with reversal of CNS lesions in dogs done before 4 months of age (77).

Biotinidase Deficiency

Biotin replacement therapy does not fully correct this syndrome (78), which must be correctly identified (79) from other defects which do respond to replacement therapy (80). Older descriptions (e.g., Omenn's syndrome) are inadequate, but patients have been corrected by DBMT (18).

Niemann-Pick Disease

A patient diagnosed as "type B," who showed initial improvement after a DBMT (81), is now showing some evidence of neurological lesions. Her defect is being fully evaluated and while it still shows many features of Type B, the neurological developments suggest that the initial diagnosis will have to be changed; there may be even more variants in this group.

Fanconi's Syndrome

The underlying defect is a failure to repair DNA, so excess somatic mutations occur throughout life which can end with neoplastic transformation; the tissues are also much more susceptible to test doses of irradiation or cyclophosphamide, whereby challenge tests enable early diagnosis to be made, before over-transfusion, and so on. Late patients with aplasia have responded to ordinary bone marrow transplants, although procarbazine is the preferred induction drug (82,83). Fatal GVHD occurred in some 60% of patients over the age of 6 years (84), but the success rate is now approaching 50% (85), and while HS donors have had poor results, two VUD bone marrow transplants have been successful (86). In our first patient (82) neoplastic epithelia around the eye and in the bladder normalized post-transplant, so the repair enzyme appears transferable.

Hunter's Disease

There now appear to be "fast," "medium," and "slow" forms of this disease (87). Our two survivors had fast disease and only had their DBMT at 5 years of age, both developing severe chronic GVHD with low levels of leukocyte and enzyme. Neither has yet shown any real evidence of mental improvement, although hepatosplenomegaly has gone. It is not known whether a graft from a normal homozygote under the age of one year can achieve better results. A boy with a slow variety had a successful DBMT at 7 years of age and appears to be progressing satisfactorily (88). Assuming that random neutralization of the X-chromosome occurs for neurons, the mother's cells unable to synthesize enzyme must obtain an adequate supply from their neighbors. It remains to be seen whether an adequate supply can cross the blood-brain barrier after early DBMT.

San Filippo A Disease

Our patient grafted at 5.4 years showed marked improvement of the systemic features, but at 5 years postgraft we are disappointed by mental deterioration and would not at present graft any patient over the age of 4 years. A French child who had DBMT at 2 years is apparently doing well.

Morquio's Disease

Here again, severe and mild forms exist (87) with at least three distinct enzyme deficiencies. One of our patients with advanced disease did not receive buffy coat immunoprophylaxis and produced postgraft IgG that bound to the normal enzyme and greatly reduced its activity; that child had improvement only in liver and spleen (89) and finally died after dislocation of her odontoid process. Our second patient had HS DBMT from his father but developed severe chronic GVHD with leukopenia and low enzyme delivery, and again while the liver and spleen has improved, his orthopedic progress has been disappointing.

Maroteaux Lamy Syndrome

A 13-year-old patient who received DBMT for this disease (90) showed improvement in hepatosplenomegaly, corneal clouding, and lung function, but little progress in the joint deformities, her age precluding much new cartilage formation. In a 7-year-old boy, DBMT ensuring immunoprophylaxis not only produced the improvements noted above but also a clearly improved range of movement within 6 weeks of the graft. We are still assessing his further progress, but at least can detect no antibodies to arylsulfatase B.

Adrenoleucodystrophy

DBMT achieved normal circulating leukocytes in the first patient (91), who, nevertheless, died at + 145 days with no reduction of the lesions. Immunoprophylaxis had not been used, so it is not known if the "peroxidation corrector" reached the required sites. Since most X-linked carriers have no lesions, those neurons unable to produce enzyme must receive it from adjacent cells. Two further patients are showing improvement after somewhat better transplants.

Lesch-Nyhan Syndrome

The original patient received an MS DBMT at 21 years of age and his metabolic disease appears completely corrected, but there has been no improvement in his psychosis in the subsequent 2 years (92). Two further attempts have been made in children under 1 year of age, but alas, early post-transplant deaths have prevented evaluation.

I-Cell Disease

Biochemical improvement has followed an MS DBMT from a heterozygote (93) and the usual downhill course has been prevented. Long-term follow-up is awaited.

GM1 Gangliosidosis

By the time the infant is born, there now appears to be extensive deposition, and DBMT at 9 months and even at 3 months from a normal homozygote have been unable to reverse the inexorable progression of the disease (94).

Pompé's Disease

Three attempts at 5–6 months of age were followed by two deaths from heart failure and one from pneumonia (95). Before transplanting our patient, we kept samples of her voluntary and smooth muscle alive in tissue culture for 24 h, by which time the added donor leukocytes had completely cleared them of glycogen; that this happened *in vivo* was confirmed at postmortem, even though the graft had only just taken. We could not test heart tissue *in vitro* and it is not known if there are sufficient coated pits to allow adequate access of donated enzyme.

Niemann-Pick A Disease

In a mouse mode (96) and in a young infant (Krivit, personal communication) bone marrow transplantation has not been able to reverse the neurological damage present at diagnosis, although it appears that immunoprophylaxis was not practiced in either case. Clearly, any antibodies that bound to donor enzyme would almost certainly prevent its entry into the central nervous system, but their postgraft presence has not been sought.

Krabbe's Disease

In the Twitcher mouse model, bone marrow transplantation, which must be before the age of 11 days, greatly improves the progress (59). As this simulates the human disease, two patients have been treated, but with very disappointing results despite full engraftment (Krivit, personal communication).

Farber's lipogranulomatosis

A boy with a severe deficiency of acid ceramidase and brain lesions had a DBMT at 18 months ago from his compatible sister, who had a normal homozygous level of enzyme. This achieved 100% donor-type engraftment with only GVH grade II. The patient nevertheless showed no improvement in the progress of his disease (Dr. G. Souillet, Lyons; to be published).

FUTURE DEVELOPMENTS

While a majority of the original diseases proposed have been corrected by a properly undertaken DBMT, Tables 2 and 3 list other diseases that might be correctable through the same principles. While a bad family history guides judgment to the seriousness, it is in those very situations that future births would best be prevented, if at all possible, by studies of chorionic villus biopsies or, indeed, amniotic biopsies. In Britain, some 80% of these diseases tend to be sporadic, with no known family history, and are not preventable. For others, prenatal diagnosis is not yet possible. Some diseases seem to be intrinsic to the B-lymphocyte and, indeed, absence of IgA has been both conferred upon a BMT recipient (97) and corrected by one of our DBMTs, just as is recorded for the atopic state (98). The severe diseases indicated can render a patient's life quite miserable, and intravenous IgG has not prevented acquisition of serious viral infection and other complications. It is possible that cytokine deficiencies may underlie some of them and that recombinant peptide therapy may become the future choice as for Kostmann's. On the other hand, in some centers, the over 90% success rate for elective MS DBMT before complications occur may provide a better choice to the parents than more expensive alternatives. It is to be hoped that DNA probes and monoclonal antibodies will better identify those severe forms justifying DBMT, and for many of the currently suggested diseases it is possible to set up fibroblast cultures from affected patients in media without corrective factors (e.g., avoid fetal calf serum) and to compare these with what happens after the addition of prospective donor leukocytes or plasma (99), and extending this to more relevant tissues such as brain or heart when this becomes feasible. However, just as for gene replacement therapy, DBMT must be tested in an intact animal with all its physiologic barriers and a normal immune system. It should also be remembered that some animal successes (simple bone marrow transplant in micro-ophthalmic mice, correction in Twitcher mice) have not been transferable to the human situation.

The cost-efficiency of current DBMT is excellent and, updating old estimates (7), some 100 children born each year in England and Wales could have DBMT for £1.8 M, to achieve lifelong correction for over 60 years, as against £8 M being expended before most of them die from a miserable existence that afflicts their families. Currently, most attempts at gene therapy have only been successful in the test tube (e.g., ref. 64), but have failed in whole animals, (e.g., ref. 100). It seems initially that many will be based on harvesting autologous bone marrow from an affected animal, transfecting it with the gene, and restoring it to the host; this is doomed to failure unless DBMT is undertaken, for it is very important to remove the competition of the remaining host stem cells. There is also the problem that the basic primordial stem cells seem to be turning over in such a way that only 1:8 is ever being used at any given time; this makes them harder to eradicate, as in young infants transplanted where, rarely, a 100% donor-type bone marrow has disappeared in a year due to replacement by host cells that had persisted. Nevertheless, methods are being developed for the positive selection of the earliest bone marrow stem cells which might be totally transfectable without impairing their power to displace those of the host and avoid the risks of allogeneic bone marrow transplant. There will still remain the real danger that the host's remaining B-cells will mount an immune rejection of the new gene product. If total displacement requires an unopposed new start, there may be a return to a total body irradiation induction with its risks (7) and, of course, the always present risk of infection. It seems at present that such gene transfers would have to be undertaken with exactly the same facilities and experience that exists in those teams undertaking DBMT and initially for many of the same diseases. Clearly, there are many factors that will influence the final decision for any given patient, that will have to be made by the parents whom we must advise as best we can. At the time of writing, the initial bone marrow transplants for genetic diseases have been extended from matched siblings (1) to other family (2) and unrelated volunteer donors (4), both to replace abnormal cells and to evolve the concept of DBMT with immunoprophylaxis (7) (first put to a European Working Party in 1978), to confer a transferable component and widen the range of previously untreatable serious genetic diseases that might be corrected.

ACKNOWLEDGMENTS

Much of this review has arisen from the work of the Westminster Children's Bone Marrow Transplant Team (many of whom are named elsewhere [76]) who are grateful to the Bostic and Dobson Funds of the Westminster Medical School Research Trust and the Riverside Health Authority for their generous support. I personally thank Mrs. Rosemary Jenkinson for her excellent secretarial assistance.

REFERENCES

1. Gatti RA, Allen HD, Meuwissen HJ, Allen HD, Hong R, Good RA. Immunological reconstitution of sex-linked lymphopenic immunological deficiency. *Lancet* 1968;ii:1366–9.
2. Hobbs JR, Humble JG, Anderson IM, James DCO. The elective treatment of graft-versus-host disease following a bone marrow graft from a father to a son with severe combined immunodeficiency. *Postgrad Med J* 1976;52(Suppl 5):91–5.
3. Hobbs JR, Williamson S, Chambers JD, et al. Use of donors sharing one genetic haplotype for bone marrow transplantation. *Tokai J Exp Clin Med* 1985;10:207–14.
4. Foroozanfar N, Hobbs JR, Hugh-Jones K, et al. Bone marrow transplantation for an unrelated donor for chronic granulomatous disease. *Lancet* 1977;i:210–3.
5. Steinmuller D, Motulsky AG. Treatment of hereditary spherocytosis in Peromyscus by radiation and allogeneic bone marrow transplantation. *Blood* 1967;29:320.
6. Valdimarsson H, Holt PJL, Moss PD, Hobbs JR. Treatment of chronic mucocutaneous candidiasis with leucocytes from HL-A compatible sibling. *Lancet* 1972;i:469–71.
7. Hobbs JR. Bone marrow transplantation for inborn errors. *Lancet* 1981;ii:735–9.
8. Hobbs JR. Correction of 34 genetic diseases by displacement bone marrow transplantation. *Plasma Ther Transplant Tech* 1985;6:221–46.
9. Hobbs JR, Hugh-Jones K, Chambers JD, et al. Lysosomal enzyme replacement therapy by displacement bone marrow transplantation with immunoprophylaxis. *Adv Clin Enzymol* 1986;3:184–201.
10. Hobbs JR. Displacement bone marrow transplantation and immunoprophylaxis for genetic diseases. *Adv Intern Med* 1987;33:81–118.
11. Hobbs JR. Outcome of displacement bone marrow transplantation for inborn errors of metabolism. *Acta Paediatr Jpn* 1988;30:462–71.
12. Riches P, Weatherald L, Walker S, et al. Transition to donor-type immunoglobulin synthesis following BMT. *Bone Marrow Transplant* 1986;1(Suppl 1):244.
13. Yamamura M, Nikbin B, Hobbs JR. Standardisation of the mixed lymphocyte reaction. *J Immunol Meth* 1976;10:367–78.
14. Buckner CD, Clift RA, Sanders JE, et al. ABO-incompatible marrow transplants. *Transplantation* 1978;26:233–8.
15. Rogers TR, Joshi R, White S, et al. Severe pneumococcal infection and splenic atrophy occurring as complications of graft-versus-host disease after haplotype mismatched marrow transplants. *Exper Hematol* 1983;11(Suppl 13):123–4.
16. Levinsky RJ, Tiedman K. Successful bone marrow transplantation for reticular dysgenesis. *Lancet* 1983;i:671–3.
17. Hobbs JR, Hugh-Jones K. Immunodeficiencies better treated by transplantation. *Tokai J Exp Clin Med* 1985;10:85–97.
18. Fischer A, Friedrich W, Griscelli C, et al. Bone-marrow transplantation for immunodeficiencies and osteopetrosis: European survey 1968–1985. *Lancet* 1986;ii:1080–3.
19. Yamamura M, Newton RCF, James DCO, Humble JG, Butler LJ, Hobbs JR. Uncomplicated HL-A matched sibling bone marrow graft for combined immune deficiency. *Br Med J* 1972;ii:265–9.
20. Sorell M, Kappor N, Pahwa R, et al. Correction of combined immunodeficiency and agranulocytosis in a patient with cartilage hair hypoplasia by marrow transplantation. *Clin Immunol Immunopathol* 1984.
21. Laure F, Courgnaud V, Rouzloux C, et al. Detection of HIV1 DNA in infants and children by means of the polymerase chain reaction. *Lancet* 1988;11:538–40.
22. Markert ML, Hershfield MS, Wiginton DA, et al. Identification of a deletion in the adenosine deaminase gene in a child with severe combined immunodeficiency. *J Immunol* 1987;138:3203–6.
23. Parkman R, Remold-O'Donnell E, Kenney DM, Perrine S, Rosen FS. Surface protein abnormalities in lymphocytes and platelets from patients with Wiskott-Aldrich Syndrome. *Lancet* 1981;ii:1387–9.
24. Filipovich AH, Frizzera G, Zerbe D, Spector BD. Lymphomas in Wiskott-Aldrich syndrome (WAS): report from the Immunodeficiency Cancer Registry. *Pediatr Res* 1983;17:233A.

25. Amino N, Aozasa M, Iwatani Y, et al. Familial OKT4 lymphocyte deficiency. *Lancet* 1984;ii:94–5.
26. Touraine J-L, Betuel H, Touraine F. The bare lymphocyte syndrome. In: Griscelli C, Vassen J, eds. *Progress in immunodeficiency research and therapy.* Amsterdam: Excerpta Medica, 1984;27–34.
27. Hobbs JR, Byrom NA, Chambers JD, Williamson SA, Nagvekar N. Secondary T-lymphocyte deficiencies. In: Byrom NA, Hobbs JR, eds. *Thymic factor therapy.* Proceedings of the Serono Symposia 15. New York: Raven Press, 1984;175–87.
28. Virelizier J-L, Arenzana-Seisdedos A. Role of abnormal lymphokine production in immunological disorders. In: Griscelli C, Vossen J, eds. *Progress in immunodeficiency research and therapy.* Amsterdam: Excerpta Medica, 1984:409–16.
29. Kazmierowski JA, Elin RJ, Reynolds HY, Durbin WA, Wolff SM. Chediak-Higashi syndrome: reversal of increased susceptibility to infection by bone marrow transplantation. *Blood* 1976;47:555–9.
30. Dale DC, Graw RG. Transplantation of allogeneic bone marrow in canine cyclic neutropenia. *Science* 1974;181:83–4.
31. Camitta BM, Quesenberry PJ, Parkmann R. Bone marrow transplantation for an infant with neutrophil dysfunction. *Exp Hematol* 1977;5:109–16.
32. Rappeport JM, Parkman R, Newburger P, Camitta BM, Chusid MJ. Correction of infantile agranulocytosis (Kostmann's syndrome) by allogeneic bone marrow transplantaton. *Am J Med* 1980;68:605–9.
33. Bonilla MA, Gillio AP, Roggiero M, et al. Correction of neutropenia in patients with congenital agranulocytosis with recombinant human granulocyte colony stimulating factor *in vivo. Exp Hematol* 1988; 16:520.
34. Pahwa RN, O'Reilly RJ, Broxmeyer HE, et al. Partial correction of neutrophil deficiency in congenital neutropenia following bone marrow transplantation (BMT). *Exp Hematol* 1977;5:45.
35. Fischer A, Pham Huu Trung, Durandy A, et al. Bone marrow transplantation in two patients with granulocytopathies. *Exp Hematol* 1983;11(Suppl 13):93.
36. Virelizier JL, Durandy A, Lagrue A, Fischer A, Griscelli C. Successful bone marrow transplantation in a patient with Chediak-Higashi syndrome. *Exp Hematol* 1983;11(Suppl 13):91–2.
37. Thomas ED, Sanders JE, Borgna-Pignatti C, et al. Marrow transplantation for thalassaemia. *Lancet* 1982;ii:227–9.
38. Lucarelli G, Galimberti M, Polchi P. Marrow transplantation in patients with advanced thalassemia. *N Engl J Med* 1983;316:1050–5.
39. Giardina PJ, Ehlers K, Lesser M, et al. Improved survival in beta thalassemia major. *Pediatr Res* 1987; 21:229A.
40. Galimberti M, Polchi P, Lucarelli G, et al. Bone marrow transplantation in thalassaemia. Report on 81 cases. *Bone Marrow Transplant* 1986;1(Suppl 1):336.
41. Hobbs JR, Hugh-Jones K, Shaw PJ, Downie CJC, Williamson S. Engraftment rates related to busulphan and cyclophosphamide dosages for displacement bone marrow transplants in 50 children. *Bone Marrow Transplant* 1986;1:201–8.
42. Shaw PJ, Hugh-Jones K, Hobbs JR, Downie JC, Barnes R. Busulphan and cyclophosphamide caused little early toxicity during displacement bone marrow transplantation in fifty children. *Bone Marrow Transplant* 1986;1:193–200.
43. Hobbs JR. Bone marrow transplantation for severe genetic anaemia. *Lancet* 1988;ii:507–8.
44. Johnson FL, Look AT, Gockerman J, Ruggiero MR, Dalla-Pozza L, Billings FT. Bone marrow transplantation in a patient with sickle cell anaemia. *N Engl J Med* 1984;311:780–3.
45. Vermylen C, Fernandez Robles E, Ninane J, Cornu G. Bone marrow transplantation in five children with sickle cell anaemia. *Lancet* 1988;i:1427–8.
46. Iriondo A, Garijo J, Baro J, et al. Complete recovery of hemopoiesis following bone marrow transplant in a patient with unresponsive congenital hypoplastic anaemia (Blackfan-Diamond syndrome). *Blood* 1984;64:348–51.
47. William S, Hewett-Emmett D, Whyte MP, Yu Y-SL, Tashian RE. Carbonic anhydrase II deficiency identified as the primary defect in the autosomal recessive syndrome of osteopetrosis with renal tubular acidosis and cerebral calcification. *Proc Natl Acad Sci USA* 1983;80:2752–6.
48. Walker DG. Bone resorption restored in osteopetrotic mice by transplants of normal bone marrow and spleen cells. *Science* 1975;190:784–5.
49. Loutit JF. Bone marrow grafts in mature osteopetrotic mice. *Transplantation* 1977;24:299–301.
50. Ballet JJ, Griscelli C, Coutris C, Milhaud G, Maroteaux P. Bone marrow transplantation in osteopetrosis. *Lancet* 1977;ii:1137.
51. Sorrell M, Rosen JF, Kapoor N. Bone marrow transplant for osteopetrosis in a 10 year-old boy. *Pediatr Res* 1978;13:481.

52. Lamendin H. First case of bone resorption evoked by bone marrow transplantation in a human patient with osteopetrosis. *Mater Med Pol* 1979;11:67–8.
53. Coccia PJ, Krivit W, Cervenka J, et al. Successful bone marrow transplantation for infantile malignant osteopetrosis. *N Engl J Med* 1980;302:701–8.
54. Key L, Carnes D, Cole S, et al. Treatment of congenital osteopetrosis with high-dose calcitriol. *N Engl J Med* 1984;310:409–15.
55. Chambers TJ. The pathology of the osteoclast. *J Clin pathol (Lond)* 1985;38:241–52.
56. Hugh-Jones K. Early diagnoses in mucopolysaccharidoses. *Lancet* 1983;ii:1300.
57. Anon. Bone marrow transplantation of neurovisceral storage disorders. *Lancet* 1986;ii:788–9.
58. Shull RM, Walker WA. Radiographic findings in a canine model of mucopolysaccharidosis. I. Changes associated with bone marrow transplantation. *Invest Radiol* 1986;23:124–30.
59. Hoogerbrugge PM, Suzuki K, Suzuki K, et al. Donor-derived cells in the central nervous system of twitcher mice after bone marrow transplantation. *Science* 1988;239:1035–8.
60. Hobbs JR, Barrett AJ, Chambers JD, et al. Reversal of clinical features of Hurler's disease and bio-chemical improvement after treatment by bone marrow transplantation. *Lancet* 1981;ii:709–12.
61. Hugh-Jones K, Kendra J, James DCO, et al. Treatment of Sanfilippo B disease (MPS IIIB) by bone marrow transplant. *Exp Hematol* 1982;10(Suppl 10):50–1.
62. Svennerholm L, Mansson J-E, Nilsson O, Tibblin E. Bone marrow transplantation in the Norrbottnian form of Gaucher disease. In: Barranger JA, Brady RO, eds. *Molecular basis of lysosomal storage disorders.* New York: Academic Press, 1984;441–59.
63. Brady RO. Enzyme replacement in the sphingolipidoses. In: Barranger JA, Brady RO, eds. *Molecular basis of lysosomal storage disorders.* New York: Academic Press, 1984;461–78.
64. Sorge J, Huhl W, West C, Beutler E. Complete correction of the enzymatic defect of type I Gaucher disease fibroblasts by retroviral-mediated gene transfer. *Proc Natl Acad Sci USA* 1987;84:906–9.
65. Ginns EI, Caplan DB, Rappeport JM, Barranger JA. Bone marrow transplantation in severe Gaucher's disease: rapid correction of enzyme deficiency accompanied by continued long term survival of storage cells. In: Barranger JA, Brady RO, eds. *Molecular basis of lysosomal storage disorders.* New York: Academic Press, 1984;429–40.
66. Hobbs JR, Hugh-Jones K, Shaw P, Lindsay I, Hancock M. Beneficial effect of pre-transplant sple-nectomy on displacement bone marrow transplantation for Gaucher's syndrome. *Lancet* 1987;i: 1111–5.
67. Starer F, Sargent JD, Hobbs JR. Regression of the radiological changes of Gaucher's disease following bone marrow transplantation. *Br J Radiol* 1987;60:1189–95.
68. Lowdon AGR, Stewart RHM, Walker W. Risk of serious infection following splenectomy. *Br Med J* 1966;i:446–50.
69. Francus T, Chen YW, Staiano-Coico L, Hefton JM. Effect of age on the capacity of the bone marrow and the spleen cells to generate B lymphocytes. *J Immunol* 1986;137:2411–7.
70. Hammarstrom L, Smith CIE. Development of anti-polysaccharide antibodies in asplenic children. *Clin Exp Immunol* 1986;66:457–62.
71. Touraine J-L. Fetal liver transplantation in congenital enzyme deficiencies in man. *Exp Hematol* 1982; 10(Suppl 10):46.
72. Joss V, Rogers TR, Hugh-Jones K, et al. A bone marrow transplant for metachromatic leucodystrophy. *Exp Hematol* 1982;10(Suppl 10):52–3.
73. Bayever E, Feig SA, Philippart M, Brill N. Bone marrow transplantation in the treatment of meta-chromatic leukodystrophy. *Clin Res* 1983;31:107a.
74. Lipton M, Lockman LA, Ramsay NKC, Kersey JH, Jacobson RI, Krivit W. Bone marrow transplan-tation in metachromatic leukodystrophy. *Birth Defects* 1986;22:57–67.
75. Hobbs JR, Hugh-Jones K, Shaw PJ, et al. Wolman's disease corrected by displacement bone marrow transplantation with immunoprophylaxis. *Bone Marrow Transplant* 1986;1(Suppl 1):347.
76. Hobbs JR. The scope of allogeneic bone marrow transplantation. In: Losowsky M, Bolton R, eds. *Advanced medicine, Leeds* Bath: Pitman, 1983;378–91.
77. Taylor RM, Farrow BRH, Stewart GJ, Healy PJ. Enzyme replacement in nervous tissue after allogeneic bone marrow transplantation for fucosidosis. *Lancet* 1986;ii:772–4.
78. Wilcken B, Hammond J. Hearing loss in biotinidase deficiency. *Lancet* 1983;ii:1366.
79. Thorne J, Wolf B. Biotinidase deficiency in juvenile multiple carboxylase deficiency. *Lancet* 1983; ii:398.
80. Rosenberg LE. Disorders of proprionate and methylmalonate metabolism. In: Stanbury JB, Wyn-gaarden JB, Fredrickson DS, Goldstein JL, Brown MS, eds. *The metabolic basis of inherited disease.* New York: McGraw-Hill, 1983;471–97.

81. Vellodi A, Hobbs JR, O'Donnell NM, Coulter BS, Hugh-Jones K. Treatment of Niemann-Pick disease type B by allogeneic bone marrow transplantation. *Br Med J* 1987;295:1375–6.
82. Barrett AJ, Brigden WD, Hobbs JR, et al. Successful bone marrow transplant for Fanconi's anaemia. *Br Med J* 1977;i:420–2.
83. Auerbach AD, Adler B, O'Reilly RJ, Kirkpatrick D, Chaganti RS. Effect of procarbazine and cyclophosphamide on chromosome breakage in Fanconi anaemia cells: relevance to bone marrow transplantation. *Cancer Genet Cytogenet* 1983;9:25–36.
84. Gluckman E, Berger R, Dutreix J. Bone marrow transplantation for Fanconi anaemia. *Semin Hematol* 1984;21:20–6.
85. Deeg HJ, Storb R, Thomas ED, et al. Fanconi's anaemia treated by allogeneic marrow transplantation. *Blood* 1983;61:954–9.
86. Gordon-Smith EC, Fairhead SM, Chipping PM, et al. Bone-marrow transplantation for severe aplastic anaemia using histocompatible unrelated volunteer donors. *Br Med J* 1982;285:835–7.
87. Orii T. *Gifu University, Japan: Ministry of Education report on 850 patients with mucopolysaccharidoses, 1979–84.*
88. Warkentin PI, Dixon MS, Schafer I, Strandjord SE, Coccia PF. *Birth Defects* 1986;22:31–9.
89. Desai S, Hobbs JR, Hugh-Jones K, et al. Morquio's disease (mucopolysaccharidoes type IV) treated by bone marrow transplant. Exp Hematol 1983;II(Suppl 13):98–100.
90. McGovern MM, Ludman M, Short MP, et al. Bone marrow transplantation in Marateaux-Lamy syndrome (MPS type 6): Status 40 months after BMT. *Birth Defects* 1986;22:41–53.
91. Yeager AM, Moser HW, Tutschka PJ, et al. Allogeneic bone marrow transplantation in adrenoleucodystrophy: clinical, pathologic, and biochemical studies. *Birth Defects* 1986;22:79–100.
92. Nyhan WL, Page T, Gruber H, Parkman R. Bone marrow transplantation in Lesch-Nyhan disease. *Birth Defects* 1986;22:113–7.
93. Kurobane I, Inoue S, Gotoh Y-I, et al. Biochemical improvement after treatment by bone marrow transplantation in I-cell disease. *Tohoku J Exp Med* 1986;150:63–8.
94. Shaw PJ, Hugh-Jones K, Hobbs JR. GM1 gangliosidosis: failure to halt neurological regression by bone marrow transplantation. *Bone Marrow Transplant* 1986;1(Suppl 1):339.
95. Harris RE, Hannon D, Vogler C, Hug G. Bone marrow transplantation in type IIa glycogen storage disease. *Birth Defects* 1986;22:119–32.
96. Sakiyama T, Tsuda M, Owada M, et al. Bone marrow transplantation in Niemann-Pick mice. *J Inher Metab Dis* 1986;9:305–8.
97. Hammarstrom L, Lonnquist B, Ringden O, Edvard Smith CI, Wiebe T. Transfer of IgA deficiency to a bone-marrow-grafted patient with aplastic anaemia. *Lancet* 1985;i:778–81.
98. Walker SA, Riches PG, Wild G, et al. Total and allergen-specific IgE in relation to allergic response pattern following bone marrow transplantation. *Clin Exp Immunol* 1986;66:633–9.
99. Olsen I, Dean MF, Harris G, Muir H. Direct transfer of a lysosomal enzyme from lymphoid cells to deficient fibroblasts. *Nature* 1981;291:244–7.
100. Belmont JW, Caskey CT. Long term expression of the human ADA gene in haemopoietic cells of the mouse. *Exp Hematol* 1988;16:421.

DISCUSSION

Dr. Saudubray: From a theoretical point of view, you divided inborn errors in two major categories: one in which DBMT can provide a transferable component and the other when DBMT can provide normal cells. I guess this separation is really too schematic and in the list you propose at least four disorders are not really well adapted to this classification (i.e., Refsum disease, X-linked adrenoleukodystrophy, MSUD, and galactosemia). In these four disorders, if DBMT is effective, and maybe it is effective, it is because the circulating leukocytes can clear circulating toxic components. So this is another category, which is different from the one that provides a transferable component. In these four diseases it is not the transferable component that is circulating, it is the toxic compound itself. So the problem is a problem of quantitative calculation and if we can calculate that the production of branched-chain amino-acids in MSUD can be cleared, or at least a significant amount of these amino acids can be cleared through the provision of a sufficient amount of leukocytes, this procedure will work. I suggest in your classification that you add a third group, that is a list of the diseases where toxic compounds are circulating and can be cleared.

Dr. Hobbs: I quite accept that. I did start with that but it got too complicated, so I tried to simplify into two main groups. In adrenoleukodystrophy I do believe the evidence is that enzyme is delivered to the brain and to the peripheral nerves, because there are three American children and one French child whose lesions have regressed, as shown by MRI and also by peripheral nerve biopsy. As I can't see a white cell getting into a peripheral nerve axon and clearing it, I suggest that enzyme must have been transferred.

Dr. Van Hoof: If I did not misunderstand you, you do not give too much credit to experiments in animals. I was personally impressed by the work of Hoogebrugge et al. (1) on the mouse model of Krabbe's disease (deficiency of the lysosomal galactosylceramidase). This generalized enzyme deficiency profoundly affects the central and peripheral nervous system. Bone marrow transplantation had beneficial effects (presence of donor macrophages in the brain, which increased enzyme activity and caused some degree of remyelination) when performed between 7 and 12 days after birth, but not later. The development of mouse brain at birth is much less advanced than that of humans, and I am afraid that the period during which donor cells could reach the brain in humans would already have passed at birth.

Dr. Hobbs: I said that very often experimental results on animals have not been confirmed in the human situation. There are at least 18 conditions in which this is so. You have chosen Krabbe's disease in mice. This was beautiful work by Dr. P. Hoogerbrugge et al. and I have studied it well. If an affected twitcher mouse is transplanted before it is 11 days old, the disease progress is largely prevented. On the basis of that work, Professor W. Krivit in America has undertaken two transplants in children with Krabbe's disease under the age of 7 months and 9 months. In a human life of 70 years, 8 months is about 1% and in a mouse life of 730 days, 11 days is about 1.5%, so the timing corresponded reasonably well. In fact, there has been a total failure to deliver any enzyme into the human central nervous system, verified at the postmortems. Although it is delivered in the mouse it is not delivered in the human. There are other situations, such as osteopetrosis, where the work in mice held up progress for 10 years. Everybody said that in osteopetrosis all you have to do is provide the cells and they will do the work themselves. There were 18 attempts to cure osteopetrosis by infusing bone marrow cells. Every one of them failed. In the human situation you have to displace a normal marrow. In a mouse you don't have to. In a mouse all you have to do is put in the cells. So mouse osteoclasts behave differently from the human ones. They just find they own way and clear the marrow. In humans you have to do a proper transplant. All I can say is that in the end, whether we like it or not, the final experiment probably has to be done in a family and the families have to understand that. We have done 18 of the first transplants for different genetic diseases and we have two discussions with the families. We have the first one where we explain what we are trying to do and what might go right or wrong. We always let them go away and think about it before we have the final discussion, where they make up their own mind. Of course, an experimental animal does not get this advantage; he does not have any chance to think about it or any chance to go away and make up his mind.

Dr. Van Hoof: Another question about the reported correction of a Wolman patient. Did you use natural or artificial substrates to measure acid lipase? Several esterases can act on artificial substrates to give a false positive result. If the presence of enzyme activity was demonstrated biochemically on a liver sample, could you exclude the possibility that this activity belonged to the white blood cells from the donor, present in this piece of tissue?

Dr. Hobbs: I only used the methods that were avilable when we did that transplant in 1981, and those were the two activities that we measured in those days to make a diagnosis. I quite accept your point, but as a histopathologist who had some training I do not think you can clear cholesterol crystals with white cell enzymes, so something went into those liver cells that enabled the crystals to be cleared.

Dr. Van Hoof: How do you know that it was not just the antirejection drugs you gave the children that did the job?

Dr. Hobbs: That has been proven already. There have been liver transplants, with the same drugs being used, where the child did not get any correction of the Wolman's diarrhea and finally died, with typically diseased gut still present.

Dr. Mowat: Do the long-term survivors develop problems?

Dr. Hobbs: Some do. We have to admit that in Hurler's disease, children who have had normal physical activity for 8 years are now suffering from bone problems. Two of our oldest children have trouble with walking. This is due to problems in the hip joint, and one of them has just had an osteotomy which helped. We don't think that the problem is totally solved. We think that the correction in Hurler's disease has been well worthwhile for the first 9 years, but we still don't know what their brains will be doing when they are 12 years old. At 6–9 years of age the five survivors are all at normal school, but we have this bone problem, which may perhaps be due to the cartilage getting thicker with age and becoming more difficult to penetrate. I hope one day we may see that when the diaphyseal cartilage has disappeared from the bones the problem corrects itself. We don't have all the answers. All we can say is that the present management of Hurler's disease with a transplant is much more satisfactory than the alternative of letting them slowly die for 10–20 years.

Dr. Mowat: Have you been able to do any biochemical studies on the bones at 9 years old?

Dr. Hobbs: We have taken biopsies. The superficial cartilage is beautiful, looking just like normal cartilage. The cells line up for about the first six or seven layers. Then I guess they run out of enzyme. They probably only had 4–10% of the normal amount and when that runs out they revert to the natural diseased state. There are three areas that have been difficult to penetrate: (a) cartilage, (b) the heart in Pompé's disease (all three patients who have died after transplant still had excess glycogen in the heart whereas it had gone from the other tissues), and (c) brain (in half the conditions where this treatment has been tried, brain lesions have not been adequately corrected).

Dr. Brodehl: After the first displacement therapy with the cytotoxic drugs, do you need any continuous treatment with drugs?

Dr. Hobbs: We use cyclosporin A after a matched sibling transplant for only 6 weeks–3 months. Nobody has yet developed a proven test of immune tolerance. We are trying to and we would like this to guide us. At present most of our patients are transplanted from matched siblings, and are off all drugs by 3 months of age, except that they all have ampicillin throughout the first year. They are reassessed in subsequent years to see if they are able to make antibodies. If necessary they stay on ampicillin for much longer periods (e.g., 3–5 years)—it can take a long time to recover. If the transplant is from an unrelated volunteer or from a half-match donor, we have to continue cyclosporin A for a year, after which we measure neopterin daily. Neopterin is a very sensitive indicator of immunologic activity. If neopterin values rise, the patient goes back on cyclosporin A; if they remain low, the patient stays off the drug. But when we initially stopped cyclosporin A at 1 year without such monitoring, we lost two transplants. Thus in a nonperfect match situation you have to use cyclosporin A for about a year. All our recent children have only had it for 1 year, but some will be found who need it for longer.

Dr. Brodehl: What is the dose of cyclosporin?

Dr. Hobbs: About 20 mg/day. And it does not seem to cause any renal problems in the older children. In the young infants this can be a very serious problem and we have sometimes have to abandon the drug because of renal complications. Then we get into trouble.

Dr. Wang: We have done marrow transplantation to correct thalassemia. I quite appreciate that you don't have particular trouble with infections, especially CMV. But we have a lot of CMV infections in Taiwan. Do you have any solutions for the improvement of early detection of infections?

Dr. Hobbs: CMV is our biggest problem as well. Our 20 thalassemic transplants have been largely done for the Asian population in Great Britain, and they have been very badly maintained: according to the Pesaro grading they would be class 3 patients. When you do class 3 patients the survival is only 60%. If you can do them at 1–2 years of age when they are class 1 patients, you can expect a 93% survival, exactly the same as in our other patients. So the answer is that you must do them before these complications occur. The only other advice with regard to cytomegalovirus is that the current opinion is that most of the reactivation occurs from the infusion of CMV-positive white cells in support therapy. Some centers give CMV-negative products to all patients, even if the mother, donor, or child is CMV positive. We haven't got that sophisticated and it is expensive, and in the British population CMV is quite frequent, so there are not enough CMV-negative donors. By a new process that reduces the remaining white cells, we give "leukocyte-poor" platelets. The dose of CMV in transfusion support, which is the major problem in thalassemia, is thus going to be much lower and this should lead to less trouble. We don't have statistics but I think this will turn out to be one of the new advances. As you know it is the thalassemics that are now the largest genetic group being transplanted. Over 400 children have now had transplants for thalassemia and around the world, with all the problems, the disease-free survival rate has been over 64%. In good centers with good selection, choosing class 1 patients under elective conditions, disease-free survival for some genetic diseases is reaching 93%. The center at Tokai university in Japan has 100% survival from their first 24 transplants. It is really quite encouraging.

REFERENCE

1. Hoogebrugge PM, Suzuki K, Suzuki K, et al. Donor-derived cells in the central nervous system of twitcher mice after bone marrow transplantation. *Science*, 1988;239:1035–8.

Inborn Errors of Metabolism, edited by
J. Schaub, F. Van Hoof, and H. L. Vis.
Nestlé Nutrition Workshop Series, Vol. 24.
Nestec Ltd., Vevey/Raven Press, Ltd.,
New York © 1991.

Liver Transplantation for Inborn Errors of Metabolism

Michel Odièvre

Hôpital Antoine BÉCLÈRE, Service de Pédiatrie, 157, rue de la Porte de Trivaux, 92140 Clamart, France

During recent years, liver transplantation has become a realistic alternative for the treatment of usually fatal types of liver disease. The list of diseases for which it has been performed has become extensive. In children, biliary atresia represents the most common diagnosis; metabolic disorders form the next largest category. Table 1 illustrates the metabolic diseases for which transplantation has been performed. The number of children who have been treated for this group of diseases at the University of Pittsburgh is shown in Table 2, indicating the relative frequency of such diseases among the first 1,000 adult and pediatric cases transplanted (1). For the most part, candidates for transplantation have cirrhosis, liver failure, and risk of developing hepatoma. Replacement of the liver cures the severely affected organ and also corrects the enzyme deficiency. Other candidates include children in whom the metabolic disorder is not associated with hepatic injury but invariably terminates in brain damage or other types of extrahepatic complications. The experience with these rare conditions remains limited.

METABOLIC DISEASES WITH LIVER DAMAGE

α-1-Antitrypsin Deficiency

α-1-Antitrypsin, the principal serum protease inhibitor, is a glycoprotein produced in the hepatocyte and secreted at a rate that maintains serum concentrations of 150–200 mg/dl. This molecule shows a remarkable degree of genetic heterogeneity and at least 75 variants have been identified by isoelectric focusing and other techniques. The most common form is type M; the best studied variant is type Z. Individuals with the PiZZ state have α-1-antitrypsin levels that are 10–15% of normal.

Incidence

Deficiency of α-1-antitrypsin is relatively common, occurring as an autosomal recessive inherited disorder in 1 in 1,500 to 1 in 4,000 live births (2).

TABLE 1. *Disorders of metabolism for which liver transplantation has been carried out*

With liver damage
  α-1-Antitrypsin deficiency[a]
  Wilson's disease
  Hereditary tyrosinemia
  Glycogen storage diseases types 1 and 4
  Protoporphyria
  Galactosemia
  Hemochromatosis
Without liver damage
  Crigler-Najjar syndrome type I
  Hyperoxaluria, type I[b]
  Niemann-Pick disease
  Sea blue histiocyte syndrome
  Familial hypercholesterolemia type II[c]
  Urea cycle
  Protein C deficiency
  Hemophilia
  Cystinosis

[a] Three patients treated by combined hepatic and renal transplantation.
[b] One patient treated by combined hepatic and renal transplantation.
[c] One patient treated by combined hepatic and heart transplantation.

Natural History

The natural history of α-1-antitrypsin deficiency is highly variable. A profound serum deficiency is associated with the development of emphysema in the fourth to fifth decades of life. A small percentage (10–20%) of homozygous ZZ individuals develops neonatal cholestasis which is indistinguishable from that of other forms of

TABLE 2. *Number of children under 18 years of age with metabolic diseases treated with liver transplantation[a]*

α-1-Antitrypsin deficiency	37
Wilson's disease	8
Tyrosinemia	8
Glycogen storage type I	1
Glycogen storage type IV	4
Hemochromatosis	2
Hyperlipoproteinemia	1
Protein C deficiency	1
	63 Total

[a] Among the first 1,000 adult and pediatric cases transplanted at the University of Pittsburgh. From Esquivel CO, et al. (1).

hepatobiliary disease. Jaundice usually clears before the age of 6 months, but biochemical abnormalities may persist for several months or years. In some series, 30–40% of children with neonatal cholestasis developed cirrhosis during the first years of life (3). This complication is more frequent in patients in whom a paucity of interlobular bile ducts and persistence of jaundice after 6 months of age are noted (4). On the other hand, about 10% of children with cirrhosis caused by α-1-antitrypsin deficiency have no history of neonatal cholestasis.

Children with cirrhosis frequently die in childhood or early adultlife from gastrointestinal bleeding or progressive liver failure. In some cases an unpredictable and unexplained fulminant hepatic failure occurs. An increased risk for hepatocarcinoma has been described in adults (5). The validity of the association between cirrhosis and the phenotypes MZ and SZ has been questioned, and even in PiZZ individuals the mechanisms responsible for hepatic complications are not defined.

Candidates for Transplantation

At the present time, α-1-antitrypsin deficiency is the second most common indication for liver transplantation in children. Transplantation should be considered in those patients proven to have cirrhosis. Timing of the procedure remains uncertain; in our opinion, because liver disease may decompensate rapidly, transplantation should not be delayed until manifestations of end-stage liver disease develop, and a reasonable age for transplantation seems to be 4–8 years.

Long-Term Effects

Liver transplantation leads to the acquisition of the donor phenotype and normal serum α-1-antitrypsin levels; however, it remains to be shown that chronic lung disease and other rare complications of the deficiency, such as glomerulonephritis, pancreatitis, and panniculitis, will be prevented. Theoretically, the heterozygous phenotype PiMZ, found in about 5% of the population, could be a risk factor for emphysema in young adults, so that it would be better to use a liver graft from donors having not this phenotype. In fact, recent studies show that the risk for the development of emphysema is related to a serum level of α-1-antitrypsin below 80 mg/dl, a concentration that is only seen in subjects with PiSZ or ZZ (6).

Wilson's Disease

In this condition, biliary excretion of copper and incorporation into ceruloplasmin are both severely impaired. The basic lesion underlying these two disturbances is not yet known. Defective biliary excretion leads to accumulation of copper in the liver with progressive liver damage and subsequent diffusion into the blood and accumulation in other sites, such as cerebral nervous system, kidneys, and eyes.

Incidence

Inheritance is autosomal recessive. The prevalence is about 1 in 30,000 to 100,000 live births (7).

Natural History

The clinical manifestations are highly variable but in children are predominantly hepatic. More often, the picture is that of a subacute or chronic liver disease resembling chronic active hepatitis or cirrhosis in which hepatic insufficiency slowly develops. Some patients present with fulminant liver failure with hemolysis and renal failure associated with very high mortality. In fact, the clinical heterogeneity of presentation is so large that Wilson's disease has to be suspected in all children over 7 years with any liver disease of unknown etiology (4). The demonstration of a serum ceruloplasmin concentration of less than 20 mg/dl and of corneal Kayser-Fleisher rings generally suffices to make the diagnosis in 85% of patients (7). Occasionally, the diagnosis may be missed: a 24-h urinary excretion of copper greater than 100 μg favors the diagnosis. The finding of persistent equivocal results is an indication for determining copper concentration in a liver biopsy specimen, but clotting abnormalities may preclude the biopsy. An elevated serum copper level has been shown to be useful is separating patients with fulminant hepatic failure due to Wilson's disease from others (8).

Treatment with penicillamine is effective. Long-term results are excellent but the 3- to 6-month lag before improvement occurs may be too long in patients with acute liver failure (9).

Candidates for Transplantation

Sternlieb (7) has identified three groups of patients to be considered for liver transplantation:

1. Patients presenting with fulminant hepatitis
2. Severely decompensated cirrhotic children who have failed to improve after 2 or 3 months of adequate chelation and nonspecific therapy
3. Effectively treated patients in whom severe hepatic insufficiency and hemolysis develop following noncompliance with chelation therapy. The latter candidates are perhaps less than ideal as their compliance with post-transplantation therapy may be suspect (10).

Patients with fulminant hepatic failure have to be transferred to the transplantation center as soon as possible, where intensive supportive care will sustain life until a suitable donor can be found. The problem in the patients belonging to the two other groups is to define the degree of severity of the liver disease in order to perform transplantation before irreversible manifestations develop (11).

Long-Term Effects

The plasma levels and urine excretion of copper and the ceruloplasmin level normalize following liver transplantation; kinetics of intravenously administered copper in five patients one or more years following transplantation have normalized to the values found in obligated heterozygotes for the gene (1). Transplantation prevents the neurologic dysfunction of Wilson's disease. Reversal of severe neurological deficits has been observed (12).

Hereditary Tyrosinemia Type I

This metabolic disorder results from a deficiency of the fumarylacetoacetase which catalyzes the last step of tyrosine degradation. Due to the enzyme defect, maleylacetoacetate and fumarylacetoacetate accumulate and are metabolized to succinylacetone, which inhibits renal tubular function and porphobilinogen synthetase (13). The liver is considered to be the main organ for tyrosine metabolism.

Incidence

The disease has autosomal recessive inheritance. It has a worldwide distribution and a high prevalence in the French Canadian population of Quebec (0.8 per 100,000 births). The prevalence in Sweden and Norway is about 1 in 100,000.

Natural History

The disorder is characterized by liver disease and renal tubular dysfunction. The course of the disease may be acute or chronic. In the acute form, the patients die of liver failure in early infancy. The chronic form is dominated by rickets and progressive cirrhosis; death is caused by liver failure and/or development of hepatocellular carcinoma. Few patients survive to adulthood (13).

Although not specific for this disorder, serum tyrosine and methionine levels are generally markedly elevated. Generalized aminoaciduria, phosphaturia, glycosuria, and renal tubular acidosis occur. Intermittent extreme elevation of blood α-fetoprotein are frequent. The diagnosis of tyrosinemia can be established by determination of succinylacetone in urine or serum and by assay of fumarylacetoacetase in lymphocytes and fibroblasts. Dietary restriction of tyrosine and phenylalanine improves the renal tubular dysfunction but does not influence the liver damage.

Candidates for Transplantation

Children with onset of liver failure would most benefit from a liver transplant as soon as it is feasible. The high risk of hepatoma formation over the age of 4 years must lead to consideration for transplantation very early in the course of the disease. The preoperative search for such a complication is mandatory in order to reduce the incidence of tumor recurrence (14). Regenerative nodules may be difficult to differentiate from hepatomas. α-Fetoprotein is not of diagnostic value in these patients, and various imaging techniques have to be used in the routine management of patients.

Long-Term Effects

Replacement of the liver corrects the enzyme deficiency in this organ, but the kidneys remain potentially affected. Some patients continue to have renal tubular dysfunction, while others are normal in this respect, suggesting a variable tissue distribution of enzymatic deficiency (15). A persistent succinylacetone excretion, about 20% of the preoperative level, has been observed in a patient, but no further deterioration of the tubular function was seen (13,16). Thus, the renal tubular dysfunction of variable severity may not be corrected by liver transplantation and must be carefully monitored, in particular because cyclosporin may cause nephrotoxicity (15). The possibility that a prolonged postoperative dietary restriction of tyrosine and phenylalanine corrects the persistent tubular dysfunction in these patients, as it does before liver transplantation, remains to be determined; otherwise, some of these patients could be potential candidates for later renal transplantation.

Glycogen Storage Diseases

These are characterized by the accumulation of glycogen mostly in the liver, muscles, and kidneys, and classified according to their specific enzyme deficiency. Types with predominant liver manifestations are IA, IIB, III, and IV (4) (Table 3).

TABLE 3. *Major types of glycogen storage diseases with liver injury*

Type	Enzyme deficiency	Metabolic disturbances	Liver damage
IA	Glucose-6-phosphatase	Severe	Adenoma, adenocarcinoma
IB	Glucose-6-phosphate translocase	Severe	Adenoma
III	Amylo-1-6-glucosidase	Moderate	Portal fibrosis, portal hypertension, adenoma
IV	Amylo-1,4-1,6-transglucosidase	No	Cirrhosis, portal hypertension, liver failure

Incidence

All these types are transmitted as an autosomal recessive trait. Among 76 patients aged more than 12 years, 19 had type 1A, three had type 1B, and 34 had type 3; no patients had type 4 (17).

Natural History

Patients affected with type 1A experience growth retardation and a variety of metabolic disturbances, including hypoglycemia and lactic acidemia with fasting, hyperlipemia, and hyperuricemia. Improvement can be obtained with frequent feedings, continuous nocturnal enteral feeding, and more recently, use of uncooked cornstarch in the diet; in some patients, the improvement is only partial and/or transient. Development of multiple hepatic adenomas is not exceptional, and there is a possibility of a malignant transformation. In addition to this symptomatology, patients with type 1B exhibit a predisposition to infection which is correlated with neutropenia.

The long-term prognosis in patients with type 3 is better, in keeping with the relatively less severe metabolic disturbances; however, myopathy, cardiomyopathy, and portal hypertension secondary to progressive portal fibrosis have been reported. Some patients also develop liver adenomas (17).

Progression to cirrhosis and liver failure is rapid in all patients with type 4, and death usually occurs before the age of 4 years.

Candidates for Transplantation

Transplantation is the only available treatment for patients with type 4 and would normally be considered at about 2 years of age. However, other affected organs, such as the heart, may further threaten life.

The indication of liver replacement in the other types depends on the response to the classical therapy. One of our patients with type 1A had undergone a portocaval shunt at 6½ years of age, and was then treated with nocturnal drip feeding until the age of 15 years; a liver transplantation was performed at that age because of persistent fasting intolerance, severe growth retardation, and very high blood cholesterol level (4.64 mmol/dl), despite good compliance with medical treatment. Two months later, cholesterolemia was 0.4 mmol/dl. Another indication for liver transplantation in this patient was prevention of malignant degeneration of the multiple adenomas present in her liver.

Miscellaneous Metabolic Diseases with Liver Injury

Protoporphyria

A relatively small fraction of afflicted patients with this disease have died in hepatic failure due to liver damage caused by protoporphyrin deposition. The biochemical abnormality reflects deficiency in ferrochelatase activity with resultant increase in protoporphyrin in erythrocytes, plasma, and feces (18).

Photosensitivity is the major clinical manifestation and is not life threatening. However, some patients develop progressive cholestasis with subsequent decreased flow of the hepatotoxic pigment into the gut and the risk of liver failure and death within a few months.

Liver transplantation is indicated in those patients who develop cholestasis (19). In one case (20), it resulted in return to normal liver function and almost complete disappearance of skin photosensitivity manifestations. However, correction of the metabolic disorder was incomplete, perhaps because the contribution of liver in protoporphyrin overproduction is small in comparison with that of the erythropoetic tissue. The long-term consequence of the persisting disorder might be recurrent liver injury, and it might be useful to propose measures for prevention.

Hemochromatosis

Hemochromatosis is another cause of cirrhosis in adult patients. Several have successfully undergone liver transplantation (1). No progression or amelioration of the nonhepatic consequences of hemochromatosis has been noted.

Two infants with congenital hemochromatosis have also received liver replacement for cirrhosis. They were alive and well 1–2 years after surgery (1).

Galactosemia and Hereditary Fructose Intolerance

Liver transplantation has been proposed in both diseases when cirrhosis is present. It has been performed for this reason in one patient with galactosemia. Early diagnosis is important in these conditions, so that the patients can be established on specific restricted diets to avoid such long-term complications.

Other Genetic Disorders

Byler's disease and cystic fibrosis are considered by some authors as metabolic in origin. Liver transplantation can be the only available treatment of cirrhosis accompanying these diseases. Several patients with Byler's disease have received a liver graft (21). The indication of transplantation in patients with cystic fibrosis is more difficult to define because the association of chronically infected pulmonary disease. A combined transplantation of liver, heart, and lungs should be considered in those patients with cirrhosis.

METABOLIC DISEASES WITHOUT LIVER DAMAGE

Crigler-Najjar Syndrome Type I

This is caused by a complete deficiency in the hepatic bilirubin-UDP-glucuronyl transferase activity.

Incidence

The syndrome is inherited in an autosomal recessive pattern. It is rare: only about 100 cases have been reported in the world literature.

Natural History

Patients with this syndrome have unconjugated serum bilirubin concentrations ranging from 20 to 40 mg/dl. As distinct from patients with type II, they do not respond to enzyme induction with phenobarbital, and severe or lethal kernicterus is a constant risk even after the neonatal period: some patients have been reported in whom irreversible neurologic damage was observed only in adolescence.

Treatment is only palliative and restricted largely to life-long phototherapy and cholestyramine in hospital and at home (22,23). Intercurrent infections are associated with further increase in unconjugated hyperbilirubinemia which may precipitate the neurologic injury, at any age.

Candidates for Liver Transplantation

Considering that the risk for neurologic impairment is permanent, all patients with Crigler-Najjar type I are potential candidates for transplantation (24). The latter should be performed when phototherapy ceases to be effective or practical, and clearly prior to the development of kernicterus.

Long-Term Effects

The serum bilirubin concentration falls postoperatively and remains thereafter normal, indicating the marked capacity of normal liver to take up bilirubin.

Familial Hypercholesterolemia Type II

A 6-year-old girl with severe hypercholesterolemia and atherosclerosis has successfully undergone combined liver–heart transplantation (25). She experienced a marked diminution in serum cholesterol to levels which, although not normal, may be compatible with long-term, complication-free survival. Another patient has undergone a liver transplantation 3 weeks after heart transplantation (26). Liver transplantation should be considered only for those patients who are unable to produce any functional LDL receptors and do not respond to other forms of therapy (27).

Hyperoxaluria Type I

In this disease the abnormal glyoxylate metabolism leads to diffuse oxalate deposits in many organs, but mainly the kidney. Liver transplantation corrects the enzyme deficiency and should be proposed in young patients before advanced renal and systemic damage. A combined hepatic and renal transplantation has been performed in patients with renal failure (28).

Miscellaneous Disorders

A child with homozygous protein C deficiency has been treated at age 20 months by liver transplantation; there was a complete postoperative reconstitution of protein C activity and resolution of the thrombotic condition (29).

Several patients with hemophilia have been transplanted for postnecrotic cirrhosis and liver failure due to replacement therapy with clotting factors. The survival patients were well 3 years after transplantation without any clinical evidence of residual clotting dysfunction (30).

Liver transplantation should be considered in several other metabolic diseases, such as some aminoacidopathies and various disorders of the urea cycle; unfortunately, these disorders are almost invariably responsible for severe and irreversible brain damage in the first days of life, too early to be amenable to transplantation. However, one child aged 20 months with carbamylphosphate synthetase (CPS) deficiency has been transplanted; there was a complete correction of hyperammonemia, but plasma citrulline remained low, suggesting that citrulline originates from the gut rather than the liver (31). It would be necessary to continue citrulline supplementation after liver transplantation for CPS and ornithine transcarbamylase deficiency. In another group of metabolic diseases, in particular lysosomial and peroxisomial diseases, extrahepatic organs are involved and liver transplantation may not affect the extrahepatic dysfunction.

CONCLUSION

In conclusion, hepatic transplantation for metabolic diseases of the liver produces a definitive cure of the liver disease and also cures the underlying metabolic abnormalities of the genetic disease. It is indicated not only for patients with evident liver damage but also for those in whom the deficiency is based exclusively within the liver. Several recent reports indicate that replacement of the liver is not always followed by complete cure of the metabolic disease in those patients in whom the deficiency is also present in extrahepatic tissues. In any case, the recipient will remain an obligate carrier of the disease and will transmit the trait to all offspring.

REFERENCES

1. Esquivel CO, Marino IR, Fioravanti V, Van Thiel DH. Liver transplantation for metabolic disease of the liver. *Gastroenterol Clin N Am* 1988;17:167–75.
2. Sveger T. Liver disease in alpha-1-antitrypsin deficiency detected by screening of 200,000 infants. *N Engl J Med* 1976;294:1316–21.

3. Alagille D. Alpha-1-antitrypsin deficiency. *Hepatology* 1984;4:11–14s.
4. Alagille D, Odievre M. *Liver and biliary tract disease in children.* New York, Paris: Wiley-Flammarion, 1979:234.
5. Erikson SG. Liver disease in alpha-1-antitrypsin deficiency. Aspects of incidence and prognosis. *Scand J Gastroenterol* 1985;20:907–11.
6. Hubbard RC, Crystal RG. Alpha-1-antitrypsin augmentation therapy for alpha-1-antitrypsin deficiency. *Am J Med* 1988;84(suppl 6A):52–62.
7. Sternlieb I. Wilson's disease: indications for liver transplants. *Hepatology* 1984;4:15–17s.
8. Rakela J, Kurtz SB, McCarthy JT et al. Fulminant Wilson's disease treated with postdilution hemofiltration and orthotopic liver transplantation. *Gastroenterology* 1986;90:2004–7.
9. Danks DM. Hereditary disorders of copper metabolism in Wilson's disease and Menke's disease. In: Stanbury JB, Wyngaarden JB, Fredrickson DS, Goldstein JL, Brown MS, eds. *The metabolic basis of inherited disease.* New York: McGraw-Hill, 1983;1251–68.
10. Schenker S. Medical treatment vs transplantation in liver disorders. *Hepatology* 1984;4:102–6s.
11. Gottran F, Razemon M, Otte JB, Vigier JE, Farriaux JP. Indications de la transplantation hépatique au cours d'une maladie de Wilson. *Arch Fr Pediatr* 1988;45:187–8.
12. Zitelli BJ, Malatack JJ, Gartner JC, Shaw BW Jr, Iwatsuki S, Starzl TE. Orthotopic liver transplantation in children with hepatic-based metabolic disease. *Transplant Proc* 1983;15:1284–7.
13. Flatmark A, Bergan A, Sodal G, et al. Does liver transplantation correct the metabolic defect in hereditary tyrosinemia? *Transplant Proc* 1986;18:67–8.
14. Starzl TE, Zitelli BJ, Shaw BW Jr, et al. Changing concepts: liver replacement for hereditary tyrosinemia and hepatoma. *J Pediatr* 1985;106:604–6.
15. Tuchman M, Freese DK, Sharp HL, Ramnaraine MLR, Ascher N, Bloomer JR. Contribution of extrahepatic tissues to biochemical abnormalities in hereditary tyrosinemia type I: study of three patients after liver transplantation. *J Pediatr* 1987;110:399–403.
16. Kvittingen EA, Jellum E, Stokke O, et al. Liver transplantation in a 23 year old tyrosinaemia patient: effects on the renal tubular dysfunction. *J Inher Metab Dis* 1986;9:216–24.
17. De Parscau L, Guibaud P, Labrune P, Odievre M. Evolution à long terme des glycogénoses hépatiques. Etude rétrospective de 76 observations. *Arch Fr Pediatr* 1988;45:641–5.
18. Bloomer JR, Sharp HL. The liver in Crigler-Najjar syndrome, protoporphyria and other metabolic disorders. *Hepatology* 1984;4:18–21s.
19. Vierling JM. Epidemiology and clinical course of liver diseases: identification of candidates for hepatic transplantation. *Hepatology* 1984;4:84–94s.
20. Samuel D, Boboc B, Bernuau J, Bismuth H, Benhamou JP. Liver transplantation for protoporphyria. Evidence for the predominant role of the erythropoetic tissue in protoporphyrin overproduction. *Gastroenterology* 1988;95:816–9.
21. Paradis KJG, Freese DK, Sharp HL. A pediatric perspective on liver transplantation. *Pediatr Clin N Am* 1988;35:409–33.
22. Shevell MI, Bernard B, Adelson JW, Doody DP, Laberge JM, Guttman FM. Crigler-Najjar syndrome type I: treatment by home phototherapy followed by orthotopic hepatic transplantation. *J Pediatr* 1987;110:429–31.
23. Odievre M, Trivin F, Eliot N, Alagille D. Case of congenital non haemolytic jaundice. Successful long-term phototherapy at home. *Arch Dis Child* 1978;53:81–2.
24. Kaufman SS, Wood RP, Shaw BW Jr, et al. Orthotopic liver transplantation for type I Crigler-Najjar syndrome. *Hepatology* 1986;6:1259–62.
25. Starzl TE, Bilheimer DW, Bahnson HT, et al. Heart–liver transplantation in a patient with familial hypercholesterolaemia. *Lancet* 1984;1:1382–3.
26. Valdivielso P, Escolar JL, Cuervas-Mons V, Pulpon LA, Chaparro MAS, Gonzalez-Santos P. Lipids and lipoprotein changes after heart and liver transplantation in a patient with homozygous familial hypercholesterolemia. *Ann Int Med* 1988;108:204–6.
27. Bilheimer DW, Goldstein JL, Grundv SM, Starzl TE, Brown MS. Liver transplantation to provide low-density-lipoprotein receptors and lower plasma cholesterol in a child with homozygous familial hypercholesterolemia. *N Engl J Med* 1984;311:1658–64.
28. Watts RWE, Calne RY, Rolles K, et al. Successful treatment of primary hyperoxaluria type 1 by combined hepatic and renal transplantation. *Lancet* 1987;ii:474–5.
29. Casella JF, Lewis JH, Bontempo FA, Zitelli BJ, Markel H, Starzl TE. Successful treatment of homozygous protein C deficiency by hepatic transplantation. *Lancet* 1988;i:435–7.
30. Lewis JH, Bontempo FA, Spero JA, Ragni MV, Starzl TE. Liver transplantation in a hemophiliac (letter to the editor). *N Engl J Med* 1985;312:1189.

31. Tuchman M. Persistent acitrullinemia after liver transplantation for carbamylphosphate synthetase deficiency (letter to the editor). *N Engl J Med* 1989;320:1498–9.

DISCUSSION

Dr. Hobbs: Has any center transplanted patients with the nul-gene defect? The ZZ is ideal to transplant, since it is a single amino acid defect and there is already some protein present, so I don't think you will get antibodies. But for the nul-gene I think you would certainly get antibodies.

Dr. Odièvre: I do not know whether any nul-gene defect patients have been transplanted but I think that the number of children with this type of phenotype in the world is very low.

Dr. Van Hoof: The ZZ phenotype of α-1-antitrypsin deficiency corresponds to an anomaly of the glycan content of the protein. The abnormal protein accumulates in the cisternae of the endoplasmic reticulum, and this causes liver damage. Most probably nul-gene will not raise the same problem and will therefore not be classified among disorders with liver damage. May I ask Dr. Odièvre the reason for classifying the diseases according to the fact that they are or are not accompanied by liver damage. A more logical classification would have been to separate the generalized enzyme deficiencies from the group in which the missing enzymatic step is located completely or predominantly in the liver. Only in the latter group could a complete correction of the disease be expected.

Dr. Odièvre: In the first group with liver damage there is no discussion about the necessity of a transplantation because if we don't perform it the child will die. Concerning the group without liver damage we are obliged to discuss the risk of surgical procedure in a child who is apparently in a good condition. From the physiological or pathogenic point of view you are right.

Dr. Sokal: I have a question about the tyrosinemia. You pointed out that these patients still excrete succinylacetone and all patients have high levels of urinary δ-aminolevulinic acid after transplantation. So would it be necessary to give to these patients detoxifying compounds as was suggested during Dr. Duran's presentation? Is there any evidence that this may be responsible for malignancies in these patients?

Dr. Otte: I think this classification is quite useful in the clinical situation for several reasons. The main reason you mentioned is regarding the balance between the risk of dying for the child and the risk of liver transplantation: you mentioned 15 to 20%. So you should balance that against the risk of dying from the disease. When the patient is going to die within a matter of weeks or days, there is not much of an ethical problem. So I think this classification is quite useful in day-to-day practice. But there is another reason why it will be useful in the future. This concerns the technique. So far we have unfortunately to do an orthotopic transplantation with removal of the native liver. There is, of course, a technique of heterotopic partial liver transplantation but at present this technique does not work particularly well, especially when the recipient liver is normal. You know maybe that the team of Rotterdam has started doing heterotopic partial liver transplantation again and they have obtained quite good results in adult patients with cirrhosis. But when they have used the technique for fulminant hepatitis, for example, they have been unable to obtain a success. From experimental studies one might extrapolate that it is unlikely that heterotopic liver transplants would work when normal recipient liver remains because there is some kind of competition. So in the future surgeons have to do a better job. Experiments are continuing to try to find a way eventually to replace only part of the liver by transplant. But for the time being there is no successful technique and the only way we have is to replace the whole liver.

Dr. Odièvre: In tyrosinemia the phenylalanine- and tyrosine-restricted diet results in disappearance of tubulopathy, while the liver disease is hardly influenced at all. Perhaps it would be interesting to continue the diet therapy after liver transplantation in those patients who have persistent urinary excretion of succinylacetone in order to see if the excretion improves, and with the hope of avoiding a further renal transplantation.

Dr. Saudubray: This raises the more general question as to whether we have to restrict this type of therapy to inborn errors that are mainly or completely restricted to the liver, or whether we can extend the therapy to inborn errors affecting not only liver but other tissues as well. I shall give two examples. In propionic and methylmalonic acidemia, we know that the enzyme defect is present in every tissue. But we also know from physiological studies and from the C13 turnover of propionate and methylmalonate that the main site of production of the toxic compound is muscles, while the main site for their catabolism is the liver. Although I don't often recommend performing liver transplantation in propionic aciduria, I would like to emphasize that from a metabolic point of view liver transplantation could be a therapeutic procedure for this kind of disorder, because the liver may well be able to clear every toxic metabolite. This is one example. On the other hand, the principal concern is for glycogenosis type 1B. In this disease you have two main sites for the defect. One is the liver, giving all the classical clinical symptoms due to glycogenosis type 1, but in addition you have defective transport of glucose-6-phosphate within leukocytes, leading to the other group of symptoms, namely recurrent infections. Is liver transplantation a suitable procedure for the therapy of glycogenosis type 1B?

Dr. Odièvre: Recurrent infections in type 1B glycogen storage disease with granulopenia are classical but not constant. I am personally following six patients with this type of disease and only one has problems with infections.

Dr. Mowat: I think one of the problems is the heterogeneity of all these disorders. A good example of this is type 4 glycogen storage disease, where recently a patient has been reported with as much as 10% of normal activity for the deficient enzyme and with no progression of the liver disease over a period of follow-up of 5 years. I think we need to know much more about many of these conditions before we make generalized statements.

Dr. Brodehl: I think the indication for a liver transplantation in glycogen storage disease type 1 is not enzyme replacement but the development of adenomas which become malignant. At least this was the reason for performing a transplantation in one case in out institute. The same is true for tyrosinemias, which have a high rate of malignancy in the later stage. This should be another indication for liver transplantation in these patients.

Dr. Odièvre: In tyrosinemia the risk of hepatoma is so high that we propose liver transplantation for all patients at about 2 years of age. In glycogen storage type 1A, 1B, and type 3 many patients develop liver adenoma. It has been claimed that the adenomata can disappear with nocturnal enteral nutrition; it is not my experience. Malignant transformation of liver adenomata is rare during childhood; this risk, however, justifies repeated evaluation of α-1-fetoprotein in blood.

Dr. Schaub: I would like to put a question concerning the long-term results in the transplanted liver. Is it clearly demonstrated that, for instance, in Wilson's disease the transplanted liver is free of copper deposit and free of fibrosis or will storage of copper and fibrosis in the transplanted liver again develop?

Dr. Brodehl: Our experience in Wilson's disease is only very limited. I would not expect the copper to accumulate again because the defect is located in the liver. Of course, initially you have a high storage of copper within the body and there could be a mobilization and spillover into the liver, but later, as far as I know from the literature, there is no further accumulation of copper in transplanted Wilson's disease. The story with cystinosis is different. The transplanted kidney accumulates cystine again but in a different fashion from the original kidneys. Cystine comes from the macrophages and leukocytes from the blood, which invade the transplanted kidney, although the cells of the transplanted organ do not accumulate cystine because they possess the lysosomal transport system, which is missing in cystinosis.

Dr. Mowat: Just to add a little bit to that: in adult patients the Kayser Fleischer rings clear gradually after transplantation. It takes about 2 years for them to disappear.

Dr. Otte: Regarding α-1-antitrypsin deficiency you remind us that the risk of death from emphysema is related to the α-1-antitrypsin concentration in the plasma. Can we be sure that the normalization of the α-1-antitrypsin will protect the patient against the risk of death from emphysema in the very long term?

Dr. Odièvre: The α-1-antitrypsin deficiency represents only one of the risk factor for emphysema; smoking and living in a dusty environment are other factors. Adult specialists claim that a level of circulating α-1-antitrypsin above 150 mg per 100 ml protects the individuals.

Dr. Mowat: I would like to comment on that. Ten percent of our children with liver disease who are asymptomatic have large lung volumes and all the lung function studies suggest they have emphysema. We don't know for certain that they have emphysema because we have not biopsied the lungs. However, this raises the consideration that some patients are already on the way to developing emphysema before you transplant them. It is true that α-1-antitrypsin is also produced in monocytes and macrophages. It may be that the tissue concentration of is more important in inhibiting tissue-damaging proteases than the serum concentration. I have reservations about whether our patients who are transplanted will avoid emphysema. We should also remember that the lungs of most patients with liver transplantation have a very stressful time in the intensive care unit, which may well aggravate or initiate lung damage.

Dr. Hobbs: I did, in fact, suggest that there might be enough α-1-antitrypsin synthesized in white cells for a bone marrow transplant to work. In fact, that has been tested and it does not work. We have tested the Pi-types in our transplant patients and I can assure you that although we have transferred marrows with different Pi-type, the patients practically never get a reasonable serum level of the donor Pi-antitrypsin.

Inborn Errors of Metabolism, edited by
J. Schaub, F. Van Hoof, and H. L. Vis.
Nestlé Nutrition Workshop Series, Vol. 24.
Nestec Ltd., Vevey/Raven Press, Ltd.,
New York © 1991.

Indications and Timing of Liver Transplantation in Metabolic Disorders

David C. van der Zee, Eric van Melkebeke, Jean de Ville de Goyet,
Etienne Sokal, Jean-Paul Buts, Jacques Rahier,
Bernard de Hemptinne, François Van Hoof, and
[1]Jean-Bernard Otte

*Department of Pediatric Surgery, University of Louvain Medical School, Cliniques
Universitaires Saint-Luc, Avenue Hippocrate 10, 1200 Brussels, Belgium*

There are several metabolic disorders which are known to evolve toward end-stage liver failure and which nowadays are generally accepted as indications for orthotopic liver transplantation (1–15). Complete cure of the basic pathology can be expected only in those metabolic disorders that are primarily restricted to the liver. Reports on liver transplantation for metabolic disorders, although still sparse, are promising (3,5,7–10,13–16).

The metabolic diseases form only a small but still important group among the patients in whom liver transplantation is indicated (Table 1). In an update to 31.12.1988, the European Liver Transplantation Registry (11) reported a frequency of 5% of metabolic diseases in 2962 patients transplanted in 55 centers throughout Europe (Table 2). Within the group of metabolic disorders, the pediatric patients evidently comprised the majority (14.6% versus 3%). In this chapter we review our experience with 23 patients who received a liver graft for various inborn errors of metabolism in order to evaluate the indications, the timing, and the results that can be obtained in this group.

PATIENTS

From 1984 to 1988, 210 patients underwent liver transplantation at the University of Louvain Medical School in Brussels. There were 117 children and 93 adults (Table 1). Metabolic disorders represented 15.4% of the indications for liver transplantation in children and 5.3% in adults (Table 2). The different indications for liver transplantation in metabolic disorders are listed in Table 3. There were three patients with α-1-antitrypsin deficiency. Wilson disease was encountered in seven patients,

---

[1] Corresponding author.

TABLE 1. *Indications for orthotopic liver transplantation (1984–1988)*

	Children (n = 117)	Adults (n = 93)
Chronic liver failure		
Biliary atresia	86	
Ductular paucity	4	
Sclerosing cholangitis	2	2
Primary biliary cirrhosis		20
Secondary biliary cirrhosis		1
Posthepatitic biliary cirrhosis		13
Cryptogenic cirrhosis	3	19
Alcoholic cirrhosis		5
Autoimmune cirrhosis		3
Fulminant hepatitis		9
Liver tumors	3	14
Metabolic disorders	18	5
Miscellaneous		
Congenital liver fibrosis	1	
Vitamin A intoxication		1
Hemosiderosis		1

TABLE 2. *Liver transplantation in inborn errors of metabolism[a]*

	Total	Inborn errors
ELTR	2,962	147 (5%)
Adults	2,462	74 (3%)
Children	500	73 (14.6%)
UCL	210	23 (10.9%)
Adults	93	5 (5.3%)
Children	117	18 (15.4%)

[a] ELTR, European Liver Transplant Registry (55 centers); UCL, University of Louvain Medical School, Brussels.

TABLE 3. *UCL experience in inborn errors of metabolism*

	Adults	Children	Total
α-1-Antitrypsin deficiency	1	2	3
Wilson's disease	3	4	7
Crigler-Najjar syndrome type I	—	2	2
Glycogen storage disease types I and IV	—	2	2
Tyrosinemia	—	2	2
Byler disease	1	6	7
	5	18	23

TABLE 4. *UCL experience*

	No.	Age	Age OLT (years)
α-1-Antitrypsin deficiency	3	2–5 months, 14 years	5, 10, 26
Wilson's disease	7	<1 month, 11–23 years	11–24
Crigler-Najjar syndrome type I	2	<1 month	2, 8
Glycogen storage disease types I and IV	2	5 months	1, 7
Tyrosinemia	2	3, 8 months	1, 4
Byler disease	7	1–12 months	1–6, 14, 15

while two children had a Crigler-Najjar syndrome type I. There was one patient with glycogen storage disease type I and one with type IV glycogen storage disease. Tyrosinemia was encountered in two children and Byler disease in seven patients.

The age of onset of symptoms and the age of transplantation are listed in Table 4. In two of the three patients with α-1-antitrypsin deficiency, onset of symptoms was within the first year of life. On the other hand, in patients with Wilson's disease the onset of symptoms was mainly in the second decade. As expected in patients with Crigler-Najjar syndrome type I, onset of symptoms was within the first months of life, while the two patients with a glycogen storage disease displayed first symptoms at 5 months. Symptoms associated with tyrosinemia were first encountered at 3 and 8 months, respectively. Finally, Byler disease usually started within the first year of life. The actuarial survival rate, as displayed in Fig. 1, is 76% at 5 years.

CASE HISTORIES

α-1-Antitrypsin Deficiency

Between 1984 and 1988, three patients with α-1-antitrypsin deficiency underwent orthotopic liver transplantation (OLT). The first patient (OLT 2) presented with onset

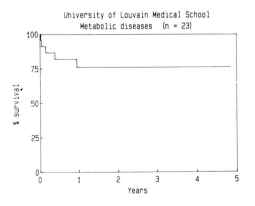

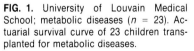

FIG. 1. University of Louvain Medical School; metabolic diseases (*n* = 23). Actuarial survival curve of 23 children transplanted for metabolic diseases.

of symptoms at 5 months. The parents and later also a younger brother appeared to be heterozygote PiMZ. The patient was phenotyped as PiZZ. At the age of 10 years, there was a sudden liver deterioration and liver transplantation was performed. There was a reintervention for biliary obstruction, after which liver function normalized. There was a postoperative phenotype switch to PiMM and α-1-antitrypsin levels normalized. He is now 4.8 years post-OLT and doing well.

The second patient (OLT 53) displayed a neonatal hepatitis during the first 2 months of life. α-1-Antitrypsin deficiency was diagnosed as his twin brother died at age of 3 years. He was transplanted at the age of 5 years. There was a prolonged elevation of liver enzymes postoperatively because of a stenosis of the hepatic artery. At 6 months post-OLT, he presented with an Epstein-Barr virus infection with transient liver dysfunction. At 2 years and 4 months post-OLT, he is doing well.

In these two young patients there have been no pulmonary manifestations of the disease. This is different in the third patient (OLT 70), who presented primarily with emphysema with diffusion disturbances. At the age of 26, she suffered from an acute deterioration of liver function, indicating urgent liver transplantation. The postoperative course was troubled by several rejection episodes finally resulting in chronic rejection. She was retransplanted after 4 months, but suffered from thrombosis of the hepatic artery 5 weeks later. Ultimately she developed multiple organ failure complicated by hepatic abscess. She died while waiting for retransplantation.

Wilson's Disease

The first patient (OLT 13) had a "Wilson-like" liver disease that started during the first year of life; he was later diagnosed as having copper intoxication. He was transplanted at the age of 19.5 years and is doing well 4 years after transplantation.

The second patient (OLT 20) presented with first symptoms at the age of 23 years. One year after first onset of symptoms, she suffered from severe variceal hemorrhage with rapidly progressing liver failure and encephalopathy with coma grade I. She underwent urgent liver transplantation and is doing well 3.5 years post-OLT.

The third patient (OLT 50) had onset of symptoms at the age of 13 years. After the diagnosis was made, the patient was treated initially with D-penicillamine but suffered from acute hepatic failure after discontinuance of chelating therapy with grade I coma status. This patient underwent urgent liver transplantation and is doing well 2.5 years post-OLT.

The fourth patient (OLT 73) presented with first symptoms at the age of 11 years. He did not respond to chelating therapy and suffered from fulminant liver failure with grade III coma status. He underwent emergency transplantation with an ABO-incompatible liver graft, experiencing substantial blood losses during the operation in spite of venovenous bypass. Ten days later he had to be retransplanted with a reduced size liver because of severe graft dysfunction. The postoperative course was complicated by an aspergillus pneumonia, which eventually led to his death.

The fifth patient (OLT 81) presented with liver enzyme abnormality during routine checkup at the age of 17 years. Before further diagnosis could be performed, she underwent urgent admission for fulminant liver failure with coma grade IV. Because of onset of multiple organ failure, she underwent combined hepatorenal transplantation. The postoperative course was complicated by a superinfection with aspergillosis and cholangitis. This patient had to be retransplanted 3 days later, and although liver function improved, there was a disturbance of the patient's cerebral condition. She eventually died of multiple organ failure.

The sixth patient (OLT 92) had onset of symptoms at the age of 10.5 years. He responded only temporary to D-penicillamine treatment and was transplanted with reduced size liver. The postoperative course was complicated by thrombophlebitis of the cerebral sinus, inducing convulsions. He also developed a coagulopathy resulting in intracerebral bleeding and death. A sister of this patient later also appeared to have Wilson's disease.

The last patient (OLT 175) first presented with a fulminant liver failure and underwent emergency transplantation with an ABO-incompatible liver. This patient had to be retransplanted after occurrence of arterial thrombosis of the graft during reintervention for an obstructive ileus. The course thereafter was uneventful.

Crigler-Najjar Syndrome Type I

Two patients were transplanted for a Crigler-Najjar type I glucoronyl transferase deficiency. The first child (OLT 14) thrived fairly well on phenobarbital until he had an ENT infection at 4 years of age. He thereafter developed progressive psychomotor retardation. He was transplanted at the age of 8 years with an uneventful postoperative course. At 4 years post-OLT liver function is normal but the child still displays some fine motor coordination disturbances.

The second child (OLT 77) remained clinically stable on phototherapy and cholestyramine medication. He was transplanted electively at the age of 2 years and 5 months. There were many postoperative complications because the donor liver turned out to be from a patient that had died of generalized tuberculosis. The patient is now 2 years post-OLT with normal liver function.

Glycogen Storage Disease Types I and IV

One patient (OLT 37) had a type I glucose-6-phosphatase deficiency presenting with recurrent episodes of hypoglycemic convulsions and therapy-resistant metabolic acidosis. He was therefore transplanted at the age of 7 years. The postoperative course was complicated by thrombosis of the hepatic artery at day 10 necessitating re-transplantation with an ABO-incompatible liver graft. Apart from two rejection episodes he is doing well 3 years post-OLT with normal liver function.

The other patient (OLT 136) had a type IV branching enzyme deficiency with progressive hepatic insufficiency. He underwent a reduced size liver transplantation at the age of 14 months. The decision for transplantation was influenced by the death of an older brother from glycogenosis type 4 at the age of 20 months. The postoperative course was uneventful with full restoration of liver function. At 9 months post-OLT the child developed cardiomyopathy related to abnormal glycogen deposits. He died of cardiac decompensation complicated by pulmonary infection 11 months post-OLT, while awaiting cardiac transplantation.

Tyrosinemia

The first patient (OLT 143) presented primarily with progressive hepatic insufficiency and cirrhosis at the age of 8 months. Creatinine clearance was not impaired. He underwent reduced size liver transplantation at 1 year of age. He was reoperated 2 days later for a twisting of the hepatic artery. Two rejection episodes evolved toward chronic rejection; he was re-transplanted 15 months after the first transplant but died of complications due to an Epstein-Barr infection.

The second patient (OLT 232) had a brother who had died of tyrosinemia. Diagnosis was made at the age of 3 months. She developed acute liver insufficiency and had elevated α-fetoprotein levels. She was urgently transplanted at the age of 5 with a split liver graft. No tumor was found at pathological examination of the recipient liver, and the patient is now 6 months post-OLT with normal liver function. Aminolevulinate levels have also normalized.

Byler Disease

Byler disease was diagnosed in seven patients. Pruritus was a dominant symptom in all patients and started shortly after onset of jaundice. Bilirubin levels and liver enzymes, with the exception of the gamma-GT, were increased.

The first patient (OLT 43) developed an acute decompensation of his liver function at the age of 1 year and underwent urgent reduced-size liver transplantation. The child is now 2.5 years post-OLT with normal liver function.

The second patient (OLT 46) was transplanted electively for cirrhosis at the age of 4 years and 10 months. A reconstruction of the biliodigestive anastomosis was carried out 4 months post-OLT. He is now 2.5 years post-OLT with normal liver function.

The third patient (OLT 61) presented with icterus at the age of 2 years. He was transplanted at the age of 6 years and is now more than 2 years post-OLT with slightly raised liver enzymes due to a non-A, non-B hepatitis.

The fourth patient (OLT 90) was transplanted at the age of 2 years. The postoperative course was complicated by thrombosis of the hepatic artery and bile duct obstruction, necessitating reintervention. She is now 1 year and 9 months post-OLT with normal liver function.

The fifth patient (OLT 154) was transplanted at the age of 5.5 years. He is now 10 months post-OLT and doing well, with normal liver function.

The sixth and seventh patients were sister and brother (OLT 197, 217) who were transplanted at the age of 15 years and 14 years, respectively. Both have normal liver function 6 months and 3 months post-OLT, respectively.

DISCUSSION

Liver transplantation for inborn errors of metabolism comprises only a small group of patients. According to the European Liver Transplant Registry, which has assembled all the data from 55 centers in 12 European countries, 147 patients (5%) underwent liver transplantation for inborn errors of metabolism (11). Of these 147 patients, 23 (15.6%) were transplanted at the University of Louvain Medical School in Brussels (UCL).

It was the aim of this study to evaluate the results regarding indication, timing, and outcome of liver transplantation for inborn errors of metabolism. Liver transplantation should be considered in those metabolic disorders where the disease is threatening life or the central nervous system; or in those instances where the disease is responsible for a poor quality of life. It is important, however, to take into consideration whether the metabolic disorder is restricted to the liver (i.e., whether complete cure of the disorder can be obtained by transplantation). The timing is important because it is evident that recovery is possible only if transplantation is performed before irreversible extrahepatic manifestations develop.

Complete cure of inborn errors of metabolism can be expected when the defective protein is normally excreted by the liver, when the defective enzyme is located exclusively in the liver, or when the defective membrane receptors are located mainly in the liver.

α-1-Antitrypsin deficiency is a hereditary disorder affecting the transfer of the glycan moiety of the glycoprotein, resulting in accumulation of insoluble material within the endoplasmic reticulum. This accumulation, observed in the phenotype PiZZ, is responsible for hepatocyte dysfunction, resulting in cirrhosis, portal hypertension and liver failure (4,12). After transplantation there is a phenotype switch to PiMM of the donor. Pulmonary lesions, as observed in one of our patients, can be expected to be prevented or halted by liver transplantation. An association between α-1-antitrypsin-deficiency-related cirrhosis and primary liver carcinoma has been described. Therefore, liver transplantation should be performed before onset of pulmonary lesions or gastrointestinal bleeding precipitating liver failure.

Crigler-Najjar syndrome type I is a hereditary disorder with a glycuronyl transferase enzyme deficiency leading to kernicterus in the first 18 months of life (4,17, 18), although in some instances, for example in one of our patients, progressive brain damage may be delayed. Palliative therapy consists of long hours of phototherapy, putting a heavy burden on both patient and parents. Liver transplantation is indicated when phototherapy cannot maintain serum bilirubin levels below 15 mg %, which in most cases will be during early childhood. Since the enzyme deficiency is restricted to the liver, transplantation brings complete cure.

Wilson's disease is a hereditary disorder of Cu metabolism in which there is a defective mobilization of Cu from hepatocellular lysosomes for excretion in the bile (7,12,19). The toxic accumulation of Cu results in liver and brain damage. The chronic form of Wilson's disease usually responds to chelating therapy with D-penicillamine, which promotes Cu excretion in the urine (4,7,12,20). In contrast, acute Wilson disease presents as a fulminant hepatic failure with renal impairment and massive nonimmune hemolysis with a high mortality. In our series, six patients rapidly progressed toward hepatic failure necessitating urgent or emergency transplantation. We therefore underline the conclusions of Schenker (14) and Sternlieb (21) that liver transplantation should be performed as soon as possible in patients presenting with a clinical picture of fulminant hepatitis. It should furthermore be considered in young cirrhotic patients who have failed to respond to chelating therapy with D-penicillamine or in patients effectively treated but who relapse after cessation of chelating therapy. This is a problem especially encountered in young adolescents who are sometimes difficult to motivate to continue their chelating therapy.

Hereditary tyrosinemia is a deficiency of the liver enzyme fumaryl acetoacetate fumaryl hydrolase and is characterized by progressive hepatocellular damage, tubular dysfunction, and hypophosphatemic rickets (1–4,7,12,13,22,23). In the neonatal form, presenting in the first 3 months of life, death from liver failure usually occurs by 8–12 months of age. Both our patients presented with their first symptoms within 2 months after birth, and a brother of one of them had died in the neonatal period of tyrosinemia. In the more chronic courses, hepatocellular carcinoma is responsible for about 60% of the mortality in these patients (2,7), so α-fetoprotein should be monitored in these patients. In our series we observed no hepatoma.

Because of the course of the disease and the risk of hepatoma formation, patients with tyrosinemia should be transplanted during early childhood or even in infancy when presenting symptoms in the neonatal period. With current new techniques of reduced- and split liver transplantation in children under 1 year of age becomes feasible (24,25) despite the shortage of small donors.

Byler disease is a hereditary disorder in which there is an inborn error of bile acid metabolism with difficulties in excreting bilirubin and bile acids. The disease ultimately leads to cirrhosis, portal hypertension, and death due to hepatic failure usually before the age of 15 years. Liver transplantation completely cures this disease, as was demonstrated in our patients.

Familial hypercholesterolemia is a hereditary disorder resulting from the absence of LDL cell membrane receptors with accumulation of lipoproteins and cholesterol in the plasma. Patients ultimately die of myocardial infarction before the age of 20 years because of severe artherosclerosis. Because of the extrahepatic manifestation of this disease, combined heart–liver transplantation might be necessary to cure these patients (7,10,26–28).

In *inborn errors of metabolism with extrahepatic manifestations*, usually involving the kidney, that have no life-threatening consequences, liver transplantation may significantly improve the patient's condition. Glycogen storage disease type I is a hereditary disorder with glucose-6-phosphatase deficiency (4,7,29). In patients in whom metabolic acidosis does not respond adequately to medical treatment, liver transplantation may be considered (4,7,12,13,29). One of our patients with a glycogenosis type I benefited well from liver transplantation. In glycogenosis types III and VI, liver transplantation would only be indicated in case of concomitant liver tumor. Another group of metabolic disorders that could significantly benefit from liver transplantation are those in which toxic metabolites could be removed by the grafted liver. Examples are methioninemia, homocystinuria, and maple syrup urine disease. So far, however, no cases of liver transplantation have been described for these indications. Finally, there is a group of inborn errors for which liver transplantation could be beneficial but would not be curative because the disorder affects organs other than the liver. Glycogenosis type IV is a branching enzyme deficiency affecting other organs such as muscle, including the heart, brain, and leukocytes (12, 15,30). One of our patients with a glycogenosis type IV initially benefited from liver transplantation but later died from cardiac failure. Hyperoxaluria type I is a hereditary disorder of the glyoxylate metabolism and patients ultimately die from renal failure. Watts et al. (31) described a successful combined hepatorenal transplantation in a patient with hyperoxaluria type I. The role of liver transplantation in protoporphyria is uncertain. This is a highly variable autosomal disorder characterized by photosensitivity and elevated levels of protoporphyrin in erythrocytes, plasma, and feces. When jaundice complicates the liver disease, death is probable within a few months. Successful liver transplantation was described in the short term, but it is uncertain whether excessive protoporphyrin will be deposited in the grafted liver and cause progressive liver damage (4,32,33).

CONCLUSION

In conclusion, with a 76% actuarial survival rate, liver transplantation has become an accepted mode of therapy in a number of inborn errors of metabolism. In metabolic disorders in which the liver is the primary affected organ, complete cure can be obtained. Otherwise, prognosis is determined by the extrahepatic extension of the disease. Timing of liver transplantation should, if possible, be elective. However, when patients present with symptoms of fulminant hepatitis or acute liver failure, rapid decision making is obligatory.

With improved prognosis in liver transplantation, new indications come to light. With the development of alternative techniques, such as auxiliary liver transplantation, perhaps in the future other modes of treatment for some inborn errors of metabolism will become available.

REFERENCES

1. Dindzans VJ, Schade RR, Gavaler JS, Tarter RE, van Thiel DM. Liver transplantation. A primer for practicing gastroenterologists, part I. *Dig Dis Sci* 1989;94:2–8.
2. Esquivel CO, Mieles L, Marino JR, et al. Liver transplantation for hereditary tyrosinemia in the presence of hepatocellular carcinoma. *Transplant Proc* 1989;21:2445–6.

3. Marsh JW, Makowka L, Todo S, et al. Liver transplantation today. *Postgrad Med* 1987;81:13–16.
4. Mowat AP. Liver disorders in children: the indication for liver replacement in parenchymal and metabolic diseases. *Transplant Proc* 1987;19:3236–41.
5. Otte JB. *La transplantation hépatique: indications et résultats chez l'enfant.* Brussels: Académie Royale Belge de Médecine, 1987.
6. Pichlmayr R, Ringe B, Burdelski M, Lauchart W, Schmidt E. Liver transplantation in metabolic diseases. *Z Gastroenterol* 1987;22:57–60.
7. Polson RJ, Williams R. Application to inborn errors of metabolism. In: Calne R, ed. Liver transplantation. *The Cambridge–Kings College Hospital experience*, 2nd ed. London: Grune & Stratton, 1987.
8. Schade RR. The changing indications for liver transplantation. *Transplant Proc* 1987;19(suppl 3):2–6.
9. Scharschmidt BF. Human liver transplantation: analysis of data on 540 patients from four centers. *Hepatology* 1984;4:95–101S.
10. Shaw BWJ, Wood RP, Kaufman SS, Williams L, Antonson DL, Van der Hoof J. Liver transplantation therapy for children: part 1. *J Pediatr Gastroenterol Nutr* 1988;7:157–66.
11. Bismuth H, Castaing D, eds. *European Liver Transplantation Registry. Update: 31-12-1988.* Villejuif, France: Hôpital Paul Brousse, 1989.
12. Alagille D, Odièvre M. *Maladies du foie et des voies biliaires chez l'enfant.* Paris: Flammarion Médecine Sciences, 1987.
13. Martinez Ibanez V, Margarit C, Tormo R, et al. Liver transplantation in metabolic diseases. Report of five pediatric cases. *Transplant Proc* 1987;19:3803–4.
14. Schenker S. Medical Treatment vs transplantation in liver disorders. *Hepatology* 1984;4:102–6S.
15. Tizard EJ, Pett S, Pelham AM, Mowat AP, Barnes ND. Selection and assessment of children for liver transplantation. In: Calne R, ed. *Liver transplantation*, 2nd ed. London: Grune & Stratton, 1987.
16. Rothfus WE, Hirsch WL, Malatack JJ, Bergman I. Improvement of cerebral CT abnormalities following liver transplantation in a patient with Wilson disease. *J Comput Assist Tomogr* 1988;12(1):138–40.
17. Pett S, Mowat AP. Crigler-Najjar syndrome types I and II. Clinical experience, King's College Hospital, 1972–1978. Phenobarbitone, phototherapy and liver transplantation. *Mol Aspect Med* 1987;9(5):473–82.
18. Shevell MI, Bernard B, Adelson JW, Doody DP, Laberge JM, Guttman FM. Crigler-Najjar syndrome type I: treatment by home phototherapy followed by orthotopic hepatic transplantation. *J Pediatr* 1987;110:429–31.
19. Gottrand F, Razemon M, Otte JB, Vigier JE, Farriaux JB. Indications for liver transplantation in Wilson's disease. *Arch Fr Pediatr* 1988;45:187–8.
20. de Bonjt B, Moulin D, Stein F, Van Hoof F, Lauwerys R. Peritoneal dialysis with D-penicillamine in Wilson disease. *J Pediatr* 1985;107:545–7.
21. Sternlieb I. Wilson's disease: transplantation when all else had failed. *Hepatology* 1988;8(4):775–6.
22. Dehner LP, Snover DC, Sharp HL, Ascher N, Nakhleh R, Day DL. Hereditary tyrosinemia type I (chronic form): pathological findings in the liver, *Human Pathol* 1989;20:149–58.
23. Tuchman M, Freese DK, Sharp HL, Ramnaraine ML, Ascher N, Bloomer JR. Contribution of extra-hepatic tissues to biochemical abnormalities in hereditary tyrosinemia type I: study of three patients after liver transplantation. *J Pediatr* 1987;110:399–403.
24. Otte JB, de Ville de Goyet J, Sokal E, et al. Size reduction of the donor is a safe way to alleviate the shortage of size-matched organs in pediatric liver transplantation. *Ann Surg* 1990;211:146.
25. Otte JB, de Ville de Goyet J, Alberti D, Balladur P, de Hemptinne B. The concept and technique of the split liver in clinical transplantation. Surgery, 1990;107:605–12.
26. Bilheimer DW. Portocaval shunt and liver transplantation in treatment of familial hypercholesterolemia. *Arteriosclerosis* 1989;9:1158–63.
27. Cienfuegos JA, Pardo F, Turrion VS, et al. Metabolic effects of liver replacement in homozygous familial hypercholesterolemia. *Transplant Proc* 1987;19:3815–7.
28. Valdivielso P, Escolar JC, Cuervas-Mons V, Pulpon LA, Chaparro MAS, Gonzalez-Santos P. Lipids and lipoprotein changes after heart and liver transplantation in a patient with homozygous familial hypercholesterolemia. *Ann Int Med* 1988;108:204–6.
29. Coire CI, Qizilhash AM, Castelli MP. Hepatic adenomata in type Ia glycogen storage disease. *Arch Pathol Lab Med* 1987;111:166–9.
30. Servidei S, Riepe RE, Langston C, et al. Severe cardiopathy in branching enzyme deficiency. *J Pediatr* 1987;111:51–6.
31. Watts RWE, Rolles K, Morgan SH, et al. Successful treatment of primary hyperoxaluria type I by combined hepatic and renal transplantation. *Lancet* 1987;ii:474–5.
32. Polsen RJ, Lim CK, Rolles K, Calne RY, Williams R. The effect of liver transplantation in a 13-year old boy with erythropoietic protoporphyria. *Transplantation.* 1988;46:385–9.

33. Samuel D, Bobor B, Bernuau J, Bismuth H, Benhamou JP. Liver transplantation for protoporphyria. Evidence for the predominant role of the erythropoietic tissue in protoporphyria overproduction. *Gastroenterology* 1988;95:816–9.

DISCUSSION

Dr. Mowat: Concerning the number of children who die very early in life, who have metabolic disorders with disastrous effects in the first week of life, do you see any possibility of liver transplantation in newborn infants?

Dr. Otte: From the technical point of view we would easily perform a transplant in a patient with metabolic disease. An operation on a child with Crigler-Najjar is an easy operation technically, although we have to use a sophisticated technique. So from the technical point of view that is possible. Surgeons must be trained in pediatric surgery, and in microvascular surgery. The second question is: How easily do these small children tolerate surgery, and how easily do they tolerate the post-transplantation period? I must confess that at the beginning, when we started the program, I was not convinced myself that very small children should be transplanted. Basil Zitelli of Pittsburgh (USA) was one of the pediatricians who convinced me that I had to change my mind, and that small children did well. This has turned out to be true. The main problem is the donor, since very small donors are extremely scarce. We don't use donors less than 1 month of age because the liver is not mature. Therefore, we often have to use a reduced-size liver from an older donor. There is an increased incidence of thrombosis if the donor is very young. In conclusion my answer is yes, but these very small children should be taken care of by extremely specialized teams having experience with such children.

Dr. Casaer: When you have a child with Crigler-Najjar syndrome on the waiting list and you would like to have a neurological variable to assess any bilirubin toxicity that might still be reversible, I would suggest that you do regular brain stem evoked responses. Bilirubin toxicity for the eight cranial nerve and its brain stem nuclei has been well established in young infants; it could therefore be useful in these children, especially since you ask for a variable that could almost predict the moment at which damage to nervous system tissue occurs.

Dr. Otte: I am not the right person to answer the question, except that as a clinician I am only interested in some way of predicting the time when brain damage is going to develop. When the first child with Crigler-Najjar and brain damage was put on the waiting list, we had a lot of discussion and some people hypothesized that the damage might be reversible, but it is not since it is caused by necrosis. We have not been presented since then with another child having encephalopathy. I don't know what I would do. We would discuss it with the parents. But the other children had no encephalopathy. The transplantation was successful in the first child, but he has neurologic sequelae and the quality of his life has not been improved as much as we hoped. I think that liver transplantation is a too major a procedure to be offered to a child as a palliation. It should be curative. So if the child has complications of his disease which are not reversible after liver transplantation, the balance between the advantages and the disadvantages is doubtful.

Dr. Odièvre: In the Crigler-Najjar disease, the problem is relatively simple. We can maintain patients in good condition for many years by controlling the index of bilirubin saturation of albumin and thus adjust the daily duration of phototherapy in order to maintain this index under 60%. The problem is when these patients develop acute infectious disease; the investigations then have to be repeated several times a week because the index may increase to 70 or 80%, necessitating 14 or 15 h of phototherapy each day instead of 12 h. Because of these problems, the patients should be transplanted when they are 5 years of age or sometimes earlier.

Dr. Otte: Maybe this is an aspect of importance. You have to choose the age when the transplantation has to be performed. I think it should be done before the age of 6, when the child enters school.

Dr. Mowat: It is also very important for us as pediatricians to make sure that the parents of potential donors have the opportunity of providing organs for transplantation.

Inborn Errors of Metabolism, edited by
J. Schaub, F. Van Hoof, and H. L. Vis.
Nestlé Nutrition Workshop Series, Vol. 24.
Nestec Ltd., Vevey/Raven Press, Ltd..
New York © 1991.

Approaches to Human Gene Therapy

Theodore Friedmann

*Center for Molecular Biology and Department of Pediatrics, University of California,
San Diego, School of Medicine, La Jolla, California 92093, USA*

Current therapies for most human genetic diseases are unsatisfactory. Even with
the application of modern tools of molecular biology, there continue to be major
temporal and conceptual gaps between an understanding of mechanisms of disease
and truly effective treatment. No doubt, as even traditional diagnostic and analytic
tools become more sophisticated and as understanding of pathogenesis grows, these
gaps will close with increasing speed. However, it is evident that the application of
molecular genetics techniques has already begun to predict conceptually powerful
new therapeutic approaches based on the introduction of normal genetic information
into defective cells to complement genetic defects and correct disease phenotypes.
Studies toward such "gene therapy" have become increasingly commonplace and
compelling during the past several years, and while there are still many technical,
medical, and ethical problems, many of the uncertainties of just a few short years
ago about the feasibility and desirability of gene therapy have dissipated. The use
of genetic correction for otherwise intractable or even untreatable disorders now
seems to be inevitable and possibly even imminent (1).

The most common current view of gene therapy involves the efficient introduction
of functional foreign genetic information into suitable defective target cells *in vitro*
followed by introduction of the genetically modified cells into an organism to provide
a new and required function. Many workers have used modified defective viruses
to act as efficient vectors for the foreign sequences, since several classes of tumor
viruses have evolved to do precisely this job (i.e., introduce new genes efficiently
and functionally into mammalian cells without killing the host cell). For the complementation of genetic defects in mammalian cells and the correction of a disease
phenotype *in vivo*, a virus vector must be capable of introducing genes efficiently
into cells and of expressing transduced genes stably without causing deleterious
effects in cells either *in vitro* or *in vivo*. Retrovirus vectors satisfy these criteria and
have therefore been particularly useful recently. Their mechanisms of infection, integration, and gene expression are well understood; they have broad host ranges,
are easily manipulated, do little if any metabolic damage in infected cells; and genes
transduced by them can be expressed stably during the lifetime of the cell. Using
these agents, a number of laboratories have reported successful gene transfer, gene

275

expression, and the complementation of genetic defects *in vitro*, first with selectable drug resistance markers and later with human-disease-related genes, such as those for hypoxanthine guanine phosphoribosyltransferase (HPRT). More recently, many other genes have been expressed *in vitro*, and several studies have reported varying degrees of efficiency of expression *in vivo*, particularly in bone marrow of mice and recently in nonhuman primates. While methods for transduction and transgene expression have been reasonably efficient *in vitro*, *in vivo* expression of transgenes from retrovirus vectors has often been inefficient and transient. Furthermore, because retrovirus vectors require cell replication for infection, their usefulness seems limited in neurons, hepatocytes, and other fully differentiated postmitotic or non-replicating cells.

Progress has been made recently to solve some of these technical problems, such as the generally poor expression of retroviral vectors in disorders of bone marrow stem and of early progenitor cells. The situation with many other classes of genetic disease is also changing rapidly. During the past few years, several workers have begun to develop approaches to the genetic modification of organs other than the bone marrow. Possibly the simplest target organ would be the skin, since skin fibroblasts or keratinocytes are easily accessible from an individual and can be cultured and manipulated *in vitro* and returned to the skin with little difficulty. Indeed, several workers have suggested the use of these cells to provide circulating functions such as insulin and blood coagulation proteins such as factor IX (2). Our laboratory has developed a method that allows retroviral transduction and gene expression in primary hepatocytes (3), and the use of retrovirally infected hepatocytes to complement a defect *in vivo* now awaits the development of efficient methods to reintroduce genetically modified hepatocytes into an intact animal. Published evidence suggests that implanted hepatocytes may provide a new metabolic function *in vivo*, and the phenotypic correction of a number of liver defects can now be attempted. Furthermore, increasing knowledge of the genetic mechanisms of tumorigenesis have begun to suggest that the replacement of recessively acting oncogenes, the shutdown of recessively acting oncogenes such as the retinoblastoma gene, or efficient vector-mediated delivery of antineoplastic agents may eventually play a significant role in improved and specific cancer therapy (4).

Serious conceptual and technical problems remain with studies of a genetic approach to disorders of the CNS. The presumed target cells, neurons, and other CNS cells are relatively inaccessible, and in the case of the nonreplicating neurons, not susceptible to infection with retrovirus vectors. One potential solution to the problem of foreign gene delivery to the CNS is through the use of cells infected *in vitro* and subsequently implanted into the CNS. We have proposed and used this indirect method to deliver new genetic functions to CNS neurons by combining *in vitro* transduction with transplantation to the CNS (5), and we have demonstrated phenotypic effects *in vivo* by such a procedure (6,7). However, for the study and treatment of many other, more global disorders of the CNS as well as diseases of liver and muscle, there is a clear need for new approaches to modification of the CNS.

To satisfy that need, it is vital to develop vectors that can transduce foreign genetic material into postmitotic cells. To that end, we and others are investigating the potential of vectors derived from herpes simplex virus type 1 (HSV-1), a ubiquitous and generally benign human virus. This virus is a very attractive candidate for development as a vector for a number of reasons. It is capable of establishing a latent, life-long noncytopathic infection in neurons. There is no conclusive evidence that HSV carries an oncogene or other unique transforming sequences and it does not integrate into the host genome, reducing the potential for tumorigenesis and insertional mutagenesis. HSV has a wide host and cell-type range and can grow lytically in fibroblasts, facilitating both its genetic manipulation and scope of use. Features required for the replication and packaging of the HSV genome are reasonably well understood, and the entire 155-kilobase nucleotide sequence has been determined, permitting rational vector design and construction. Finally, the intact HSV genome can be expanded without interfering with packaging, and since many of the viral genes are dispensable for growth in tissue culture, even larger insertions of foreign sequences are feasible.

One group has inserted human HPRT cDNA into a replication-competent HSV genome and detected expression of the human gene, under control of the HSV thymidine kinase (TK) promoter, during lytic infection of an HPRT-deficient rat neuroma cell line (8). Using a plasmid-vector approach, others transferred the *E. coli* β-galactosidase gene (lacZ) into rat sympathetic and sensory neurons *in vitro* (9). In these studies, vectors were based on wild-type virus and a single point mutation in the helper virus, respectively, and are thus not suitable for long-term gene transfer because infected cells will eventually lyse due to wild-type virus replication. However, these reports are an encouraging indication of the potential usefulness of these and further modified HSV vectors for transferring and expressing foreign genes in cells for purposes of correcting genetic defects.

There are several very attractive new disease models for gene therapy, involving disorders for which current therapy is unsatisfactory and for which the genes have been or are soon to be isolated. Our initial work to establish conditions for efficient retrovirus vector-mediated gene transfer into differentiated hepatocytes has permitted us and others to begin to study genetic aspects of the pathogenesis of model defects of liver function and to develop genetic approaches toward their therapy. We have been particularly interested in a genetic approach to hypercholesterolemia, and have demonstrated that retrovirus-mediated transfer of the human LDLR gene into cells from the Watanabe rabbit complemented the LDLR defect and even corrected the associated defect in cholesterol esterification (10), and recent work in other laboratories has also shown LDLR expression in Watanabe hepatocytes (11). The isolation of the gene encoding the A-I apolipoprotein and the recognized role of A-I-containing HDL in the regulation of serum cholesterol levels also indicates that over-expression in some cells and secretion of A-I into the circulation may have an ameliorative effect on some kinds of hypercholesterolemia. Such cells need not be hepatocytes, the ordinary site of synthesis and expression of A-I, but might instead include fibroblasts and endothelial cells with intimate contact with the circulation. Several studies have recently shown that endothelial cells lining some of the large blood vessels can be genetically modified through infection with retrovirus vectors, and the possibility exists that the introduction of foreign genes into such cells *in vivo* would provide an ideal method of delivering new metabolites, such as coagulation factors and other serum proteins, directly into the circulation. Retroviruses have also been used *in vitro* to complement genetic defects of other liver disorders, including the phenylalanine hydroxylase defect in PKU (12), argininosuccinate synthetase deficiency in citrullinemia (2), and factor IX deficiency in hemophilia B (13).

The recent isolation and characterization of the dystrophin gene and its role in the pathogenesis of Duchenne's and Becker's muscular dystrophy (14), as well as an applicable and relevant mouse model, the *mdx* mutant (15), and a dog model, makes this an intriguing model for gene therapy despite the enormous size of the gene and an incomplete understanding of the role of the gene product in muscle physiology. Recent work demonstrating a beneficial phenotypic effect of implanted wild-type cells in muscle of *mdx* mice (16) lends support to the argument that the reasonably efficient genetic modification of even some defective cells *in vivo* may result in a beneficial effect on muscle function. Mechanisms of muscle-specific gene expression are coming to be better understood through studies of the regulated expression of a number of muscle-specific genes, and at least some of the regulatory sequences that drive muscle-specific expression of actin, creatine kinase, and other genes have been identified by *in vitro* transfection studies and in transgenic mice.

The recent isolation of the gene responsible for cystic fibrosis makes this disorder a very attractive target disease for gene therapy. Biochemical work has identified a cell function that is deficient in CF, although present evidence does not allow one to say unambiguously that this defect represents the primary gene defect. Cystic fibrosis is associated with a reduced Cl permeability of apical epithelial cell membranes in sweat gland ducts and intestinal and airway epithelial cells. There is reasonably good evidence that the CF gene product is involved in the function of a cyclic AMP–dependent cell surface chloride channel. The chloride impermeability affects the physical properties of the secretions and is associated with a great increase in their viscosity. Whether the CF gene encodes the channel itself, some intracellular inhibitor of the channel of other components needed for channel integrity and function is not yet clear. Current evidence at the moment is that the defect in this disease, the most common lethal genetic disease in the Caucasian population in this and many other "developed" societies, involves the expression of an epithelial cell surface chloride channel in multiple cell types of the exocrine system, and the physiology of the disease suggests that the organs in which aberrant physiology is expressed and which would presumably be suitable target organs for genetic correction are epithelial cells of the airway, pancreas, and other organs of the gastrointestinal tract.

These and other model systems currently being developed are all examples of new approaches to disease treatment that are relatively straightforward conceptually and ethically. They are directed toward the correction of defects in somatic cells and the rationalization for the use of new molecular genetic tools and techniques has come to be largely accepted in a growing number, although certainly not all, biomedical communities. Most scientific, governmental, public policy, and religious bodies have concluded that therapeutic uses of genetic tools aimed at somatic target cells poses few if any new kinds of ethical dilemmas and is ethically defensible. The rapidly developing positive attitudes toward somatic cell gene therapy has recently led in the United States to approval by the Director of the National Institutes of Health and by the Food and Drug Administration of the first experiments aimed at introducing genetically modified cells back into human patients. These experiment involve the introduction *in vitro* of an antibiotic resistance marker into tumor infiltrating lymphocytes (TIL cells) derived from tumors of terminally ill people followed by the reintroduction of those cells into the donor patients. These studies have no immediate therapeutic goals, but rather are meant simply to answer the question of whether TIL cells are in fact targeted to tumors. The real effect of these studies will be to encourage additional applications to those regulatory bodies for truly therapeutic experimental studies, and we can probably expect to see several such proposals in the relatively near future.

A rather surprising result from these and many additional studies in laboratories throughout the world is the realization that biomedical science has already undergone a quiet but profound revolution, one that is not yet fully tested and certainly not over. But the idea that it may become possible to treat some human human diseases, finally, at the point of the defect, the gene defect, has progressed from being a rather unrealistic dream to being a very widely accepted and reasonable goal. It is really quite remarkable how straightforward it all seems now in retrospect, and quite amazing how rapidly it has all come. Most extraordinary of all is the fact that it is really just beginning.

REFERENCES

1. Friedmann T. Progress toward human gene therapy. *Science* 1989;244:1275–81.
2. Palmer TD, Thompson AR, Miller AD (1989). Production of human factor IX in animals by genetically modified skin fibroblasts: potential therapy for hemophilia B. *Blood* 1989;73:438–45.
3. Wolff JA, Yee J-K, Skelly HF, et al. Expression of retrovirally transduced genes in primary cultures of adult rat hepatocytes. *Proc Nat Acad Sci USA* 1987;84:3344–8.
4. Haung H-JS, Yee J-K, Shew J-Y, et al. Suppression of the neoplastic phenotype by replacement of the RB gene in human cancer cells. *Science* 1988;242:1563–6.
5. Gage FH, Wolff JA, Rosenberg MB, et al. Grafting genetically modified cells to the brain: possibilities for the future. *Neuroscience* 1987;23:795–807.
6. Rosenberg MB, Friedmann T, Robertson RC, et al. Grafting genetically modified cells to the damaged brain: restorative effects of NGF expression. *Science* 1988;242:1575–8.
7. Wolff JA, Fisher LJ, Xu L, et al. Grafting fibroblasts genetically modified to produce L-dopa in a rat model of Parkinson disease. *Proc Nat Acad Sci USA* 1989;86:9011–4.
8. Palella TD, Silverman LJ, Schroll CT, et al. Herpes simplex virus-mediated human hypoxanthine-guanine phosphoribosyltransferase gene transfer into neuronal cells. *Mol Cell Biol* 1988;8:457–60.
9. Breakefield XO, Geller AI. Gene transfer into the nervous system. *Mol Neurobiol* 1987;1:339–71.
10. Miyanohara A, Sharkey MF, Witztum JL, Steinberg D, Friedmann T. Efficient expression of retroviral vector-transduced human low density lipoprotein (LDL) receptor in LDL receptor-deficient rabbit fibroblasts *in vitro*. *Proc Natl Acad Sci USA* 1988;85:6538–42.
11. Peng H, Armentano D, MacKenzie-Graham L, et al. Retroviral-mediated gene transfer and expression of human phenylalanine hydroxylase in primary mouse hepatocytes. *Proc Natl Acad Sci USA* 1988;85:8146–50.
12. Wood PA, Herman GE, Chao CY, O'Brien WE, Beaudet AL. Retrovirus-mediated gene transfer of

argininosuccinate synthetase into cultured rodent cells and human citrullinemic fibroblasts. *Cold Spring Harbor Symp Quant Biol* 1986;51:1027–32.

13. Kunkel LM, Beggs AH, Hoffman EP. Molecular genetics of Duchenne and Becker muscular dystrophy: emphasis on improved diagnosis. *Clin Chem* 1989;35(Suppl B):B21–4.
14. Bulfield G, Siller WG, Wight PAL, Moore KJ. X chromosome-linked muscular dystrophy (mdx) in the mouse. *Proc Natl Acad Sci USA* 1984;81:1189–92.
15. Partridge TA, Morgan JE, Coulton GR, Hoffman EP, Kunkel LM. Conversion of mdx myofibres from dystrophin-negative to -positive by injection of normal myoblasts. *Nature (Lond)* 1989;337:176–9.
16. Weissman BE, Saxon PJ, Pasquale SR, et al. Introduction of a normal human chromosome 11 into a Wilms' tumor cell line controls its tumorigenic expression. *Science* 1987;236:175–80.

DISCUSSION

Dr. Van den Berghe: You mentioned the problem of the stability of the gene product inside the recipient. This has been reported for several enzymes, for example adenosine deaminase transfer in monkeys.

Dr. Friedmann: It is not a question of the stability of the gene product. It is a question of the stability of the gene. The gene is integrated into the chromosome of the host cell and for all intents and purposes we might hope that the new gene looks like an ordinary cellular sequence. In fact, it does not. We know that the bits of foreign genes rearrange; they shut down for genetic and epigenetic reasons. We don't know yet how to control that stability. One can image all kinds of manipulations of the vector itself, designed to prevent these rearrangements, but no one to my knowledge has been able to deduce the rules for producing a stable vector. Anything that one does to the vector may modify the stability, but there is no rule yet for stability.

Dr. Saudubray: What about the other target organs, for example muscles? Can you give some comments on the future?

Dr. Friedmann: Muscles are a wonderful target and we are certainly working on that as well. The target disorder that we have in mind at the moment is Duchenne muscular dystrophy, of course. The problem with Duchenne is that the gene for dystrophin is so enormous that it does not fit into these vectors. One has to design new kinds of vectors. There are other genes, other disorders of muscles that might be approachable. A possible approach is to remove muscle cells from a muscle, manipulate them *in vitro,* and then return them to a muscle. One knows now that myocytes can be put back into muscle and become incorporated in the functional myotubes. On the other hand, one can also learn how to target the vector directly to the muscle. I don't have any doubt that muscle disorders will be a suitable target. How effective the approach will be, I don't know. One can image all kinds of additional target organs, and with the success of a couple of weeks ago in the case of cystic fibrosis one can imagine airway cells, the epithelial cells, to be targets for similar kind of manipulations.

Dr. Widhalm: Could you explain a little bit more about the Watanabe rabbit? You showed that the infection with the virus was able to reduce LDL receptor activity. Is it also possible to reduce HMG CoA reductase activity, and which gene did you use, because there are several different genes for LDL receptor activity?

Dr. Friedmann: Our gene was full-length human cDNA,

Dr. Widhalm: And was it possible to show an effect of the HMG CoA reductase activity?

Dr. Friedmann: We have not studied it.

Dr. Leroy: I did not hear completely what was said about the osteosarcoma cell. Was this cell strain derived from a donor who had retinoblastoma before? In other words, was this a secondary tumor in a retinoblastoma patient, or was this an osteosarcoma of a totally different nature that happened to be cured by introducing the retinoblastoma gene?

Dr. Friedmann: That was an established osteosarcoma cell line. It was an existing osteosarcoma cell from a patient who had survived a retinoblastoma. So it is a osteosarcoma cell with a defect in RB gene. There are other osteosarcomas without defects in RB gene, but this was one in which an RB defect was present.

Dr. Leroy: Have you done studies on those osteosarcoma lines that do not have the defect?

Dr. Friedmann: The gene was introduced into osteosarcoma cells that have their own expressed RB gene. Those cells were not modified in any apparent way by the introduction of the gene. They continue to grow, and their morphology is unchanged.

Dr. Hobbs: Tissue culture and experiments in the nude mouse are very privileged situations because there is no host immune system. One of the problems with the introduction of the gene and the production of a gene product is that some of the patients are going to have products that they recognize as foreign.

Dr. Friedmann: We are aware of the immunological problems. The ability of the human to raise an immune response to gene product that he has not seen before is certainly a major concern. The immune response will depend on whether or not there is cross-reacting gene product present in the defective cell. At the moment we are not concerned with the immune response, but obviously it is something we are going to worry about later. We are most concerned with gene transfer at the moment and how effectively that can be done.

Dr. Hobbs: That would have to be before 10 weeks of pregnancy.

Dr. Saudubray: How many kilobases can you insert in your vector?

Dr. Friedmann: The retrovirus will accept approximately seven or eight kilobases. That is enough for most cDNAs but it is not enough for very large genes such as dystrophin. There are other vectors that we are working on, for instance the herpes-based vectors, which may have a much larger capacity.

Dr. Mowat: One approach that has intrigued me is the use of the asialoglycoprotein receptor, which is found only on the surface membrane of hepatocytes to target genetic material to the liver. Asialoglycoprotein has been successfully combined with a retrovirus, DNA, and appropriate promoters to get a bacterial enzyme to function in the liver of intact rats. They produced specific mRNA for some weeks (1). For the hepatocyte to do this in its own milieu seems a particularly important advance. I would like to have your comments.

Dr. Friedmann: This is very attractive as well. We would like very much to learn other target materials for the liver without the *in vitro* step, and that is one way to do it.

Dr. Hobbs: Certainly it is much more attractive in genetic disease because you don't have to infect 100% of the cells. The problem with tumors is much more difficult if you have an osteosarcoma in a patient. You are only going to have one or more cells that do not accept the regulator gene, and they will go on growing and kill the patient. That is a much harder target. I would encourage you to go to the genetic disease. There are just as many. In fact, there are more children dying of genetic disease than dying of cancer. It takes me a long time to persuade the childhood organizations in Britain that we can use their money a lot better than the cancer people can.

Dr. Friedmann: I do agree that treatment of tumors is difficult and presumably one wants to hit every cell in a tumor. It is a different problem in this sort of manipulation, learning how to produce enough virus to infect every cell of an existing tumor *in vivo*. But I think that perfection may be too much to ask of any therapy, including this therapy at an early and primitive stage of its development. So I think even the ability to infect a high percentage of cells will be helpful.

REFERENCE

1. Wu GY, Wilson JM, Wu CH. Targeting genes: delivery and expression of a foreign gene driven by an albumin promoter *in vivo*. *Hepatology* 1988;8:1251.

Inborn Errors of Metabolism, edited by
J. Schaub, F. Van Hoof, and H. L. Vis.
Nestlé Nutrition Workshop Series, Vol. 24.
Nestec Ltd., Vevey/Raven Press, Ltd.,
New York © 1991.

Closure Remarks

Jürgen Schaub

Department of Pediatrics, University of Kiel, Schwanenweg 20, 2300 Kiel 1, Federal Republic of Germany

Ladies and Gentlemen, dear friends, the 24th Nestlé Nutrition Workshop on inborn errors of metabolism has certainly maintained the high scientific standard established by previous symposia in this series. Once again the Nestlé Company has provided us with a program that presented new results as well as a comprehensive overview of the various aspects of metabolic diseases. This strategy has proved more successful in giving physicians, biochemists, and geneticists the means to improve both their basic and clinical approaches to a better understanding of metabolism.

The first session reminded participants of the extreme diversity of diseases of fatty acid oxidation. Our knowledge about whether children with the various types of these abnormalities will derive long-term benefits from dietetic or drug therapy is poor. Very important is the relation between the sudden infant death syndrome and metabolic diseases. We learned especially that metabolic diseases of fatty acid oxidation may be the cause of this syndrome. Further epidemiological metabolic studies are necessary to evaluate the true incidence of this relation.

Session 2 on amino acids, ammonia, and neurotransmitter diseases updated previous information in this large field of metabolic disorders. Protecting fetuses of pregnant mothers with PKU will be a challenge to all physicians engaged in this disease. In neurotransmitter metabolism we expect to discover further defects as we have in the last 10 years. The development of new techniques might eventually lead to the detection of common defects such as Parkinson's disease.

The third session gave a good overview on disorders of carbohydrate metabolism. For many years galactosemia seemed to pose no problem for pediatricians dealing with this disease. However, the most recent enquiries by American and European colleagues have revealed disastrous long-term results with conventional dietetic therapy. Thus new prospective studies and stringent clinical and biochemical controls are necessary for this disease, which no longer seems to be easy to treat.

The final session on transplantation and on gene therapy was a fascinating demonstration of recent data on surgical, immunological, and genetic treatment modalities. This session opened up new aspects and promised interesting developments.

I now wish to express thanks on behalf of all participants to the organizers of this 24th Nestlé Nutrition Workshop. The results of basic research and careful clinical studies are surely important contributions to our knowledge of metabolic diseases. I warmly thank Madame Dr. Dufour and Dr. Guesry, who was not able to attend the meeting, and their co-workers in Nestec in Switzerland for the excellent symposium program, and the local organizers, M. de Prelles and his co-workers, for their kind welcome to their guests. I would also like to express thanks on behalf of the children whom we all take care of in the hope that Nestlé will continue with their valuable support of research in nutritional and metabolic disorders. Thank you very much.

Subject Index